Readings in Psychology

A Debate and Issues Approach

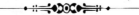

Lee D. Merchant, M.A., M.F.T.

Modesto Junior College

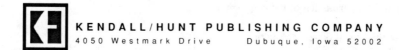

KENDALL/HUNT PUBLISHING COMPANY
4050 Westmark Drive   Dubuque, Iowa 52002

❧ Contents ❧

Children

∽ Preface ∽

Active learning is one of the seven standards of good teaching practice in undergraduate education. This book is designed to promote an active approach to learning in the introductory psychology course and other more discipline specific psychology courses. By incorporating the debate process into the psychology curriculum, students will develop critical thinking skills, become informed about current controversial issues, and increase their ability to present information to an audience in an organized and convincing manner.

The purpose of this book is to add excitement to introductory psychology courses through debate. Our students are more informed and more interested in controversy than ever before. They are the generation exposed to extensive media debate through programs such as 60 Minutes, Dateline, 2020, Day One, Meet the Press, and many others. Today's student has often watched countless hours of talk show format with Jenny Jones, Oprah, Maury Povich and the ultimate in controversial programming, The Jerry Springer Show. Today students expect to share their opinions and deal with challenging issues in debate format. Organized debate creates a lively learning experience in the college classroom.

The feature that distinguishes this book is the emphasis on the debate process. There are guidelines included in this text, for both the student and the instructor, to assist in creating meaningful discourse in the classroom. The disparate points of view in this book represent current thinking on controversial issues in psychology and in life. These topics are provocative and enlightening and they are intended to engage students through argumentation. This unique debate approach has added measurably to the interest in college psychology courses. Rather than presenting articles to students for an individual response, this book uses the articles as a starting point for active learning though research and class presentation. The debating process fosters skills in:

Critical thinking

Research

Presentation

I created this book because I am thrilled with the enhancement of my teaching experience through the debate process. I believe in interactive learning and the use of controversial topics to stimulate students to think, research, and present is an ideal way to facilitate their involvement in the class.

With information available at their fingertips through the internet and a cultural standard of discourse that supports debate, your students need only a starting point for a controversy for a great class experience and you will find that foundation in this text. When you teach your students to debate timely, controversial issues in an informed and responsible manner you will find debate days in your course will become a favorite teaching experience!

Preparing this manuscript has been a pleasure because I have had excellent assistance from Charles Borgquist, Jayne Nunes, and Michelle Keener. This book represents my enthusiasm for the learning process and I want to express gratitude to my professors, Dr. Thomas Kimlicka, Dr. Jamie McCreary, and Dr. Mack Goldsmith for being superb mentors and role models and inspiring me to express the love I have for teaching.

I want to dedicate this book to my husband and colleague, Fred Fernandez, with whom I share the language of psychological science and to my children Brittany, Bret, and Brad for sharing their mom with this process.

Introduction

The Debate Process in the Psychology Course

Overview of the Debate Process

The debate process in the psychology curriculum is a rewarding and challenging experience. Students often comment that they really enjoy the debates as audience members because they look forward to hearing views of fellow students as well as sharing their own. Debate presenters are pleased with their accomplishment when they successfully express their points derived from researching the topic.

I have designed this book to facilitate success in the presentation of clear and informed ideas and facts to maximize the audience experience during debates. Students will be well prepared to state points incorporating fact and opinion.

It is important to note that the focus of this text is an informal debate process. Students do not need experience with formal debate procedures or prior speech coursework. The format includes the use of note cards with points in support of one side of the issue obtained from research articles related to the topic. Students from opposing sides of the controversy alternate making points from their cards. When the presenters are finished, the audience can begin to get involved. Students are not required to make direct counter-points or to further support their main statement.

Of course, some students are uncomfortable with the idea of making a statement on a controversial topic in front of the class. This is a valid concern shared by a majority of people. Successful people have found a way to overcome this fear and the experience of making one point in a college course is a good beginning. These students should recognize the goal of such a presentation is to prepare them for future courses where more extensive presentations are required as well as to help them develop skills in communicating information and ideas that will be valuable in their future professions. Right now, imagine a situation in your future where being able to present ideas with confidence would be an asset to your personal and professional life.

The debate process described in this text is designed to minimize the anxiety associated with public speaking and maximize success in conquering this discomfort. Even students who have initially had a great deal of angst about debating often write enthusiastic evaluations of this experience at semester's end. In fact, the most consistent comment on course reviews is the enjoyment of each debate day in class!

Preparing to Debate

The process begins with the student's selection of their debate topic from a list prepared by the instructor containing the issues and two columns indicating a "yes" and "no" position. This list includes the debates from this text selected for a particular course. The instructor can use any number of debates during the semester depending on time available for the process and relevance of the topics to the course content. Instructors may schedule debate topics when they coincide with course content or they can choose to add topics to the class at any time by selecting preferred issues from this text. At least one extra debate can be scheduled in case students miss a class when a debate occurs. This way, there is no missing score or make-up assignment needed.

Students will usually present on at least one topic and be audience members for approximately five to ten other topics. Signing up for a debate to present is accomplished by listing names under the topic and on the specific side of the debate the student chooses to support. See appendix for an example debate sign-up sheet.

It is very important to select a debate on a topic that you care about. You will find that it is much easier to invest time into research and preparation for your debate if you have chosen a controversy that affects you or that you have a strong opinion about. Take your time evaluating the topics available for debate and make your choice based on your interest.

Students can be asked to consider debating on the side of the issues they actually do not support. Many students are quite willing to engage in an attempt to present facts in opposition to their own position. If there are not enough presenters for one side of the debate, volunteers can be recruited for extra credit and the instructor can join the under-represented side.

Dates for debates can be listed in the course outline along with due dates for each debate preparation and response. To ensure that students are prepared as presenters, research sources and points to be made can be submitted in advance.

Debate Presentations: Guidelines for Presenters

Your mission, as a debate presenter, is to gather reliable and valid information from credible sources to support your side of the debate. The student who does a thorough search for the most convincing facts is one who will be confident on the day of his or her debate. The sources can include this text, your class text, the internet, journal articles, books, and in some selected cases, interviews.

Interviews with individuals who are knowledgeable on your topic can be an asset to your presentation. Try to interview experts who have general knowledge about the issue due to their professional activity or scholarly background. One individual with a personal experience does not provide useful information for an academic debate. You may obtain an anecdote that would interest the audience, but not convince them of your point of view because you are citing only the results of a single case. The credibility of your source may be questioned by fellow debaters and audience members.

Audience members are likely to ask presenters to cite their sources, especially when information is highly controversial or difficult to support with research. Be prepared to cite information from sources that you believe are convincing because they are based on good research or well-informed views.

The internet is an expansive, comprehensive, and useful research tool. All students should use this network to find the most current research outcomes and scholarly discourse on their topic. Be cautioned that not everything posted to a website represents truth. Try to confirm your facts and propositions with secondary sources whenever possible.

The internet and the opposing articles contained in this text are good sources to help you consider potential opposing arguments and try to develop counter-points to them. In most cases you will not be required to present counter-arguments, but having these points ready will allow you to refute some points made by the opposing side and gain an advantage for your side of the debate.

Your instructor may give you guidelines for a specific number of references to obtain from each type of source. If not, a suggestion would be to compile at least three points from varying types of sources. Note that fellow debaters, on your side of the debate, may make points similar to yours. Being prepared with several facts allows you to make a unique contribution.

To contribute the most convincing arguments in your debate, you need to commit your points to memory. The 3" by 5" cards should serve only as prompts during the debate. It is not effective to read, word for word, from your cards or your paper. Hopefully, after researching your topic thoroughly and discovering many facets to the arguments related to the issue, you will find yourself quite knowledgeable on the topic. Most prepared students become passionate about presenting their points because they feel confident about knowing their information! This enthusiasm allows for ease of memorization of material because the arguments become meaningful to the student. Whether the facts come from great quotes or good information, the messenger is the catalyst for persuasion of the audience.

Occasionally sources provide comments that are powerful and worthy of quotation. Quoting an author requires that you give him or her credit. In addition to reading the quote, you should elaborate on the point, made by the author of the quote, in your own words.

I urge you to invest yourself in the research process. You will benefit by becoming somewhat of an expert on the topic you choose to debate. You can enjoy being well informed about the entire issue. Stretch yourself to support the opposing side and see what insights develop as a result of this challenge. You will be surprised at the number of occasions on which you may bring up the topic with people outside the classroom if you have chosen an issue you care about and developed a wealth of knowledge about it!

Instructors will have various criteria for evaluating the success of your debate presentation and resources. If you are in an introductory psychology course you may need to prepare at least three reference sources, with content in your own words, and make at least one point during the debate. If your course is more advanced, your instructor may increase these criteria to include more references, sources of specific types, and more arguments made during the debate. The most advanced students may be required to develop counter-points and employ a more sophisticated argumentation format.

At the end of each chapter in this book you will find a worksheet for organizing the content for your debate presentation paper. In general, you need to include complete bibliographic information for each source, properly cited, and a summary of the information obtained in your own words. Many of you have learned to develop this type of annotated bibliography in prior English coursework. Your paper can be written on the form in this book according to the requirements of your instructor. The forms at the end of each issue can serve as your rough draft if you type your report.

In summary, follow these steps to ensure your success as a debate presenter.

1. Sign up for a debate on a topic that is meaningful to you so you will be invested in the research for your presentation and become an enthusiastic debater.

2. Conduct a thorough search for the most convincing points from credible sources to support your side of the controversy. Consider opposing arguments and prepare to refute them.

3. Fill out the Debate Presenter form at the end of the chapter related to your debate, including reference citation details, and points you plan to make, written in your own words.

4. Create 3" by 5" cards with points and references to use as cue cards during the debate.

5. Commit your points to memory and practice presenting your material in a convincing manner.

Debate Presentations: Guidelines for Audience Preparation

As an audience member you will prepare by reading both sides of the issue in this text. As you read, you will formulate your own opinion on the controversy and then you will answer three questions about your views and reading.

A form is included at the end of each set of arguments for each issue to help you organize your responses to the reading. Be sure to give complete answers and turn in the form when instructed to do so. This form is usually due on the day of the debate.

The form asks you for five aspects of your views. First, you are to describe the general controversy related to the issue in your own words. Try to present a summary of the topic in a non-biased manner.

Second, you are asked to identify two points from each side of the debate. Select the two points you believe to be the most important arguments for each side.

Third, write your own opinion about the topic. State which side of the debate you support, and why. Fourth, discuss how your views developed and what influenced you to believe as you do. Reflect on people such as parents, teachers, peers, church friends and leaders and the media as sources of influence on your views.

Last, discuss what information might be necessary to change your views. Imagine learning something during the debate that could influence your opinion. Write about the way in which your views could be changed through exposure to new information.

Debate Presentations: Guidelines for Audience Response

During the debate you will be listening for a poignant comment from a presenter. This statement will be one that catches your attention for some reason. It may be because you heartily agree with the presenter or you may, in fact, seriously disagree with what has been said. The presenter might provoke you to think about some aspect of the controversy that you had not previously considered. For whatever reason, a statement from a presenter will stand out in your mind. Write down the exact quote during the debate and prepare to comment on it later. Ask the presenter to repeat the statement if your need clarification.

There is an audience response form included at the end of each chapter. State the quote, discuss why you felt this quote to be important and state your opinion about it.

The second part of the audience response form asks you to discuss which side of the debate you felt was more convincing. Consider the side that makes the most reliable and valid points to be the most convincing. Try to differentiate between emotional appeals and appeals to logic. Although emotional appeals may be persuasive, they are not as potent as logical arguments. Evaluate the "winning" side according to logic and credible factual information.

The last portion of the audience response asks you to write about the way in which your views have been influenced by listening to the debate. Review the part of your audience preparation that asked for potential information that might change your opinion. Compare your answer to this question with the experience you had during the debate. If you found your views changed, write about the statements that influenced you. Finally, if your view has strengthened, discuss the information that caused you to deepen your convictions.

The audience response form is usually due during the class following the debate. Try to convince your instructor that you were an active listener during the debate and that you are open to information that might influence your position on a topic.

I S S U E 1

Is There a Significant Moral Decline in America?

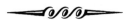

YES James Patterson and Peter Kim, *The Decline and Fall: An Alarmed Perspective*

NO Everett C. Ladd, *The Myth of Moral Decline*

James Patterson and Peter Kim assert that America is in a moral decline. They support this claim by identifying the social institutions where deterioration in values can be observed: the community, the family, religious practices and beliefs, the workplace, public and political institutions, and our morally deficient leaders.

Everett Ladd suggests that people have always thought the moral fiber of America to be in decline. If, in fact, this were the case, we would be completely morally bankrupt at this point in history! He goes on to cite many areas exemplifying our progress in obtaining higher moral ground: race relations, higher standards for our behavior in relation to each other, persisting strength of religious beliefs and practices, reduced academic cheating, fewer extramarital affairs, less stealing and lying, and individualism.

Applications

1. Do you think America is in a state of moral decline? What is the evidence for your answer?

2. Discuss an example of moral decline.

3. Discuss an example of current high moral standards.

4. Do you think your own standards exceed or fall short of your parent's beliefs? What about your practices in comparison to your parent's practices?

Issue 1

YES

The Decline and Fall
An Alarmed Perspective

James Patterson
Peter Kim

Americans have become increasingly alienated from family, church, calling, community, and nation. By the late 1980's, we were living our lives as isolated individuals, islands unto ourselves, detached and self-interested.

Social institutions to which individuals have traditionally looked for moral support and guidance—community, family, religion, work-place, public and political institutions, and our leadership—are less central to everyday American life than they once were.

Community

The prospects for community—in both the moral and sociological sense—are in serious jeopardy. Seventy-two percent of Americans don't know their neighbors well; 66 percent have never worked with others trying to solve community problems; 65 percent refuse to donate any time to community activities; Americans rate their level of community activity a "3" on a scale of "1" to "10"; two-in-three cannot name their local member of Congress.

When asked what traits contemporary Americans are more likely to embody than Americans of the past, our respondents selected such negative adjectives as materialistic, greedy, selfish, criminal, phony, mean, devious, and skeptical. On the other hand, when asked to select traits that Americans of 30 years ago were more likely to embody, they selected neighborliness, civic-mindedness, patriotism, volunteerism, religiousness, honesty, morality, hard work, compassion, and charity. In short, all of the traits we generally associate with community were associated with the past, while the traits we associate with selfishness, narcissism, calculation, and anti-social behavior are associated with the present.

Family

The American family is crumbling. Over 50 percent of Americans assert that there is no need for people living together ever to marry; 60 percent of Americans who were married have considered divorce or been divorced; 39 percent of Americans believe that "till death do us part," is an outdated concept; 31 percent of currently married Americans have cheated on their spouses; 43 percent of married respondents aren't sure they would marry the same person if they had it to do over; 25 percent would abandon their families for $10 million.

Religion

Religion has little impact on the moral life of the majority of Americans. Most Americans aren't sure of their church's position on the great moral issues of the day—from school busing, capital punishment, book-banning, affirmative action, birth control, homosexuality, teaching creationism in the schools, pornography, and premarital sex to civil rights. Eighty-four percent of Americans report being willing to violate the teachings of their own faith if those teachings conflict with their own personal sense of right and wrong. And although we are a predominately Christian nation, only 11 percent report believing in all 10 of the Ten Commandments (42 percent of African-Americans report believing in five or fewer).

Work

The work ethic has given way to hedonism, and the spirit of capitalism has gone awry. Sixty-four percent of Americans confess to malingering, procrastinating, or abusing alcohol or drugs in the workplace; 33 percent conduct personal chores on company time; fewer than one in four Americans report giving their maximum effort at work. Americans report goofing-off about 20 percent of the time while at work; only 24 percent of Americans report that they work in order to realize their full potential (the rest do it for the money); 13 percent regularly leave work early and 10 percent regularly arrive late.

Public Institutions

Our public institutions have lost much of their legitimacy. From 1973/74 to 1989, the proportion of Americans expressing a great deal of confidence in each of the institutions below declined by the amount shown:

- organized religion (-55 percent);

- organized labor (-50 percent);

- educational institutions (-39 percent);

- television (-39 percent);
- the press (-35 percent);
- the executive branch (-31 percent);
- the Congress (-26 percent);
- major companies (-23 percent).

Leadership

We face a serious crisis in leadership. Seventy-two percent of Americans do not think that any public figure provides moral leadership; 68 percent cannot name a single American leader they admire; 70 percent do not think America has any more heroes; 68 percent do not think there are any adequate role models in public life for their children to follow.

The Age of Moral Ambiguity

More and more, the isolated individual, disconnected from external moral reference points, has come to view himself/herself as the sole arbiter of moral life. In fact, 93 percent of all Americans report that they alone determine what is moral in their lives.

As a consequence of this lack of external structures of moral support, Americans are increasingly coming to view the great moral issues of the day as "gray" issues without a clear right and wrong. More than a third of Americans believes there is no clear right or wrong position when it comes to the following issues: affirmative action (54 percent); creationism in schools (52 percent); premarital sex (52 oercent); the right to die (44 percent); school busing (44 percent); homosexuality (43 percent); flag burning (38 percent); pornography (38 percent); capital punishment (37 percent).

Crime and Punishment in a Post-Moral Society

One need no longer read Dostoevsky, Camus, or Genet to probe the significance of crime and punishment in everyday life. One is tempted to speculate that a decline of moral support-structures and the rise of the self have led to a society in which it is increasingly difficult to maintain social order. If individuals no longer believe in the moral legitimacy of the community, what is there to keep them from flouting its rules? We found that systematic rule-breaking was one such consequence.

Crime has become so rampant, as to be a part of everyday life: fully 60 percent of Americans have been the victim of a least one crime in their lifetimes, and fully 35 percent have been victimized more than once; 39 percent of Americans readily confess to having committed some kind of crime themselves.

Violence has become so commonplace as to have become "normalized" to an extent. Sixty-four percent of Americans believe the use of physical force is sometimes justified, 59 percent admit to having used physical force on another person; fewer than half (45 percent) of those who have used physical force regret it; 12 percent of Americans report having injured someone enough to send them to the hospital; 9 percent have threatened someone with a knife (6 percent used it); 9 percent have threatened someone with a gun (4 percent used it).

The End of Childhood

In our society, childhood has traditionally been a time of innocence. No one aspect stood for childhood innocence more than sexual innocence and naivete. Even Freud, who placed sexuality at the very heart of his world view, attributed a period of "dormancy" to childhood sexuality. However, today, we are facing a radically new phenomenon: we are living in a age of sexually precocious children.

Discussions of the "sexual revolution" go back to the coming of age of baby boomers in the 1960s. Indeed, our data found that baby boomers were significantly less likely to have been virgins when they married (29 percent), than either their parents' generation (42 percent) or their grandparents (41 percent). Clearly, baby boomers had disconnected sex from marriage.

However, baby boomers do not report having started sexual activity at an earlier age than either their parents or grandparents. The baby boomers and their parents both became sexually active at about the same age; the only difference is that baby boomer's parents married younger. For both baby boomers and their parents, only a relative few had become sexually active by age 13 (less than 5 percent). What is so striking about those between the ages of 18 and 24 is that more than one in five has lost their virginity by age 13 and almost two-thirds by age 16.

A Thousand Points of Darkness: The Privatization of Social Responsibility

With the end of the 1980s, we found Americans retreating into an ever-more private and isolated existence, and are becoming less willing to confront the social issues and social problems of the day. Poverty and race are being redefined as private problems, more the fault of those "afflicted" than social problems that need to be addressed by society as a whole. Forty-two percent of Americans believe that the poor are poor because they are lazy or because of other faults of their own. And when it comes to race, Americans clearly believe that the problem lies with African-Americans and not with white America: two in three believe that African-Americans have the same opportunities as whites; 68 percent believe that some races are harder working than others.

The Myth of Moral Decline

Everett C. Ladd

The moral state of the United States is the subject of enormous attention and concern. Although this has been a recurring theme throughout American history, there is some indication that concern has grown in our own time. Rushworth M. Kidder, President of the Institute for Global Ethics, recently noted in *The Public Perspective* that dozens of ethics organizations are springing up across the nation, hundreds of executive ethics seminars are conducted every year, and thousands of students are participating in character education at school. The press is now full of discussions of ethics issues. Kidder cites data showing, for example, that between 1969 and 1989 the number of stories found under "ethics" in the *New York Times* index increased four-fold.

Survey data also indicate that the proportion of the public troubled by what they perceive to be serious deficiencies in the moral state of the nation is not only large but expanding. True, throughout the span of our history for which we have survey data, large majorities have expressed dissatisfaction with such matters as the honesty and standards of behavior of their fellow citizens. Nonetheless, the proportions today are at the highest levels we have seen. For instance, in 1938, when asked if the "general morals" of young unmarried people were better or worse than they had been 10 years earlier, 42 percent of those interviewed by the Roper Organization said they were worse, compared to just 13 percent who said they were better. In 1987, 60 percent of those interviewed in a Yankelovich Clancy Shulman poll said teenagers were "less moral in their behavior at present than when (the respondents) were growing up," while only 11 percent described young people as more moral. Every time we have located a pair of queries like this from the 1930s-50s span on the one hand, and from the 1980-90s on the other, we have found the same pattern: Majorities always profess to see decline in moral standards, but the majority is larger in the contemporary period than earlier.

Again and again, polls show Americans expressing this kind of values nostalgia. But has there, in fact, been a deterioration in moral conduct in the United States, as compared to, say, the 1950s? Ethical norms and moral conduct are of great importance to the health of the American society and polity, and it certainly matters which way the great engines of contemporary society are pulling us with regard to them. Yet for all the importance of this question and the attention it has received, the data are not as clear as the polls might suggest.

There's Always So Much Wrong

One obstacle standing in the way of productive analysis involves the fact that at every point in time, in the view of many thoughtful people, ethical standards and moral conduct leave much to be desired. Michael Josephson and his colleagues have attempted empirical work on Americans' moral judgments and behavior which, they say, reveals that a "disturbingly high proportion of young people regularly engage in dishonest and irresponsible behavior." What an extraordinary way to put it! It is, after all, a little late in human history to present as a finding that a disturbingly high proportion of people variously err and sin. The Josephson study documents that many young people are struggling and stumbling ethically, but it tells us nothing about whether things are actually getting better or worse.

Is the contemporary U.S. beset with moral decline? If we had a "Morality Index," on which 100 was utopia and zero the modern equivalent of Sodom and Gomorrah, and found the U.S. standing at 50, that should be cause for national concern. But it would be one thing if we also found that the country's position on this mythic measure had been 80 in 1867, 70 in 1917, and 60 in 1957, quite another if we found that it had been hovering around 50 in each of those earlier years.

We don't have such an index, nor do we have the kind of imaginative and thorough data-gathering such a measure would require. We only know that moral conduct today is "deficient." I have no intention of making light of this when I note that part of the reason we think today's problems are so pressing is that they are the ones we face. Since we can do absolutely nothing about previous sins, present problems are the "worst" in the sense that they are the ones that occupy us and require our efforts at remedy....

Changing Standards and Perceptions

Assessing the moral state of the union is made more difficult by the fact that our standards keep changing. Moreover, the institutions through which the public gains a sense of the moral state of the nation now tend to portray social and political institutions in a negative light.

As to changing standards, consider the area of race relations. Surely we have made enormous strides along this dimension of national moral conduct since the 1850s. We have ended slavery and, all to belatedly, we must acknowledge, eradicated the system of gross exclusion of African-Americans from various facilities and entitlements, known as "Jim Crow." Survey data on racial attitudes and various behavioral data alike attest to the spread and strengthening of public support for extending to African-Americans the Declaration's lofty insistence that all people are created equal and possess inalienable rights.

But in assessing moral conduct, we seem largely to ignore this historical perspective. Is America now living in satisfactory accord with the norm set forth in the Declaration of Independence and in other statements of national ideals? Of course not. But today's short-comings are the ones that now occupy us—even when we recognize marked gains from times past. *We expect more of ourselves in this area than we did 50 or 150 years ago—and we come up short.*

Media studies have for some time examined the issue of political negativism or cynicism, suggesting that press bias results not so much from political preferences as from professional outlook. The press often portrays various national institutions as seamy and even unworthy of support. Austin Ranney argues that there is not so much "a political bias in favor of liberalism or conservatism, as a structural bias..." which encourages a cynical and excessively manipulative view of politics. Michael Robinson's research has supported the view that the press fosters a pervasive cynicism:

> Events are frequently conveyed by television news through an inferential structure that often injects a negativistic, contentious, or anti-institutional bias. These biases, frequently dramatized by film portrayals of violence and aggression, evoke images of American politics and social life which are inordinately sinister and despairing.

In addition to America's historic sense of creedal anxiety, then, recent factors, such as changing standards of justice and press negativism, may be encouraging an even more pessimistic view. At the very least, all these factors suggest there is reason to doubt that the apparently widespread sense of moral decline is simply a reflection of the actual progression.

What the Data Actually Show

The various factors sketched above present terrible difficulties for the literature which purports to provide thoughtful guidance on the matter of which way we are headed. As a result, analysts often seem to be led to the conclusion that deterioration is occurring, even when available information is inconclusive or flat-out says otherwise.

When we look at the status of religion in America and a number of moral norms, it is not at all clear America is in moral decline. The country's religious life, for instance, is often considered a moral barometer. A decade ago, I was asked to prepare a conference paper reviewing what surveys had to say about the religious beliefs and practices of the American people. As the Reverend Richard John Neuhaus observed at the New York Conference, the conventional wisdom had it that "America is or is rapidly becoming a secular society."

I began my paper by acknowledging that on this subject, as on so many, there are severe limits as to what polls can tell us. They are blunt instruments, unable to help us much with the searching, the ambiguity, the depth and subtlety that necessarily surround any basic set of human needs and values. Nevertheless, the story told by survey research was remarkably clear and unambiguous with regard to the general character and directions of Americans' religious life; namely, the U.S. is distinguished from most other advanced industrial democracies by the persisting strength of religious beliefs and of organized religious practice. As Seymour Martin Lipset argued in *The First New Nation*, published in 1963, "the one empirical generalization which does seem justified about American religion is that from the early nineteenth century down to the present, the United States has been among the most religious countries in the Christian world." Similarly, James Reichley concluded his examination of *Religion in American Life* with the assessment that "Americans remain, despite recent incursions of civil humanism among cultural elites and relentless promotion of egoism by advertising and entertainment media, overwhelmingly, in Justice [William O.] Douglas's words, 'a religious people'."

My own assessments of available survey information have supported these observations. Americans continue, for example, in virtually unchanging proportions to describe religion as important in their own lives. The proportion describing themselves as members of a church or synagogue, while down just a bit from the levels of the 1930–50s, has, on the whole, remained both high and constant. Surveys conducted by the National Opinion Research Center have continued to find overwhelming majorities of the public describing the Bible as either "the actual word of God ... to be taken literally, word for word," (the response of 33 percent in 1993); or as "the inspired word of God, but not everything in it should be taken literally, word for word" (49 percent stating this). Only 15 percent categorized the Bible as "an ancient book of fables, legends, history, and moral precepts recorded by men." Also, prayer remains integral to Americans, even among young adults and high-income citizens (65 percent and 69 percent of whom, respectively, agreed with the statement that "prayer is an important part of my daily life").

Perhaps most striking is the extent to which the U.S. differs religiously from other advanced industrial democracies. In 1981, Gallup conducted a series of surveys cross-nationally which found 79 percent of Americans saying they gained strength from religion, compared to 46 percent in Britain, 44 percent of West Germans, and 37 percent of the French. Similarly, 84 percent of those interviewed in the U.S. said they believed in heaven, as against 57 percent in Britain, 31 percent in West Germany, 27 percent in France, and 26 percent in Sweden.

This isn't to say that there have been no changes in the structure of American religious life. We know, for example, that over the last 30 to 40 years, while the proportion of the population which is "churched" has remained basically constant, the denominational mix has changed quite strikingly. Sociologist Benton Johnson notes that American religious groups have differed greatly in terms of membership gains and losses. He points out that evangelical churches have prospered even as main-line Protestant denominations have suffered serious membership losses during this period.

Taking a longer view of American religious experience from the eighteenth century to the present, we see many substantial shifts. Interesting enough, though, these shifts are more often than not in the opposite direction from those assumed in most commentary. That is, *the long movement over time in the U.S. seems clearly to be toward religion*, not away from it. Pointing to the decline of organized atheism and church membership gains in the nineteenth century, sociologist Theodore Caplow suggested:

> One concedes too much when one says we're just about as religious as we used to be. We may be a good deal more religious than we used to be.

Yet, while virtually all the scholars who have reviewed the systematic data which are available to us have reached the same conclusions on American religious experience, most of the group assembled at the New York conference strongly rejected the idea that American religious commitments are notably strong and enduring. For example, George Marsden, a leading student of evangelicalism and fundamentalism, dismissed most of the findings on religious belief as essentially meaningless because, as he saw it, they picked up only an insubstantial, superficial, essentially trivial commitment. "As you know," Marsden argued, "the common comment on fundamentalism is that it is just secularism in disguise. It is a way of endorsing a materialistic, self-centered lifestyle. And that's something that could be said about a lot of American Christianity."

Marsden brought up the often-cited remark which is attributed (perhaps entirely incorrectly, according to some historians) to Dwight Eisenhower. Ike is reputed to have said: "Our government makes no sense unless it is founded on a deeply religious faith—and I don't care what it (that faith) is." This hollow, instrumental approach to faith encapsulates, Marsden argued, what's wrong with religion in the U.S.

Political scientist Stanley Rothman had a perspective similar to Marsden's:

> In a public opinion survey people are asked, "Do you believe in hard work?" Sure, everyone may mouth that. But there's a difference between saying that and actually doing it... And I would say the same thing about religious attitudes among the population as a whole. Modernization of the west has led to the erosion of the traditional structures and beliefs...now there is evidence that people no longer take religion so seriously, unless they redefine it in some ways. I think there has been a general redefinition, not among the whole population, but among substantial segments of the population, so as to fit religion into their own wishes and desires... Unfortunately this cannot be proven with data.

And so it went. Most of the participants were convinced that in a deeper sense, whatever the numbers seem to show, religious belief is in precipitous decline in modern America.

Nor is religion the only area in which our perceptions of deterioration conflict with other measures of experience. While there are important areas where Americans are in deep disagreement about what constitutes the proper moral or ethical standards—the case of abortion is certainly a prime example—far more often than not the data point to broad agreement on the norm. As Table 1 shows, norms condemning various forms of cheating, lying, and

Table 1
Professed Norms Are Strong and Conventional

Tax Fraud

Question: Do you feel it is wrong if...
a taxpayer does not report all of his
income in order to pay less income tax?

Wrong: 94%   Not Wrong: 4%

Source: Survey by NORC for the
International Social Survey Program
(ISSP), Feb.–April 1991.

Question: Have you ever cheated on
your federal income taxes, or not?

No: 95%   Yes: 4%

Source: Survey by the Gallup
Organization, March 28–30, 1991

Lying

Question: Do you think is is sometimes
justified to lie to friends or to family
members or do you think lying is never
justified?

Never: 73%   Depends: 10%
Justified: 18%

Source: Survey by CBS News/New York
Times, December 7–9, 1992.

Extramarital Affairs

Question: Do you think it is always wrong
or sometimes okay for...a married person
to have sex with someone other than
his/her spouse?

Always Wrong: 87%   Sometimes OK: 11%

Source: Survey by Yankelovich Clancy
Shulman for Time/CNN, June 4–5, 1991.

Question: (If ever married) Have you ever
had sex with someone other than your
husband or wife while you were married?

No: 83%   Yes: 17%

Source: Survey by NORC-GSS,
February–April 1993.

Stealing

Question: The...eighth commandment
is...Do not steal...Does the way you live
these days completely satisfy...or not at all
satisfy the commandment?

Completely: 86%   Not at all: 2%

Source: Survey by Barna Research Group,
January 1992.

stealing seem firmly entrenched across most of the population. If we are going to hell in a handbasket, it's not because the preponderance of Americans have abandoned their attachment to many of the older verities.

But does this simply suggest that hypocrisy is on the rise—that we have become more inclined to act contrary to our professed standards? Not necessarily. Take the case of cheating. A lot of people, including many educators, seem to believe that cheating is on the rise—even though young Americans continue to condemn cheating. But many of the best survey data available to us say otherwise. The Gallup Youth Surveys, for example, show that many more young people describe cheating at their own schools as *more infrequent* now than three decades ago. The proportion saying that they themselves have cheated at some time or another, while high, seems to be decreasing.

We know that people often fail to live up to standards to which they express adherence. But we also know that norms matter—that is, they actually regulate conduct, if imperfectly—and that large changes in conduct rarely, if ever, take place without correspondingly large changes in professed norms. Consider, for example, premarital sexual relations. Behavior has clearly shifted mightily in the "sexual revolution" of the last several decades, but so too has the professed norm. When there is a problem, as in the latter area, the survey findings readily pick it up.

One of the things that seem to be bothering Americans most is the sense that the old-time standards-setting, which was centered around the institutions of family and church, is being replaced by new ones, centered in remote and morally vacuous institutions, such as popular music, TV, and movies. Data presented in Table 2 demonstrate this concern clearly. But as we see in the figure, other data show that most of us say that, for us personally, the old order of standards-setting still holds. Furthermore, a Roper Organization survey for *Good Housekeeping* in 1991 found that 86 percent of women shared the values of their parents, 10 percent had somewhat different values, and only 4 percent had very different values. In the same survey, 85 percent of the women who were mothers thought their children would have the same values.

Once again, there is a striking tension between the perceived deterioration in moral norms and conduct nationally on the one hand, and the sense of strength and continuity drawn from personal experience on the other. We see this again and again across many areas. Thus 63 percent of respondents in the Gallup survey of November 1992 said that "religion as a whole" is losing its influence on American life, while only 27 percent described religion's influence as increasing. As we have seen, though, a great deal of the data indicates that religion in America continues to flourish.

Individualism: Strength or Weakness?

The moral shortcomings of this society often grow out of the same elements that enhance national life. The positives and negatives are frequently but flip sides of a single structure of national values. As many analysts from Alexis de Tocqueville on down to the present have observed, the core of the sociopolitical ideology on which the U.S. was founded is a uniquely insistent and far-reaching individualism—a view of the individual person which gives unprecedented weight to his or her choices, interests, and claims. This distinctive individualism has always enriched the moral life of the country in important regards and posed serious challenges to it in yet others....

Table 2
Where Do Today's Values Come From?

Question: What do you think (has/should have) the most influence on the values of young people today?

	Has	Should Have
TV & Movies	34%	1%
Parents	20	74
Young People	19	1
Musicians & Music Videos	10	0
Celebrities, Athletes	6	1
Teachers	5	9
Political Leaders	2	1
Religious Leaders	1	11
Military Leaders	1	0

Source: Survey by Mellman & Lazarus for Massachusetts Mutual Life Insurance Co., September 1991.

Question: What do you feel has been the single most important factor in influencing your beliefs about what is right or wrong?

Parents	47%
Religion	28%
Personal Experience	8%
Other	8%
Not Sure	8%

Source: Survey by Yankelovich Clancy Shulman for Time, January 19–21, 1987.

An abundance of data from our own time show that this dynamic sense of individual responsibility and capabilities has continued. Philanthropy has also increased dramatically: in 1955, individuals gave more than $5 billion to charity; this amount rose to $102 billion in 1990 (a rate of increase that outpaced inflation significantly). Surveys suggest that, in recent years, the proportion of the populace giving of its time for charitable and social service activities has actually been increasing. The moral life of the nation is thus strengthened.

Individualism has contributed much historically to the vitality of American family life and created a distinctively American type of family. Children, nineteenth century visitors often remarked, didn't occupy a subordinate place—"to be seen and not heard"—like their European counterparts, but were exuberant, vociferous, spoiled participants. Similarly, visiting commentators often remarked on the effects of America's pervasive individualism on the status of women. Bryce, for example, saw women's rights more widely recognized in the U.S. than in Europe. This had resulted, he argued, because "the root idea of democracy cannot stop at defining men as male human beings, anymore than it could ultimately stop at defining them as white human beings.... Democracy is in America more respectful of the individual... than it has shown itself in Continental Europe, and this regard for the individual enured to the benefit of women."

But just as the country's demanding individualism has liberated individuals to achieve productive lives for themselves and contribute to a dynamic public life, so it has also been a source of distinctive problems. Many analysts have argued that these problems with the American ideology are evident not so much in the fact that these ideals are sometimes unachieved, as that their achievement may create terrible difficulties....

Present-day critics of the "dark side" of individualist America charge that individualism has come to emphasize the gratification of the self over the needs of various important social institutions including, above all, the family. In *Habits of the Heart: Individualism and Commitment in American Life*, Robert Bellah and colleagues grant that "our highest and noblest aspirations, not only for ourselves, but for those we care about, for our society in the world, are closely linked to our individualism." Moreover, America cannot abandon its individualism, for "that would mean for us to abandon our deepest identity."

Still, Bellah *et al.* insist, "some of our deepest problems both as individuals and as a society are also closely linked to our individualism." It has become far too unrestrained. Historically in the U.S., the natural tendencies within individualism toward narrow self-service were mitigated by the strength of religion and the ties of the local community. No longer. In their view, individualism has been trans-mogrified by a radical insistence upon individual autonomy, so profoundly corrosive of the family and other collective institutions that depend upon substantial subordination of individual claims for social goods.

The recent historical record suggests that neither the boosters nor the knockers of individualism quite have it right. On the positive side, factors like the continued strength of voluntarism in America signal the degree to which individualism strengthens moral conduct by stressing individual responsibility and encouraging the view that "what I do" can really matter. Also, the individualistic ethic in America has fueled important advances for women and African-Americans under the banner of the "inalienable rights" to "Life, Liberty and the pursuit of Happiness." On the other hand, that ethic constantly runs the risk of leaving the individual far too radically autonomous. It suggests that whatever serves a person's sense of his/her rights and entitlements is, miraculously, good for the society or, at the least, something which the society may not lightly challenge.

But the down-side of contemporary individualism does not quite play itself out in the way that recent arguments suggest. Individualism does not necessarily equal "selfishness." Rather, it seems to be that Americans are construing their own self-interest too narrowly. Hence, many of the men and women implicated in the rise in divorce and single-parent households—which has posed difficulties for many children and communities—would seem to have a "narrow" sense of self-interest, which is not serving them or their children very well. They need to be reminded, as Tocqueville argued, that self-interest is only justified when it is "properly understood" in a communal context, which is to say that individuals can only flourish in robust communities....

Has there been a deterioration of moral conduct? Probably not. But we have been given ample proof that extending commitment to our national idea, which centers around a profound individualism, is by no means an unmixed blessing. As the U.S. has progressed in recognizing the worth and the claims of people previously excluded from the Declaration's promise, it has also encouraged tendencies which have destructive possibilities, liable to see the individual as too radically autonomous and leave him too narrowly self-serving. In seeking to improve the moral conduct of the nation, earlier generations of Americans have had to build on the positive elements of the country's individualist ethic, so as to curb its dark side. Ours is surely no exception.

Debate Presenter Form

Follow the guidelines for debate presenters contained in the introduction of this text and those given to you by your instructor. Use the format below to organize the material for your debate. Remember to include all relevant citation information and to present the related information in your own words. Give credit to authors when you cite a quote and be as thorough as possible when writing about your points so you will be prepared for your debate.

Reference citation #1:

Author: _____

Title: _____

Date: _____

Source: _____

_____

Content from reference citation #1: _____

_____

_____

_____

_____

_____

_____

_____

_____

_____

_____

_____

_____

Reference citation #2:

Author: _____

Title: _____

Date: _____

Source: _____

_____

Content from reference citation #2: _____

_____

_____

_____

_____

_____

_____

Reference citation #3:

Author: _____

Title: _____

Date: _____

Source: _____

_____

Content from reference citation #3: _____

_____

_____

_____

_____

Audience Preparation Form

Follow the guidelines for preparing to be an informed audience member on the day of the debate included in the introduction to this text. After reading both sides of the debate from this chapter, answer the following questions. Be as thorough as possible so that you will be able to make a contribution to the debate by asking informed questions or making provocative comments. This form is usually due on the day of the debate.

State the issue in your own words. Do not plagiarize the text. Demonstrate that you understand the topic and it's relevant arguments.

_____

_____

_____

_____

_____

Discuss two points on the "yes" side of the debate.

Point #1: _____

_____

Point #2: _____

_____

Discuss two points on the "no" side of the debate.

Point #1: _____

_____

Point #2: _____

_____

What is your opinion on this topic?

_____

_____

_____

_____

_____

_____

_____

What has contributed to the development of your views about this topic?

_____

_____

_____

_____

_____

_____

_____

_____

What information would be necessary to cause you to change your thinking about this topic?

_____

_____

_____

_____

_____

Debate Response Form

Follow the guidelines for responding to the debates in the introductory chapter of this text. Complete this form and submit your answers at the class following the debate. Try to be thorough and convince your instructor that you were an active listener during the debate.

List a quote from a debate presenter that you think was important and explain why you think this comment was significant.

_____

_____

_____

_____

Which side of the debate do you think made the most convincing arguments, why?

_____

_____

_____

_____

_____

After hearing the debate, in what way has your thinking been affected?

_____

_____

_____

_____

_____

_____

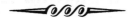

Social Issues

I S S U E   2

Is Physician Assisted Suicide a Psychologically Valid Choice?

 YES H.S. Cohen, *Euthanasia as a Way of Life*

 NO Herbert Hendin and Gerald Klerman,
Physician-Assisted Suicide: The Dangers of Legalization

   This issue focuses on the **psychological** reasons for physician-assisted suicide. This emphasis differs from medically based decisions and decisions that reside with the person's family. The central question addresses the psychological condition of the person choosing to die and the controversy surrounds the legitimacy of allowing an individual to choose to end his or her life as a psychologically valid option.

   Herbert Hendin and Gerald Klerman assert that the individual choosing to die with the assistance of a physician is most likely to have a treatable mental illness such as depression. This depression can result from such tragedies as having a terminal illness or being elderly and fearful of burdening one's family.

   Terror of illness and hopelessness at the end of the life cycle are not legitimate reasons to end one's life according to these authors. They suggest that treatment for depression be the solution, not death. These authors also have great concerns for the potential abuses a legal sanction for physician-assisted suicide would bring to our society.

In the counter-argument, H.S. Cohen cites the potential psychological benefits to having the right-to-die with physician assistance. He has witnessed changes in terminally ill patients that he describes as "tranquility," "acceptance," and "radiating peace" as the psychological reasons for conducting euthanasia. He comments that the patient actually grows emotionally and psychologically during the period when the assisted death is being negotiated.

Cohen supports the positive effects of the prospect of physician-assisted suicide on healthy individuals. The terror associated with anticipation of a prolonged illness or uselessness that comes with age is diminished with the knowledge that one has the power to avoid these circumstances if one chooses.

Finally, Cohen addresses the biblical considerations of euthanasia. He supports the right of individuals to conduct a dignified ending to their lives based on their beliefs, not to be restricted from doing so by the beliefs of others.

Applications

1. Would you consider a physician-assisted suicide? If yes, why, if no, why not?

2. Do you think it should be an individual's right to choose physician-assisted suicide or do you believe a standard of disallowing physician-assisted suicide serves humanity best? Explain.

3. Identify the conditions under which you would support physician-assisted suicide. If there are no such situations, explain why.

Euthanasia as a Way of Life

— H.S. Cohen —

In this contribution I shall concentrate on a not so straightforward, but fascinating question: What is the effect of the option of euthanasia before it is performed? More specifically on the life of patients, relatives, doctors, nurses, volunteers and on society as a whole. That such an influence exists and is profound indeed, I hope to demonstrate.

Let me first concentrate on individuals who have a considerable stretch of life and suffering waiting for them, e.g., patients with AIDS and those severely handicapped by multiple sclerosis. (The use of the word "patient" does not suggest a kind of inferior race. It just means you and me somewhere in the future when we shall be not as healthy as we are now.) Anybody with bedside experience must have noted the change that comes over these patients when a request for euthanasia is being seriously negotiated and the end of life is no longer a conversational topic to be hushed up. After becoming aware of it, this effect can be observed more often and more clearly. I cannot offer any proper scientific evidence in this field, just observations and speculations. To describe this change in the sick person, which of course is different for every individual, I would use words ranging from "acceptance," and "tranquility" up to "radiating peace" and "happiness." In careful euthanasia the decision-making process usually takes weeks or even months. In my memory it is the patient himself or herself who grows and matures in this period and gradually provides relatives with support and consolation. Euthanasia takes away the fear of unknown suffering in unknown intensity for an unknown period.

But I want to stress a second point, i.e., that euthanasia forces us to communicate about life and death in a very direct way, without the usual social chitchat and niceties. A tendency towards non-verbal communication comes quite naturally. Hugging and kissing are not inappropriate. Doctors should not discuss euthanasia, standing at the foot of the bed, in a white coat, mumbling Latin incantations. The least is to sit down, hold hands, and speak only if silence does not speak for itself. This kind of attitude is bound to be catching in the family and will improve the closeness and warmth and understanding between relatives and friends. I'm convinced that in fact a substantial part of the bereavement is experienced before the patient passes away. Of course there is grief afterwards as well. But, in my experience grief of a "healthy" kind, often mixed with sincere relief and cheerfulness. Dr. Admiraal has often stated that the performance of euthanasia is part of good medical care. In this line the option of euthanasia might well be considered part of spiritual care.

The paradox that euthanasia is good for life goes further. Can it even prolong life, that is, an acceptable form of life? Let's consider an AIDS patient who is determined to commit suicide before the going gets too rough. He'll have to execute his plans while he still has the strength to do so himself. In this situation the promise of assisted suicide or euthanasia takes away the urgency of executing his intention. Euthanasia can indeed prolong life by offering a humane way of dying.

In a well-known experiment, published [recently] in the *Lancet*, Dr. Spiegel of Stanford University offered psycho-social group therapy to women with breast cancer. He found that these patients lived for a average [of] 36 months. The matched control group lived for 19 months only. The gained life-span of 17 months is attributed to the psycho-social treatment. Other research also suggests that social interventions (and why not euthanasia?) in fact may prolong not only the quality, but the quantity of life as well.

In postgraduate courses for nurses or doctors quite often the questions pops up whether it is appropriate for a doctor or nurse to take the initiative in bringing up the subject of euthanasia. This is a tricky dilemma of course. It could be misunderstood as a sign of impatience on the part of the doctor. Still I want to answer that question in the affirmative. In terminal care time runs faster and the future is nearer than one might hope. To have plenty of time to discuss the subject leisurely, without being pressed by the progress of disease, creates circumstances for careful preparation and, as I have mentioned, contributes to the quality of life.

Does euthanasia affect the life of healthy people, like you and me, the patients of the future? Does it affect those who have witnessed the process, in the first place the volunteers of the Dutch Members Aid Service, but also relatives, doctors and nurses? Speaking for myself it has indeed. The subjects of death and illness and aging have lost much of their terror. The fountain of youth does not exist and I don't mind anymore. We rather avoid thinking of ourselves as mortals. That seems to be one reason for the shortage of organ-donors for transplantation. It could also explain the small membership of euthanasia societies in contrast to the majorities in favor in opinion polls. It has taught me to approach patients with a warm heart and a clear head. After those moments of closeness and sharing one realizes how much time is lost in polite conversations and good manners. On the other hand it is most important not to be carried away by emotions, but to remain firmly in charge of oneself and the situation. Our efforts in this field are properly rewarded with personal growth and maturing.

So much for individuals, now about society: Let me quote Joseph Fletcher in a milestone article on 'The courts and euthanasia': "Poll after poll of public opinion shows a clear and growing majority in favor of the right to choose to die, and to have medical help in doing so. The taboo is simply dying away, as most taboos do sooner or later. The hurdle in the way is a psychological or visceral one, not logical or ethical, as we break through the conventional wisdom." The polls result indeed in astonishing numbers: Sometimes over 80% of the population and 50% of the doctors [are] in favor. The last bulletin of the Belgian Euthanasia Society written by professor Kenis presents a clear review. But taboos are still with us. Even in Holland, which to many of you must appear to be Utopia. The foremost one is still the fear of death and dying. And indeed our real adversaries are not the pope or the archbishop of Canterbury but the makers of television commercials, brainwashing us with the notion that only youth makes life worthwhile.

Euthanasia forces society to reconsider the limits of tolerance: Will those opposed allow the other side to practice euthanasia? Will those in favor respect the freedom of conscientious objectors to not be involved? In respect of the latter, the qualification "voluntary" goes not only for the patient's request but for the cooperation of doctors and nurses as well. The usual arguments in the debate clearly demonstrate that tolerance is still a sapling in need of a lot of care and nursing.

There is the rather easy mud [s]linging and character defamation: people in favor of euthanasia must be cruel, lazy, atheist doctors. Or greedy, careless relatives. Let anybody prove such an allegation! As an experienced colleague of mine remarked: "If you want the best care and the most attention from your doctor, just ask for euthanasia."

The second class of objections is of [a] religious or philosophical nature: "We are the stewards of life, not the owners." "Thou shalt not kill," or in the new English translation "You must not commit murder." The Bible seems to offer great support to any opinion whether it be in favor or against. These considerations must carry much weight for believers and may in fact wholly determine their conduct. But they do not regard those of differing convictions. Legislation or the attitude of society in general are political subjects! Most of our societies are permissive enough to let citizens [be] free to indulge in drinking, to have twenty children, to take part in motor-races. All rather unhealthy activities, but tolerated. Euthanasia is more unobtrusive than any of those.

What does affect us are the slippery slope type arguments: the idea that use will be followed by abuse. The fear that safeguards will shrink to a shoddy routine. It is a very human reaction to resist any change and to feel secure in the trusted routines. All parents observe that in their children. I do take this argument as an incentive to keep my eyes open. Those involved in euthanasia themselves should be the guardians of this slippery slope and watch closely for strict observance of all safeguards. And it works in [my] country. In the hundreds of cases that have been examined by judicial authorities no trend of laxity has been detected. On the contrary. I do not advocate to transplant the Dutch system of guidelines to every country in the world. We are fortunate to have a health care system that is available for every citizen. So euthanasia does not have to be a substitute for lack of medical care. And secondly our medical establishment is not commercially inclined. I can easily imagine the necessity of stricter safeguards and checks in many other communities.

I'm consulted two to four times a week on euthanasia. These consultations of today differ markedly from those five years ago. There is much improvement in the knowledge of principles and procedures involved. Panic situations have become exceptional. Effective medical interventions are rarely overlooked. And to my great satisfaction, growing skills in terminal and palliative care are evident.

Still a lot of work is to be done, even in Holland. Quite separate from the matter of legislation, euthanasia is still not fully integrated in our culture. It does not have a firm place in the curriculum of all medical and nursing schools. It is not discussed in high schools as is contraception or voting rights. It deserves such a place because euthanasia, by its sheer existence as an option stimulates terminal care, makes patients aware of their rights. And generally speaking it has a very healthy influence on the attitude of doctors.

Issue 2

NO

Physician-Assisted Suicide
The Dangers of Legislation

Herbert Hendin
Gerald Klermen

There are situations when helping a terminally ill patient end his or her life seems appropriate. For centuries physicians have helped such patients die. Why should we not protect them and at the same time make it easier for the terminally ill to end their lives by legalizing physician-assisted suicide? The movement to do so represents such a drastic departure from established social policy and medical tradition that it needs to be evaluated in the light of what we now know about suicide and terminal illness.

We know that 95% of those who kill themselves have been shown to have a diagnosable psychiatric illness in the months preceding suicide. The majority suffer from depression, which can be treated. This is particularly true of the elderly, who are more prone than younger victims to take their lives during the type of acute depressive episode that responds most effectively to modern available treatments. Other diagnoses among the suicides include alcoholism, substance abuse, schizophrenia, and panic disorder; treatments are available for all of these illnesses.

Advocates of physician-assisted suicide try to convey the impression that in terminally ill patients the wish to die is totally different from suicidal intent in those without terminal illness. However, like other suicidal individuals, patients who desire an early death during a terminal illness are usually suffering from a treatable mental illness, most commonly a depressive condition. Strikingly, the overwhelming majority of the terminally ill fight for life to the end. Some may voice suicidal thoughts in response to transient depression or severe pain, but these patients usually respond well to treatment for depressive illness and pain medication and are grateful to be alive.

From *American Journal of Psychiatry*, vol. 150, no. 1, pp. 143–145, 1993. Herbert Hendin and Gerald Klerman. Copyright © 1993, the American Psychiatric Association. Reprinted by permission.

Studies of those who have died by suicide have pointed out the nonrational elements of the wish to die in reaction to serious illness. More individuals, particularly elderly individuals, killed themselves because they feared or *mistakenly* believed they had cancer than killed themselves and actually had cancer. In the same vein, preoccupation with suicide is greater in those awaiting the results of tests for HIV antibodies than in those who know that they are HIV positive.

Given the advances in our medical knowledge and treatment ability, a thorough psychiatric evaluation for the presence of a treatable disorder may literally make the difference between choosing life or choosing death for patients who express the wish to die or to have assisted suicide. This is not an evaluation that can be made by the average physician unless he or she has had extensive experience with depression and suicide.

Even the highly publicized cases that have been put forward by the advocates of legalizing assisted suicide dramatize the dangers and abuses we would face when those who are not qualified to do so evaluate such patients or when we accept at face value a patient's assertion that he or she prefers death. Perhaps the first such case was featured in a front-page story more than a decade ago. It concerned a woman who, after being diagnosed as having breast cancer, brought together her friends and her husband (who was a psychologist), filmed her farewells, and took a lethal overdose. For years, the woman had been an advocate of the "right to suicide." Her film became a television documentary, and media stories portrayed her as something of a pioneer. A pioneer for what? Does her story contain a message we wish to send to the thousands of women facing possible breast surgery? The woman was not terminally ill; her cancer was operable. Although her psychologist husband supporter her decision and felt it was appropriate, surely he was not the person to evaluate her. Was her choice as rational as everyone claimed?

Suicidal individuals are prone, just as this woman was, to make conditions on life: "I won't live if I lose by breast," "if this person doesn't care for me," "if I don't get this job" or "if I lose my looks, power, prestige, or health." Depression, often precipitated by discovering a cancer, exaggerates the tendency toward rigid thinking, toward seeing problems in black-and-white terms.

More recent cases are equally troubling. In the *New England Journal of Medicine*, a physician published the case of a woman who he helped to commit suicide. The woman had a past history of both alcoholism and depression and had recently been diagnosed as having acute leukemia. Her chances of surviving painful chemotherapy and radiation were assessed as one in four. She told her doctor that "she talked to a psychologist she had seen in the past" and implied that the psychologist supported her decision to commit suicide. The physician helped her to implement her decision to end her life. He then published an account of what transpired in an attempt to persuade the medical community of the need for legal sanction for his actions.

The fact that this or any patient may find relief in the prospect of death is not necessarily a sign that the decision is appropriate. Many who are depressed and suicidal appear less depressed after deciding to end their lives. It is coping with the uncertainties of life and death that agitate and depress them. One would need a far more extended examination by someone knowledgeable about suicide to evaluate this woman.

Depression, which is often covert and can coexist with physical illness, is, together with anxiety and the wish to die, often the first reaction to the knowledge of serious illness and possible death. This demoralizing triad can usually be treated by a combination of empathy, psychotherapy, and medicine. The decision whether or not to live with illness is likely to be different with such treatment.

The publications of groups like the Hemlock Society, who advocate a more general "right to suicide," make clear that physician-assisted suicide for patients who have less than 6 months to live (as in the recently defeated California and State of Washington proposals) is but a first step in their campaign. Only a small percentage of the people they are trying to reach are terminally ill. The terminally ill, in fact, constitute only a small portion (less than 3%) of the total number of suicides. Right-to-suicide groups have been joined in their efforts by well-meaning physicians concerned with the plight of the terminally ill.

Discussions of the right to suicide or the rationality of suicide in particular cases have tended to ignore the potential of abuse were physician-assisted suicide to be legalized. Particularly vulnerable potential victims would be the elderly, those frightened by illness, and the depressed of all ages.

The elderly are often made to feel that their families would prefer that they were gone. Societal sanction for physician-assisted suicide for the terminally ill is likely to encourage family members so inclined to pressure the infirm and the elderly to collude with uninformed or unscrupulous physicians to provide such deaths. Some advocates of changing social and medical policy toward suicide concede that such abuses are likely to occur but feel that this is a price we should be willing to pay.

Those whose terror of illness persuades them that quick death is the best solution may be willing victims of physicians who advocate assisted suicide. A woman in the early stages of Alzheimer's who was fearful of the progress of the disease was seen briefly by Dr. Jack Kevorkian, a retired pathologist in Michigan with a passionate commitment to promoting assisted suicide and the use of his "suicide machine." After a brief contact he decided she was a suitable candidate. He used the machine to help her kill herself. Is he the person who should be making such a determination? No Michigan law prohibits assisted suicide (19 states do not have such laws), but Dr. Kevorkian was admonished by the court not to engage in the practice again. Disregarding the admonition, he subsequently provided machines to two more women who were seriously but not terminally ill. They used the machines to kill themselves. Dr. Kevorkian's license to practice medicine has since been "summarily suspended," but a Michigan judge ruled that he could not be prosecuted for murder in the absence of a state law assisting a suicide.

Societal sanction for physician-assisted suicide is likely to encourage assisted suicide by nonphysicians, rendering those who are depressed, with or without physical illness, vulnerable to exploitation. Such abuse already exists. For example, a young man gave a depressed young woman he knew a lethal quantity of sleeping pills. He sat with her and fed them to her as she ate ice cream. While she was doing so, he persuaded her that, since she was going to die, she should write out a will leaving him her possessions. He went home and told his roommate what he had done; the roommate called the police and the young woman was saved. The young man went unpunished because he did what he did in a state with no law prohibiting assisted suicide....

Surely there is a price to be paid for current policy where physicians, patients, and family members must act secretly or may be unwilling to act even in situations where it seems appropriate. The protection of the honorable physician does not now warrant legalizing physician-assisted suicide in a society where the public is relatively uninformed of present abuses involving assisted suicide and the potential for much greater abuses if legalization occurs. It took us several decades to become knowledgeable about when it may be appropriate to withdraw life support systems. We are not close to that point with physician-assisted suicide.

Nor by itself can evaluation of the patient by psychiatrists knowledgeable about suicide, depression, and terminal illness provide us with a simple solution to a complex social problem. Certainly, the individual physician confronted with someone requesting assisted suicide should seek such consultation. There is still too much we do not know about such patients, too much study yet to be done before we could mandate psychiatric evaluation for such patients and define conditions under which assisted suicide would be legal. We are likely to find that those who seek to die in the last days of terminal illness are a quite different population from those whose first response to the knowledge of serious illness is to turn to suicide.

Not all problems are best resolved by a statute. We do not convict or prosecute every case in which someone assists in a suicide, even in states where it is illegal. Given the potential for abuse, however, to give assisted suicide legal sanction is to give a dangerous license.

In some cultures (the Alorese are perhaps the most famous example), when people become seriously ill, they took to their beds, stopped eating, and waited to die. How we deal with illness, age, and decline says a great deal about who and what we are, both as individuals and as a society. The growing number of people living to old age and the increasing incidence of depression in people of all ages present us with a medical challenge. Our efforts should concentrate on providing treatment, relieving pain for the intractably ill, and, in the case of terminal illness, helping the individual come to terms with death.

If those advocating legalization of assisted suicide prevail, it will be a reflection that as a culture we are turning away from efforts to improve our care of the mentally ill, the infirm, and the elderly. Instead, we would be licensing the right to abuse and exploit the fears of the ill and depressed. We would be accepting the view of those who are depressed and suicidal that death is the preferred solution to the problems of illness, age, and depression.

Debate Presenter Form

Follow the guidelines for debate presenters contained in the introduction of this text and those given to you by your instructor. Use the format below to organize the material for your debate. Remember to include all relevant citation information and to present the related information in your own words. Give credit to authors when you cite a quote and be as thorough as possible when writing about your points so you will be prepared for your debate.

Reference citation #1:

Author: _____

Title: _____

Date: _____

Source: _____

_____

Content from reference citation #1: _____

_____

_____

_____

_____

_____

_____

_____

_____

_____

_____

_____

_____

Reference citation #2:

Author: _____

Title: _____

Date: _____

Source: _____

_____

Content from reference citation #2: _____

_____

_____

_____

_____

_____

_____

Reference citation #3:

Author: _____

Title: _____

Date: _____

Source: _____

_____

Content from reference citation #3: _____

_____

_____

_____

_____

_____

Audience Preparation Form

Follow the guidelines for preparing to be an informed audience member on the day of the debate included in the introduction to this text. After reading both sides of the debate from this chapter, answer the following questions. Be as thorough as possible so that you will be able to make a contribution to the debate by asking informed questions or making provocative comments. This form is usually due on the day of the debate.

State the issue in your own words. Do not plagiarize the text. Demonstrate that you understand the topic and it's relevant arguments.

_____

_____

_____

_____

_____

Discuss two points on the "yes" side of the debate.

Point #1: _____

_____

Point #2: _____

_____

Discuss two points on the "no" side of the debate.

Point #1: _____

_____

Point #2: _____

_____

What is your opinion on this topic?

_____

_____

_____

_____

_____

_____

_____

What has contributed to the development of your views about this topic?

_____

_____

_____

_____

_____

_____

_____

What information would be necessary to cause you to change your thinking about this topic?

_____

_____

_____

_____

_____

Debate Response Form

Follow the guidelines for responding to the debates in the introductory chapter of this text. Complete this form and submit your answers at the class following the debate. Try to be thorough and convince your instructor that you were an active listener during the debate.

List a quote from a debate presenter that you think was important and explain why you think this comment was significant.

_____

_____

_____

_____

Which side of the debate do you think made the most convincing arguments, why?

_____

_____

_____

_____

_____

After hearing the debate, in what way has your thinking been affected?

_____

_____

_____

_____

_____

_____

Psychological Treatment

ISSUE 3

Does Maximizing Time in Prison Decrease Crime?

An enduring challenge in any society is effective consequation of behavior. Psychologists and criminologists debate what would be the most powerful means for decreasing criminal acts. The first author, Morgan Reynolds believes that catching, convicting, and fully sentencing more criminals would reduce crime. D. Stanley Eitzen suggests that prison does more harm than good and that alternatives such as house arrest and job corps be used.

Reynolds describes the expected time in prison as alarmingly low. He sees a clear relationship between expected sentence duration and crime rate. If criminals were sentenced to the full extent of the law, crime would decrease. If a criminal views the cost/benefit ratio in favor of crime, then he or she behaves illegally because there is no fear of sanction being worse that the rewards of crime. The most effective deterrent to crime occurs prior to the creation of the criminal according to Eitzen. He supports the implementation of programs to prevent, not consequate, crime. He believes we should reduce the number of handguns in general, and especially in the hands of juveniles, restructure the criminal justice system to engender fear and respect in adults and children, concentrate on effective rehabilitation of criminals, and legalize drugs in order to reduce crime. His article concludes with numerous ideas for long-term crime preventive measures.

Applications

1. What do you think potential criminals think about the probability of being caught, convicted and sentenced to the full extent to the law?

2. How would you change our system of preventing or consequating crime if you were in charge?

3. How does your experience with convicted criminals, even traffic and drunk driving violators, or being the victim of crime affect your views on this issue?

Issue 3
YES

Crime Pays, but So Does Imprisonment

Morgan O. Reynolds

America is burdened by an appalling amount of crime. Even though the crime rate is not soaring as it did during the 1960s and 1970s, we still have more crimes per capita than any other developed country.

- Every year nearly 6 million people are victims of violent crimes—murder, rape, robbery or assault.

- Another 29 million Americans each year are victims of property crimes—arson, burglary and larceny-theft.

- There is a murder every 25 minutes, a rape every six minutes, a robbery every minute and an aggravated assault every 35 seconds.

- There is a motor vehicle theft every 22 seconds, a burglary every ten seconds, and a larceny-theft every four seconds.

Although the number of crimes reported to the police each year has leveled off somewhat in the 1980s, our crime rate today is still enormously high—411 percent higher, for example, than it was in 1960.

Why is there so much crime?

The Expected Punishment
for Committing a Crime

The economic theory of crime is a relatively new field of social science. According to this theory, most crimes are not irrational acts. Instead, crimes are freely committed by people who compare the expected benefits of crime with the expected costs. The reason we have so much crime is that, for many people, the <u>benefits outweigh the costs</u>. For some people, a criminal career is more attractive than their other career options. Put another way, the reason we have so much crime is that crime pays.

Because criminals and potential criminals rarely have accurate information about the probabilities of arrest, conviction and imprisonment, a great deal of uncertainty is involved in the personal assessment of the expected punishment from committing crimes. Individuals differ in skill and intellect. The more skillful and more intelligent criminals have better odds of committing successful crimes. Some people overestimate their probability of success, while others underestimate theirs.

Despite the element of subjectivity, the economic theory of crime makes one clear prediction: Crime will increase if the expected cost of crime to criminals declines. This is true for "crimes of passion" as well as economic crimes such as burglary or auto theft. The less costly crime becomes, the more often people fail to control their passions.

The economic theory of crime is consistent with public opinion, and with the perceptions of potential criminals. It is supported by considerable statistical research. According to the theory, the amount of crime is inversely related to expected punishment. What follows is a brief summary of the punishment criminals can expect.

Expected Time in Prison

What is the expected punishment for committing major types of serious crime in the United States today?... [T]he expected punishment is shockingly low.

- Even for committing the most serious crime—murder—an individual can expect to spend only 2.3 years in prison.

- On the average, an individual who commits an act of burglary can expect to spend only 7.1 days in prison.

- Someone considering an auto theft can expect to spend only 6.3 days in prison.

Figure 1
Crime and Punishment

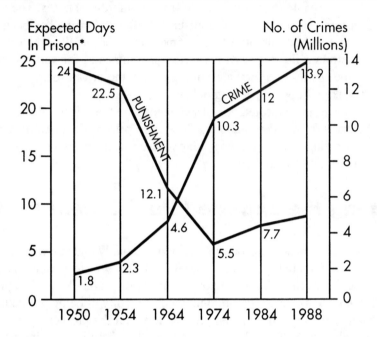

*Median prison sentence for all serous crimes, weighted by probabilities of arrest, prosecution, conviction, and imprisonment.

The Decline in Expected Imprisonment and the Rise in Crime

...On the average, those crimes with the longest expected prison terms (murder, rape, robbery and assault) are the crimes least frequently committed, comprising only about 10 percent of all serious crime. The remaining 90 percent carry an expected prison term of only a few days. When expected punishment is weighted by the frequency of types of crimes, the picture is even more shocking: On the average, a perpetrator of a serious crime in the United States can expect to spend about eight days in prison.... [T]his overall expectation has changed over time.

- Since the early 1950s, the expected punishment for committing a serious crime in the United States (measured in terms of expected time in prison) has been reduced by two-thirds.

- Over the same period, the total number of serious crimes committed has increased sevenfold.

The "Prices" We Charge for Crime

It is virtually impossible to prevent people from committing crimes. The most that the criminal justice system can do is impose punishment after the crime has been committed. People are largely free to commit almost any crime they choose. What the criminal justice system does is construct a list of prices (expected punishments) for various criminal acts. People commit crimes so long as they are willing to pay the prices society charges, just as many of us might risk parking or speeding tickets.

Viewed in this way, the expected prison sentences...are the prices we charge for various crimes. Thus, the price for murder is about 2.3 years in prison; the price of burglary is 7.7 days; the price for stealing a car is 4.2 days. Since these prices are so low, it is small wonder so many people are willing to pay them.

Calculating the Expected Punishment for Crime

Five adverse events must occur before a criminal actually ends up in prison. The criminal must be arrested, indicted, prosecuted, convicted and sent to prison. As a result, the expected punishment for crime depends upon a number of probabilities: The probability of being arrested, given that a crime is committed; the probability of being prosecuted, given an arrest; the probability of conviction, given prosecution; and the probability of being sent to prison, given a conviction. As Table 1 shows, the overall probability of being punished is the result of multiplying four probabilities.

Even if each of the separate probabilities is reasonably high, their product can be quite low. For example, suppose that each of these probabilities were 0.5. That is, one-half of crimes result in an arrest, one-half of arrests lead to prosecution, one-half of prosecutions lead to conviction, and one-half of convictions lead to a prison term. In this case, the overall probability that a criminal will spend time in prison is only 6.25 percent.

Table 1 also depicts recent probabilities in the case of burglary. Note that burglars who are sent to prison stay there for about 17 months, on the average.... But someone considering an act of burglary will surely be influenced by the fact that the probability of being arrested is only 14 percent. Although the probabilities of prosecution and conviction following an arrest are high, the criminal's probability of going to prison is less than one in three after being convicted. When all factors are taken into account (including the probability that the crime will never be reported), the overall probability that a burglar will end up in prison is less than one percent. The expected punishment prior to committing the crime is only 7.1 days.

Table 1
Circulating the Expected Punishment for Potential Criminals

Expected Time in Prison	= Probability of arrest	x Probability of prosecution given arrest
	x Probability of conviction, given prosecution	x Probability of imprisonment, given conviction
	x median sentence	

Example: Expected punishment for burglary

Expected Time in Prison	= 14% (Probability of arrest)	x 88% (Probability of prosecution, given arrest)
	x 81% (Probability of conviction given prosecution)	x 25% (Probability of imprisonment, given conviction)
	x 1/2 (Adjustment for unreported crimes)	x 17 months (median sentence)
	= 7.1 days	

*Approximately one-half of all burglaries are not reported to the police. Law enforcement agencies "clear" (or solve) an offense when at least one person is arrested, charged with the offense, and turned over for prosecution.

Probability of Arrest

...The striking fact...is the degree to which arrest rates have declined over the past 40 years, even for the most serious crimes. For example:

- Since 1950, the probability of being arrested after committing a murder has fallen by 25 percent.

- The probability of arrest for rapists has fallen 35 percent, for robbers 42 percent and for burglars 53 percent.

On the average, during the 1980s, only about 21 percent of all crimes in the United States were cleared by arrest. In Japan, by contrast, the clearance-by-arrest rate is 50 percent. Moreover, Japan with a population of 122 million has fewer murders each year than New York City with a population of seven million.

Probability of Prosecution, Conviction and Imprisonment

Although there are 13 million arrests each year in the United States, including 2.8 million for serious (Index) crimes, annual admissions to prison only topped 200,000 in 1986. In other words, only eight of every 100 arrests for Index crimes results in imprisonment after defense attorneys, prosecutors and courts complete their work.

Overall Probability of Going to Prison

A criminal's overall probability of imprisonment has fallen dramatically since 1950...:

- Since 1950, the percent of crimes resulting in a prison sentence has declined by at least 60 percent for every major category of crime.

- This includes a 60 percent drop for murder, a 79 percent decrease for rape, an 83 percent reduction for robbery and a 94 percent plunge for auto theft.

Unreported Crimes

Based on the number of crimes reported to the police, 1.66 percent of all serious crimes are punished by imprisonment; therefore 98.34 percent of serious crimes are not. According to the National Crime Survey, however, only 37 percent of serious crimes are actually reported. If there are two unreported crimes for every one reported, then the overall probability of going to prison for the commission of a serious crime falls to about 0.61 percent (.37 x 1.66%). This amounts to one prison term for every 164 felonies committed.

A Possible Explanation: The Role of the Warren Court

The main factor in the decline in expected punishment over the last three decades was a virtual collapse in the probability of imprisonment. Why? We cannot point to a shrinkage in law enforcement personnel as an explanation.... [T]he number of full-time police employees has risen steadily over the past three decades. Further, total employment in the criminal justice sector increased from 600,000 in 1965 to nearly 1.5 million in 1986. Government spending on the criminal justice sector doubled as a share on GNP, rising from less than 0.6 percent to nearly 1.2 percent. During the same period, private employment in detective and protection services grew rapidly, reaching half a million persons by the end of 1989. Apparently, more people now produce less justice.

The 1960s was a turbulent decade—the Vietnam War, the counterculture, urban riots. But one policy change that lasted well into the 1970s and 1980s was the change in the criminal justice system caused by the Supreme Court. Influenced by sociologists and other intellectuals, there was a growing reluctance to apprehend and punish criminals during the 1960s. In particular, 1961 brought the first landmark decision of the U.S. Supreme Court expanding the rights of criminal defendants and making it more costly for police and prosecutors to obtain criminal convictions.

Mapp v. Ohio (1961) declared that illegally obtained evidence could not be admitted in any state criminal prosecution, imposing the so-called "exclusionary rule" on all state judicial systems. A series of related decisions followed: *Gideon v. Wainwright* (1963) required taxpayer-funded counsel for defendants; *Escobedo v. Illinois* (1964) and *Malloy v. Hogan* (1964) expanded privileges against self-incrimination, thereby impeding interrogation by the police; and *Miranda v. Arizona* (1966) went further and made confessions, even if voluntary, inadmissible as evidence unless the suspect had been advised of certain rights.

The enforcement system was transformed by these decisions. Under the exclusionary rule, according to Justice Cardozo, "The criminal is to go free because the constable has blundered." Justice White, dissenting in the *Miranda* case, warned that the decision would have "a corrosive effect on the criminal laws as an effective device to prevent crime." It appears that the "pursuit of perfect justice," as Judge Macklin put it, changed the rules and increased the time and effort required to apprehend, convict and punish the guilty....

The Cost of Crime Deterrence

If America is to succeed in lowering the crime rate to, say, the level that prevailed in the 1950s, we must create at least as much crime deterrence as existed in the 1950s. For example, [there are] three ways of raising the expected prison sentence for burglary to its 1950 level. Since the probabilities of prosecution and conviction, given an arrest, are already high, the options are:

- Increase the proportion of burglaries cleared by arrest from 14 to 42 percent; or

- Increase the percent of convicted burglars sent to prison from 28 to 84 percent; or

- Increase the median prison sentence for burglars from 17 to 51 months.

All three alternatives are expensive. A higher arrest rate requires that more money be spent on criminal investigation. A higher sentencing rate requires more court and litigation costs. All three alternatives require more prison space. Unless prison space can be expanded, little else in the way of deterrence will be of much value.

America is in the midst of the biggest prison building boom in its history. On December 30, 1989, prisons held 673,565 convicts, up from 438,830 prisoners at the beginning of 1984 and at 110 percent of design capacity. In 1988 the system added 42,967 inmates, or enough to fill 86 new 500-bed prisons.

- Today, one out of every 364 Americans is in prison—not jail, probation or parole but in prison.

- With an additional 296,000 in local jails, 362,000 on parole and 2.4 million on probation, one out of every 69 Americans is under the supervision of the corrections establishment, or one of every 52 adults.

At and annual cost exceeding $20,000 per prisoner, the total prison tab is more than $15 billion a year. That cost will surely rise. Thirty-five states are under court orders to relieve prison overcrowding and others face litigation. To increase capacity, more than 100 new state and federal prisons currently are under construction around the country. California alone is spending $3.5 billion on new prison beds and has added 21,000 beds since 1984. State governments spent some $9 billion in 1989 on new prisons. In most cases, the construction cost per prison bed exceeds $50,000.

How to Reduce Prison Costs

Much could be done to reduce the high costs of constructing and operating prisons. The most promising ways to reduce taxpayer costs exploit private sector competition and efficiency in construction and operating prisons and employing prisoners. Contracting out construction and remodeling is a proven economizer. Short of full privatization, government-operated correctional facilities should be corporatized and required to operate like private businesses, with profit and loss statements. Even within the existing system, economies are possible. What follows is a brief summary of ways to economize.

Opportunities for Reducing Costs within the Public Sector

Better Management Practices.   Although entrepreneurship in the public sector is rare, opportunities for innovation in prison construction abound. For example:

- Florida expanded an existing facility by 336 beds for only $16,000 per cell.

- South Carolina used inmate labor to reduce construction costs by an estimated 50 percent with no quality loss and some delay.

- New York City has begun using renovated troop barges and a ferry boat for detention facilities.

Early Release of Elderly Prisoners.   Although the recidivism rate is about 22 percent for prisoners age 18 to 24, among prisoners over 45 years old the recidivism rate is only 2.1 percent. Nationwide, there are at least 20,000 inmates over the age of 55. Moreover, the average maintenance cost of an elderly prisoner is about $69,000—three times the cost of a younger prisoner. Early release of elderly prisoners to make room for younger criminals makes sense and would improve crime deterrence.

Boot Camp Therapy for Young Prisoners.   Called "shock incarceration" by federal drug Czar William Bennett, boot camp therapy as an alternative to prison for youngsters (not yet hardened criminals) is being used in Georgia, Alabama, Florida, Louisiana, Mississippi, New York, Oklahoma, South Carolina and Texas. Costs are lower, although the recidivism rate is about the same as for the prison system as a whole.

Electronic Ankle Bracelets.   The cost of punishment would be greatly reduced if ways were found of punishing criminals without imprisonment. Few people would deny that imprisonment is necessary and desirable for violent crimes such as homicide, rape, robbery and assault. But less than half of U.S. prisoners have been incarcerated for such crimes. A mid-1980s survey found that:

- One-third of the prisoners were imprisoned for property offenses and another 20 percent for crimes against public order (including drug offenses).

- In Arkansas, nonviolent offenders outnumbered violent ones by a ratio of three to one.

- In Mississippi, Kentucky, Missouri and Wyoming the ratio was two to one.

A recent alternative to imprisonment is the electronic monitoring device that is worn by parolees. Judges can impose conditions of parole, including restrictions on the range and timing of activities, and they can be enforced by monitoring companies....

Productive Work for Prisoners

A recent survey commissioned by the National Institute of Justice identified more than 70 companies which employ inmates in 16 states in manufacturing, service and light assembly operations. Prisoners work as reservations clerks for TWA and Best Western, sew leisure wear, manufacture water-bed mattresses, and assemble electronic components. PRIDE, a state-sponsored private corporation that runs Florida's 46 prison industries from furniture-making to optical glass grinding, made a $4 million profit in 1987. This work benefits near-ly everyone. It enables prisoners to earn wages, acquire skills, and subtly learn individual responsibility and the value of productive labor. It also insures that they can contribute to vic-tim compensation, and to their own and their families' support....

The Cost of Not Building Prisons

Although the cost of building and maintaining prisons is high, the cost of not creating more prisons appears to be much higher. A study by the National Institute of Justice con-cluded that the "typical" offender let loose in society will engage in a one-man crime wave, creating damage to society more than 17 times as costly than imprisonment. Specifically:

• Sending someone to prison for one year cost the government about $25,000.

• A Rand Corporation survey of 2190 professional criminals found that the average criminal committed 187 to 287 crimes a year, at an average cost per crime of $2,300.

• On the average, then, a professional criminal out of prison costs society $430,000 per year, or $405,000 more than the cost of a year in prison.

The failure to keep offenders in prison once they are there is also a hazard of too little prison space, and early release often leads to much more crime. A Rand Corporation survey of former inmates found that:

• In California, 76 percent were arrested within three years of their release and 60 percent were convicted of new crimes.

• In Texas, 60 percent of former inmates were arrested within three years and 40 percent were reconvicted.

• A survey of 11 states showed that 62.5 percent of all released prisoners were arrested within 3 years, 46.8 percent were reconvicted and 41.1 percent were reincarcerated.

In California, a comparison between ex-convicts and criminals who received probation rather than a prison sentence showed a disheartening rate of failure for both. Each ex-convict committed an estimated 20 crimes. Each probationer committed 25 crimes.

A Bureau of Justice Statistics study of 22 states found that 69 percent of young adults (ages 17 to 22) released from prison in 1978 were arrested within six years—each continu-ing an average of 13 new crimes.

Conclusion

While crime continues on the high plateau, there are grounds for optimism. The number of young males began to decline in the 1980s and will continue to do so through the 1990s. Further, the odds of imprisonment for a serious offense increased in the 1980s as legislators responded to the public's "get tough" attitude. Yet we remained plagued with crime rates (per capita) triple those of the 1950s.

What can be done to build on this relatively promising recent trend? At a minimum the analysis in this report suggest three things. First, the U.S. Supreme Court should continue to reestablish the rule of law by restricting application of the exclusionary rule and other expansions of criminal privileges inherited from the Warren Court. Second, the public sector must continue raising the odds of imprisonment toward those of the 1950s in order to improve personal security. Deterrence of criminals implies building prisons and reducing prison costs by privatization. Third, the laws hampering productive employment of prisoners must be relaxed to take full advantage of the benefits of privatization.

Acknowledgement

My thanks to Dr. John Goodman, President, National Center for Policy Analysis, Dallas, Texas, for his help on this paper and his permission for reprint material from NCPA Report No. 149. Author.

Violent Crime
Myths, Facts, and Solutions

D. Stanley Eitzen

My remarks are limited to violent street crimes (assault, robbery, rape, and murder). We should not forget that there are other types of violent crimes that are just as violent and actually greater in magnitude than street crimes: corporate, political, organized, and white collar. But that is another subject for another time. Our attention this morning is on violent street crime, which has made our cities unsafe and our citizens extremely fearful. What are the facts about violent crime and violent criminals and what do we, as a society, do about them?

I am going to critique the prevailing thought about violent crime and its control because our perceptions about violent crime and much of what our government officials do about it is wrong. My discipline—sociology—knows a lot about crime but what we know does not seem to affect public perceptions and public policies. Not all of the answers, however, are always crystal clear. There are disagreements among reasonable and thoughtful people, coming from different theoretical and ideological perspectives. You may, difficult as it seems to me, actually disagree with my analysis. That's all right. The key is for us to address this serious problem, determine the facts, engage in dialogue, and then work toward logical and just solutions.

What do criminologists know about violent crime? Much of what we know is counter intuitive; it flies in the face of the public's understanding. So, let me begin with some demythologizing.

Myth 1: As a Christian nation with high moral principles, we rank relatively low in the amount of violent crime.   Compared with the other industrialized nations of the world, we rank number one in belief in God, "the importance of God in our lives," and church attendance. We also rank first in murder rates, robbery rates, and rape rates. Take homicide, for example: The U.S. rate of 10 per 100,000 is three times that of Finland, five times that of Canada, and nine times greater than found in Norway, the Netherlands, Germany, and Great Britain. In 1992 for example, Chicago, a city about one-fifth the population of the Netherlands had nine times more gun-related deaths than occurred in the Netherlands.

Myth 2: We are in the midst of a crime wave.   When it comes to crime rates we are misled by our politicians, and the media. Government data indicate that between 1960 and 1970 crime rates doubled, then continued to climb through the 1970s. From 1970 to 1990 the rates remained the same. The problem is with violent crime by youth, which has increased dramatically. Despite the rise in violent crime among youth, however, the *overall* violent crime rate actually has decreased in the 1990s.

Our perceptions are affected especially by the media. While crime rates have leveled and slightly declined during the 1990s, the media have given us a different picture. In 1993, for example, the three major networks doubled their crime stories and tripled their coverage of murders. This distortion of reality results, of course, in a general perception that we are in the midst of a crime wave.

Myth 3: Serious violent crime is found throughout the age structure.   Crime is mainly a problem of male youths. Violent criminal behaviors peak at age 17 and by age 24 it is one-half the rate. Young males have always posed a special crime problem. There are some differences now, however. Most significant, young males and the gangs to which they often belong now have much greater firepower. Alienated and angry youth once used clubs, knives, brass knuckles, and fists but now they use Uzis, AK47s, and "streetsweepers." The result is that since 1965, the murder rate for 18–24 year-olds has risen 65 percent while the rate for 14–17 year-olds has increased 165 percent.

The frightening demographic fact is that between now and the year 2005, the number of teenagers in the U.S. will grow by 23 percent. During the next ten years, black teenagers will increase by 28 percent and the Hispanic teenage population will grow by about 50 percent. The obvious prediction is that violent crime will increase dramatically over this period.

Myth 4: The most dangerous place in America is in the streets where strangers threaten, hit, stab, or shoot each other.   The streets in our urban places are dangerous, as rival gangs fight, and drive-by shootings occur. But, statistically, the most dangerous place is in your own home, or when you are with a boyfriend or girlfriend, family member or acquaintance.

Myth 5: Violent criminals are born with certain predispositions toward violence. Criminals are not born with a criminal gene. If crime were just a function of biology, then we would expect crime rates to be more or less the same for all social categories, times, and places. In fact, violent crime rates vary considerably by social class, race, unemployment, poverty, geographical place, and other social variables. Research on these variables is the special contribution of sociology to the understanding of criminal behavior.

Let's elaborate on these social variables because these have so much to do with solutions. Here is what we know about these social variables:

1. The more people in poverty, the higher the rate of street crime.

2. The higher the unemployment rate in an area, the higher the crime rate. Sociologist William J. Wilson says that black and white youths at age 11 are equally likely to commit violent crimes but by their late 20s, blacks are four times more likely to be violent offenders. However, when blacks and whites in their late 20s are employed, they differ hardly at all in violent behavior.

3. The greater the racial segregation in an area, the higher the crime rate. Sociologist Doug Massey argues that urban poverty and urban crime are the consequences of extremely high levels of black residential segregation and racial discrimination. Massey says,

    "Take a group of people, segregate them, cut off their capital and guess what? The neighborhoods go downhill. There's no other outcome possible."

    As these neighborhoods go downhill and economic opportunities evaporate, crime rates go up.

4. The greater the family instability, the higher the probability of crimes by juveniles. Research is sketchy, but it appears that the following conditions are related to delinquent behaviors: (a) intense parental conflict; (b) lack of parental supervision; (c) parental neglect and abuse; and (d) failure of parents to discipline their children.

5. The greater the inequality in the neighborhood, city, region, or society, the higher the crime rate. In other words, the greater the disparities between rich and poor, the greater the probability of crime. Of all the industrialized nations, the U.S. has the greatest degree of inequality. For example, one percent of Americans own 40 percent of all the wealth. At the other extreme, 14-1/2 percent of all Americans live below the poverty line and 5 percent of all Americans live below *one-half* of the poverty line.

When these social variables converge, they interact to increase crime rates. Thus, there is a relatively high probability of criminal behavior—violent criminal behavior—among young, black, impoverished males in inner cities where poverty, unemployment, and racial segregation are concentrated. There are about 5 million of these high-risk young men. In addition, we have other problem people. What do we do? How do we create a safer America?

To oversimplify a difficult and contentious debate, there are two answers—the conservative and progressive answers. The conservative answer has been to get tough with criminals. This involves mandatory sentences, longer sentences, putting more people in prison, and greater use of the death penalty. This strategy has accelerated with laws such as "three strikes and you're out (actually in)," and the passage of expensive prison building programs to house the new prisoners.

In my view, this approach is wrong-headed. Of course, some individuals must be put in prison to protect the members of society. Our policies, however, indiscriminately put too many people in prison at too high a cost. Here are some facts about prisons:

1. Our current incarceration rate is 455 per 100,000 (in 1971 it was 96 per 100,000). The rate in Japan and the Netherlands is one-tenth ours. Currently, there are 1.2 million Americans in prisons and jails (equivalent to the population of Philadelphia).

2. The cost is prohibitive, taking huge amounts of money that could be spent on other programs. It costs about $60,000 to build a prison cell and $20,000 to keep a prisoner for a year. Currently the overall cost of prisons and jails (federal, state, and local) is $29 billion annually. The willingness to spend for punishment reduces money that could be spent to alleviate other social problems. For example, eight years ago Texas spent $7 dollars on education for every dollar spent on prisons. Now the ratio is 4 to 1. Meanwhile, Texas ranks 37th among the states in per pupil spending.

3. As mentioned earlier, violent crimes tend to occur in the teenage years with a rapid drop off afterwards. Often, for example, imprisonment under "3 strikes and you're out" law gives life imprisonment to many who are in the twilight of their criminal careers. We, and they, would be better off if we found alternatives to prison for them.

4. Prisons do not rehabilitate. Actually, prisons have the opposite effect. The prison experience tends to increase the likelihood of further criminal behavior. Prisons are overcrowded, mean, gloomy, brutal places that change people, but usually for the worse, not the better. Moreover, prisoners usually believe that their confinement is unjust because of the bias in the criminal justice system toward the poor and racial minorities. Finally, prisoners do not ever pay their debt to society. Rather they are forever stigmatized as "ex-cons" and, therefore, considered unreliable and dangerous by their neighbors, employers, fellow workers, and acquaintances. Also, they are harassed by the police as "likely suspects." The result is that they are often driven into a deviant subculture and eventually caught—about two-thirds are arrested within three years of leaving prison.

Progressives argue that conservative crime control measures are fundamentally flawed because they are "after the fact" solutions. Like a janitor mopping up the floor while the sink continues to overflow; he or she may even redouble the effort with some success but the source of the flooding has not been addressed. If I might mix metaphors here (although keeping with the aquatic theme), the obvious place to begin the attack on crime is *upstream*, before the criminal has been formed and the crimes have been committed.

We must concentrate our efforts on high-risk individuals before they become criminals (in particular, impoverished young inner city males). These prevention proposals take time, are very costly, and out-of-favor politically but they are the only realistic solutions to reduce violent street crime.

The problem with the conservative "after-the-fact" crime fighting proposals is that while promoting criminal justice, these programs dismantle social justice. Thus, they enhance a criminogenic climate. During the Reagan years, for example, $51 billion dollars were removed from various poverty programs. Now, under the "Contract for America" the Republicans in Congress propose to reduce subsidized housing, to eliminate nutrition programs through WIC (Women, Infants, and Children), to let the states take care of subsidized school lunches, and to eliminate welfare for unmarried mothers under 18 who do not live with their parents or a responsible guardian.

Progressives argue that we abandon these children at our own peril. The current Republican proposals forsake the 26 percent of American children under six who live in poverty including 54 percent of all African American children and 44 percent of all Latino children under the age of six. Will we be safer as these millions of children in poverty grow to physical maturity?

Before I address specific solutions, I want to emphasize that sociologists examine the structural reasons for crime. This focus on factors outside the individual does not excuse criminal behavior, it tries to understand how certain structural factors *increase* the proportion of people who choose criminal options.

Knowing what we know about crime, the implications for policy are clear. These proposals, as you will note, are easy to suggest but they are very difficult to implement. I will divide my proposals into immediate actions to deal with crime now and long-term preventive measures:

Measures to protect society immediately:

1. The first step is to protect society from predatory sociopaths. This does not mean imprisoning more people. We should, rather, only imprison the truly dangerous. The criminal law should be redrawn so that the list of crimes reflects the real dangers that individuals pose to society. Since prison does more harm than good, we should provide reasonable alternatives such as house arrest, half-way houses, boot camps, electronic surveillance, job corps, and drug/alcohol treatment.

2. We must reduce the number of handguns and assault weapons by enacting and vigorously enforcing stringent gun controls at the federal level. The United States is an armed camp with 210 million guns in circulation. Jeffrey Reiman has put it this way:

   "Trying to fight crime while allowing such easy access to guns is like trying to teach a child to walk and tripping him each time he stands up. In its most charitable light, it is hypocrisy. Less charitably, it is complicity in murder."

3. We must make a special effort to get guns out of the hands of juveniles. Research by James Wright and his colleagues at Tulane University found that juveniles are much more likely to have guns for protection than for status and power. They suggest that we must restore order in the inner cities so that fewer young people do not feel the need to

provide their own protection. They argue that a perceived sense of security by youth can be accomplished if there is a greater emphasis on community policing, more cooperation between police departments and inner city residents, and greater investment by businesses, banks, and cities in the inner city.

4. We must reinvent the criminal justice system so that it commands the respect of youth and adults. The obvious unfairness by race and social class must be addressed. Some laws are unfair. For example, the federal law requires a five-year, no-parole sentence for possession of five grams of crack cocaine, worth about $400. However, it takes 100 times as much powder cocaine—500 grams, worth $10,000—and a selling conviction to get the same sentence. Is this fair? Of course not. Is it racist? It is racist since crack is primarily used by African Americans while powder cocaine is more likely used by whites. There are also differences by race and social class in arrest patterns, plea bargain arrangements, sentencing, parole, and imposition of the death penalty. These differences provide convincing evidence that the poor and racial minorities are discriminated against in the criminal justice system. As long as the criminal justice system is perceived as unfair by the disadvantaged, that system will not exert any moral authority over them.

5. We must rehabilitate as many criminals as possible. Prisons should be more humane. Prisoners should leave prison with vocational skills useful in the real world. Prisoners should leave prison literate and with a high school degree. And, society should formally adopt the concept of "forgiveness" saying to ex-prisoners, in effect, you have been punished for your crime, we want you to begin a new life with a "clean" record.

6. We must legalize the production and sale of "illicit drugs" and treat addiction as a medical problem rather than a criminal problem. If drugs were legalized or decriminalized, crimes would be reduced in several ways: (a) By eliminating drug use as a criminal problem, we would have 1.12 million *fewer* arrests each year. (b) There would be many *fewer* prisoners (currently about 60 percent of all federal prisoners and 25 percent of all state prisoners are incarcerated for drug offenses). (c) Money now spent on the drug war ($31 billion annually, not counting prison construction) could be spent for other crime control programs such as police patrols, treatment of drug users, and job programs. (d) Drugs could be regulated and taxed, generating revenues of about $5 billion a year. (e) It would end the illicit drug trade that provides tremendous profits to organized crime, violent gangs, and other traffickers. (f) It would eliminate considerable corruption of the police and other authorities. (g) There would be many fewer homicides. Somewhere between one-fourth and one-half of the killings in the inner cities are drug-related. (h) The lower cost of purchasing drugs reduces the need to commit crimes to pay for drug habits.

Long term preventive measures to reduce violent crime.

1. The link between poverty and street crime is indisputable. In the long run, reducing poverty will be the most effective crime fighting tool. Thus, as a society, we need to intensify our efforts to break the cycle of poverty. This means providing a universal and comprehensive health care system, low-cost housing, job training, and decent compensation for work. There must be pay equity for women. And, there must be an unwavering commitment to eradicate institutional sexism and racism. Along other benefits, such a strategy will strengthen families and give children resources, positive role models, and hope.

2. Families must be strengthened. Single-parent families and the working poor need subsidized child care, flexible work schedules, and leave for maternity and family emergencies at a reasonable proportion of their wages. Adolescent parents need the resources to stay in school. They need job training. We need to increase the commitment to family planning. This means providing contraceptives and birth control counseling to adolescents. This means using federal funds to pay for legal abortions when they are requested by poor women.

3. There must be a societal commitment to full and decent employment. Meaningful work at decent pay integrates individuals into society. It is a source of positive identity. Employed parents are respected by their children. Good paying jobs provide hope for the future. They also are essential to keep families together.

4. There must be a societal commitment to education. This requires two different programs. The first is to help at-risk children, beginning at an early age. As it is now, when poor children start school, they are already behind. As Sylvia Ann Hewlett has said:

> "At age five, poor children are often less alert, less curious, and less effective at interacting with their peers than are more privileged youngsters."

This means that they are doomed to be underachievers. To overcome this we need intervention programs that prepare children for school. Research shows that Head Start and other programs can raise IQ scores significantly. There are two problems with Head Start, however. First, the current funding only covers 40 percent of eligible youngsters. And second, the positive effects from the Head Start program are sometimes short-lived because the children then attend schools that are poorly staffed, overcrowded, and ill-equipped.

This brings us to the second education program to help at-risk children. The government must equalize the resources of school districts, rather than the current situation where the wealth of school districts determines the amount spent per pupil. Actually, equalization is not the answer. I believe that there should be special commitment to invest *extra* resources in at-risk children. If we do, we will have a safer society in the long run.

These proposals seem laughable in the current political climate, where politicians—Republicans *and* Democrats—try to outdo each other in their toughness on crime and their disdain for preventive programs. They are wrong, however, and society is going to pay in higher crime rates in the future. I am convinced that the political agenda of the conservatives is absolutely heading us in the wrong direction—toward more violent crime rather than less.

The proposals that I have suggested are based on what we sociologists know about crime. They should be taken seriously, but they are not. The proposals are also based on the assumption that if we can give at-risk young people hope, they will become a part of the community rather than alienated from it. My premise is this: Everyone needs a dream. Without a dream, we become fatalistic. Without a dream, and the hope of attaining it, society becomes our enemy. Many young people act in antisocial ways because they have lost their dream. These troubled and troublesome people are society's creations because we have not given them the opportunity to achieve their dreams—instead society has structured the situation so that they will fail. Until they feel that they have a stake in society, they will fail, and so will we.

Debate Presenter Form

Follow the guidelines for debate presenters contained in the introduction of this text and those given to you by your instructor. Use the format below to organize the material for your debate. Remember to include all relevant citation information and to present the related information in your own words. Give credit to authors when you cite a quote and be as thorough as possible when writing about your points so you will be prepared for your debate.

Reference citation #1:

Author: _____

Title: _____

Date: _____

Source: _____

_____

Content from reference citation #1: _____

_____

_____

_____

_____

_____

_____

_____

_____

_____

_____

_____

_____

_____

Reference citation #2:

Author: _____

Title: _____

Date: _____

Source: _____

_____

Content from reference citation #2: _____

_____

_____

_____

_____

_____

Reference citation #3:

Author: _____

Title: _____

Date: _____

Source: _____

_____

Content from reference citation #3: _____

_____

_____

_____

_____

Name _____

Section _____

Audience Preparation Form

Follow the guidelines for preparing to be an informed audience member on the day of the debate included in the introduction to this text. After reading both sides of the debate from this chapter, answer the following questions. Be as thorough as possible so that you will be able to make a contribution to the debate by asking informed questions or making provocative comments. This form is usually due on the day of the debate.

State the issue in your own words. Do not plagiarize the text. Demonstrate that you understand the topic and it's relevant arguments.

_____

_____

_____

_____

_____

Discuss two points on the "yes" side of the debate.

Point #1: _____

_____

Point #2: _____

_____

Discuss two points on the "no" side of the debate.

Point #1: _____

_____

Point #2: _____

_____

What is your opinion on this topic?

_____

_____

_____

_____

_____

_____

_____

What has contributed to the development of your views about this topic?

_____

_____

_____

_____

_____

_____

_____

What information would be necessary to cause you to change your thinking about this topic?

_____

_____

_____

_____

_____

Debate Response Form

Follow the guidelines for responding to the debates in the introductory chapter of this text. Complete this form and submit your answers at the class following the debate. Try to be thorough and convince your instructor that you were an active listener during the debate.

List a quote from a debate presenter that you think was important and explain why you think this comment was significant.

_____

_____

_____

_____

Which side of the debate do you think made the most convincing arguments, why?

_____

_____

_____

_____

_____

After hearing the debate, in what way has your thinking been affected?

_____

_____

_____

_____

_____

_____

Psychological Treatment

ISSUE 4

Are We Relying on Too Much Prozac?

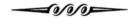

YES Mark Nichols, *Questioning Prozac*

NO Nancy Wartik, *Prozac: The Verdict Is In*

Mark Nichols cites several complications with Prozac including a possible connection to exacerbation of existing cancer tumors, violence, suicide, suicidal thinking, diminished sexual desire, nausea, nervousness, and insomnia. Of these, the potential disastrous consequence of suicide is, of course, the worst. Nichols finds it ironic that the very drug prescribed to cure depression might also cause the same patient to commit suicide.

If sadness serves a purpose, then the benefits of going through depression may be eliminated through the use of Prozac and other selective serotonin reuptake inhibitors. In addition to negating the value of angst, the use of Prozac for complaints that do not reach the level of diagnosable psychological disorders seems to Nichols to be an abuse of the medication. He concludes with the issue of allowing patients to use just Prozac for their entire treatment rather than combining this medication with psychotherapy.

Speaking in favor of Prozac, Nancy Wartik cites several reasons for the popularity of this medication. First, there are fewer side effects with Prozac than in the previous generation of antidepressants. Second, Prozac really works. Depression is lifted and angst is gone.

73

Wartik suggests that untreated depression is dangerous and those who benefit from Prozac live to extol its wonders. This medication has made it socially acceptable to have and to seek treatment for depression.

Wartik makes a powerful point regarding the concerns about the over use of Prozac. Citing a physician, Wartik concurs with the idea that there are more people who could benefit from Prozac who are not taking it than people who are on it and should not be.

Applications

1. If you were depressed, would you consider taking Prozac or one of the new selective serotonin reuptake inhibitors? Explain your answer.

2. If you were depressed, and you would take an antidepressant, would you combine it with psychotherapy or take it alone for your depression? Explain your answer.

3. Would you agree that if you were not actually depressed, but you just didn't feel great, that it would be legitimate for you to try an antidepressant to see if your mood or personality would improve? Why or why not?

4. What do you think is the impact of the high numbers of people who take antidepressants on cultural expectations about personality?

Issue 4

YES

Questioning Prozac

Mark Nichols

With more than 11 million mostly satisfied customers around the globe, it is one of the most rapidly successful drugs in history. An antidote to clinical depression, the green-and-yellow capsule, introduced six years ago, has also been extolled by some enthusiasts as just the thing to help frazzled parents cope with their kids or to make chronic loners stop fearing rejection. Prozac—brand name for the chemical fluoxetine hydrochloride—has entered pop culture, as well, becoming the stuff of cartoons and stand-up comedy routines. And it has summoned the vision of an era of so-called cosmetic psychopharmacology, in which a society of pill-poppers, seeking relief from everything from shyness to fear of crowds, will have to look no further than the nearest medicine cabinet. That day may yet come. But it raises serious medical and philosophical questions—and the first wave of them is descending upon Prozac itself. Is Prozac—non-addictive and, according to some doctors, capable of transforming personalities for the better—a nearly perfect pill? Well, not quite.

There *are* some problems. Many medical experts worry that some doctors may be overprescribing Prozac and using it to treat relatively trivial personality disorders. As a result, far too many people—including some of the estimated 200,000 Canadians currently taking Prozac—may be using a drug whose long-term effects might not be known for decades. As well, there have been reports—contradicted by manufacturer Eli Lilly and Co. of Indianapolis and U.S. health officials—suggesting that a small number of Prozac patients may become violent or prone to suicidal thinking. Even more worrisome, Dr. Lorne Brandes, a Winnipeg cancer researcher, claims to have evidence that Prozac and some other widely used drugs may promote the growth of cancerous tumors. "I'm very concerned about

Prozac," says Brandes, who reported in 1992 that rats and mice with artificially induced cancer showed an increased rate of tumor growth when they were given Prozac and another antidepressant. Brandes's findings alarmed some cancer researchers and prompted federal scientists to launch a similar study.

And although Prozac has fewer side-effects than earlier antidepressants, it does have some. Users may experience nausea, nervousness and insomnia and their sex life can suffer: a U.S. study, published in *The Journal of Clinical Psychiatry* in April (1994) found that among 160 patients taking Prozac, 54 reported that sexual desire or response diminished after they began using the drug. And even proponents wonder about the social implications of a medicine that promises to abolish angst—what would happen to the world's art and culture if future Vincent van Goghs and F. Scott Fitzgeralds were prescribed Prozac? Peter D. Kramer, a psychiatrist from Providence, R.I., who paints a largely favorable portrait of the pill in his best-selling book *Listening to Prozac*, allows: "We cannot escape entirely the fear that a drug that makes people optimistic and confident will rob them of the morally beneficial effects of melancholy and angst."

In defense of Prozac, which grossed $1.7 billion in worldwide sales last year, Eli Lilly officials say that it is one of the most thoroughly tested medications in history: more than 32,000 people took part in Prozac's clinical trials, and scientists have conducted at least 3,000 separate studies. "Nothing alarming has shown up," says Cameron Battley, corporate affairs manager for Eli Lilly Canada Inc. in Scarborough, Ont. Battley also insists that, despite reports of the drug being used to treat people who do not really need an antidepressant, "there is absolutely no indication of any inappropriate use of Prozac in Canada." Maybe, but there are signs that Eli Lilly suspects something amiss. In an advertisement that began appearing recently in North American medical publications, the company deplores the "unprecedented amount of media attention" given to Prozac and stresses that the drug is intended for use "only where a clear medical need exists."

While there are concerns about Prozac, there is also unstinting praise from doctors and patients for an antidepressant that has made it easier to treat a debilitating illness. The side-effects of older antidepressants—including a parched mouth, difficulty urinating and feelings of psychological detachment—made them hard to take. "There were serious problems involved in getting patients to tolerate those drugs in therapeutic doses," says Dr. James Brooks, a Toronto general practitioner. "With Prozac, you don't have this. I'm really pleased with Prozac."

Many patients are equally enthusiastic. Three years ago, William Pringle, Vancouver special events organizer, was flattened by a major depression. His doctor put him on Prozac. "I fell into this dark pit," says Pringle. "Prozac pulled me out and got me relaunched on my life." Pringle, 36, stopped using Prozac a year ago and says that he is still feeling fine. Maria Theresa Spagnuolo of Toronto began taking it in 1989, after three automobile accidents left her with chronic pain throughout her body—and serious depression. Married and the mother of a young son, Spagnuolo found that she "was crying about everything—spilled milk was a catastrophe." Prozac, adds the 38-year-old Spagnuolo, "gave me energy and changed my outlook so that I can cope with life. I don't think I could function without it."

Interestingly, many doctors report that the majority of their Prozac patients are women. William Ashdown, a Prozac user who is executive director of the Winnipeg-based Society for Depression and Manic-Depression of Manitoba, says that "it is more acceptable for a woman to seek help for an emotional disorder. Most men are culturally pressured into other avenues of self-medication, alcohol being a common one."

Spurred by Prozac's success, competing drug companies have begun producing similar antidepressants, including Paxil (made by Britain's SmithKline Beecham PLC) and Zoloft (by New York City-based Pfizer Inc.). All the drugs tinker with the same delicate mechanism— the brain's chemical communication system. Over the past decade, scientists have made important strides in understanding how the brain works—and how to affect the intricate chemical activity that makes some people chipper and outgoing while leaving others habitually despondent. Among the key determinants are a group of chemicals known as neurotransmitters—they include serotonin, dopamine and norepinephrine—that help to flash signals among the brain's 50 billion cells. Discharged by one cell, the neurotransmitters lock onto the receptors of neighboring cells. In this chemical interplay, serotonin plays a powerful role in modifying mood and emotion—but some people apparently don't have enough of it.

To remedy that, Prozac and similar drugs—known collectively by scientists as selective serotonin re-uptake inhibitors (SSRIs)—prevent brain cells from reabsorbing used serotonin. That leaves a pool of serotonin available for further use, which can lighten the mood and thinking of depressed people. Rose Rancourt, a 42-year-old Vancouverite, began using Paxil last fall after battling severe depressions from the age of 16. A former computer information systems supervisor, Rancourt now devotes herself to working with other depressed people. Thanks to Paxil, she says, "I feel good. I feel fine. I have peace of mind."

Despite its success in blazing the way for other SSRIs, Prozac has been embroiled in controversy almost from the start. After taking about 15 years to develop the drug, Eli Lilly began marketing Prozac in the United States in 1988 and in Canada the following year. Then, in February, 1990, Dr. Martin Teicher, a psychiatrist at the highly regarded McLean Hospital in Belmont, Mass., and two of his colleagues reported that six depressed patients began to have suicidal thoughts after using Prozac. Writing in *The American Journal of Psychiatry*, Teicher said that when they began taking the drug, none of the patients were suicidal and all were "hopeful and optimistic" about their treatment. After that, a spate of anecdotal reports told of violence and suicide among Prozac users. And the drug acquired a tenacious enemy in the Los Angeles-based Citizens Commission on Human Rights, which has ties to the Church of Scientology, a movement that, among other things, opposes some aspects of psychiatry and drug therapy.

The Scientologists claim that by Sept. 16, 1993, no fewer that 1,089 suicides had been recorded among patients taking the capsule. If that figure is correct, it works out to about .01 percent of the 11 million people who have used the drug. Eli Lilly's Battley denies that Prozac is to blame. "Sadly," he added, "it is impossible to eradicate the possibility of depressed people committing suicide, even if they are receiving medication." Hearings by the U.S. Food and Drug Administration exonerated Prozac, but the bad publicity cut into its sales and produced a flood of lawsuits against Eli Lilly. So far, U.S. courts have rejected 80 claims against the company, many alleging that Prozac caused violent or suicidal tendencies; another 170 lawsuits are pending. In Canada, five lawsuits—at least one involving violence—are pending against the company.

Prozac weathered the bad notices and soon began getting good ones. Kramer's book, published last year, describes personalities transformed by Prozac and patients made "better than well." According to Kramer, the effect Prozac will have on a patient can never be accurately predicted. "Sometimes," he writes, "you take Prozac to treat a symptom, and it transforms your sense of self." The pill seems "to give social confidence to the habitually timid, to make the sensitive brash, to lend the introvert the social skills of a salesman."

Boosted by Kramer's best-seller, Prozac took off in 1993, recording a 15-percent increase in North American sales over the previous year—and prompting concern that doctors now may be dispensing the drug too liberally. In Canada and the United States, Prozac has been approved for use in treating clinical depression, bulimia (habitual purging to lose weight) and obsessive-compulsive disorder (persistent irrational thoughts and actions). But many doctors have effectively expanded the definition of what constitutes clinical depression to include dysthmyia—chronic low-grade depression—and in some cases have prescribed Prozac to otherwise healthy patients suffering from low self-esteem or gnawing anxieties. Hubert Van Tol, an associate professor of psychiatry and pharmacology at the University of Toronto, says: "If it's a question of someone who isn't feeling so hot, or maybe a man who's nervous about addressing meetings—that's not what the drug was designed for."

As well, some psychiatrists argue that it is dangerous for Prozac or similar drugs to be used without accompanying psychotherapy sessions, which enable doctors to monitor the drug's effects. Some experts worry that general practitioners, who write the majority of Prozac prescriptions and see scores of patients a day, do not have time to do that. Others argue that far from being overprescribed, the drug has just begun to realize its potential. "In terms of sheer numbers," author Kramer told *Maclean's*, "you could probably double or triple the number of people using antidepressants, because depression is so underdiagnosed." Adds Kramer: "Prozac is not an enjoyable drug to use. It doesn't give you a high. With people who have problems but are less than clinically depressed, we would have no compunction about treating them with psychotherapy. So I don't see why we can't also treat them with a chemical that will ease their symptoms."

As compelling as that argument sounds, critics respond by insisting that any relatively new drug may have unforeseen consequences. Sidney Wolfe, director of the Public Citizen Health Research Group, a Washington-based consumer advocacy organization, compares Prozac to Valium, the popular tranquillizer that was on the market for more than 10 years before doctors discovered its highly addictive properties during the mid-1970s. "Prozac," declares Wolfe, "has become the Valium of the 1990s." Asks Dr. David Bakish, associate professor of psychiatry at the University of Ottawa: "Is there a chance that with Prozac some problem could show up in 15 or 20 years? Yes, it could happen."

Some doctors say they have seen disturbing reactions in Prozac patients. Dr. Shiva Sishta, a Fredericton psychiatrist who prescribes Prozac for people suffering from obsessive-compulsive disorders, says that one married woman who was on a fairly high dosage, "became rather promiscuous—she recognized that she was not behaving properly." Sishta took her off the drug, then resumed it later at a lower dosage with encouraging results. Dr. Randolph Catlin, a psychiatrist who is chief of the mental health service at Harvard University in Cambridge, Mass., says that "two or three" students he treated with Prozac reported "feeling split off from themselves. They feel as though they're not there anymore." Adds Catlin: "One wonders if these reports that you hear about people acting aggressively with Prozac might be cases where patients who are out of touch with their feelings act on their impulses, without having any feeling of guilt or concern."

While controversy swirls around Prozac and the other SSRIs, a new generation of drugs—with an even greater potential for brightening moods and dispelling disruptive emotions—is fast coming of age.... New York City's Bristol-Myers Squibb Co.... introduce[d] Serzone, a more finely tuned serotonin-related drug designed to help people with depression and panic disorders while causing even fewer side-effects than the current SSRIs. Effexor, a new drug produced by Philadelphia-based Wyeth-Ayerst Laboratories Co. and already on the market in the United States, controls levels of serotonin and norepinephrine to help people suffering from depression; the company claims it has even fewer side-effects than Prozac.

Early in the 21st century, the new stage of drug development may give doctors more sophisticated tools for treating mental illnesses and correcting minor personality disorders—happy pills for every occasion. Because chemical imbalances in the brain are often the result of an inherited defect, says Rémi Quirion, director of the neuroscience division at the Douglas Hospital Research Centre in Montreal. I think in 10 years' time we will be able to look at a patient's genetic background and choose the drug to use accordingly." Quirion thinks that eventually it will be possible for doctors to administer just the right mix of drugs "to fine-tune the behavior of a given person. We may be able to almost modulate personality." At that point, says the University of Toronto's Van Tol, society "will face an ethical question: do we think it's right to use drugs that change our behavior in a certain direction that we want it to go in? I don't know the answer." It is a question that society already has begun to grapple with as it struggles to come to terms with the unanswered questions about Prozac and the dawning of the age of cosmetic psychopharmacology.

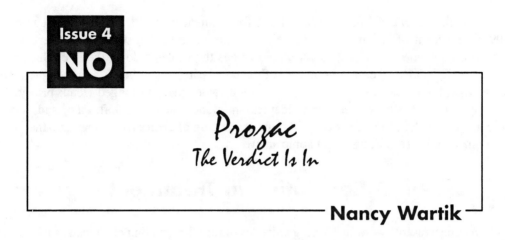

Issue 4

NO

Prozac
The Verdict Is In

Nancy Wartik

Five years ago, a traumatic sexual encounter sent Cindy Thompson, (names have been changed) now 41, plummeting into depression. "It was agonizing," recalls Thompson, a public relations consultant in Baltimore. "I wanted to kill myself every day." Thompson's psychotherapist recommended Prozac. "But I resisted," she says. "I was concerned about using a chemical to alter my mind and emotions." Finally, poised between the knife drawer and the telephone, "I called my therapist." Thompson agreed to be briefly hospitalized-and to try Prozac. "I figured I'd hit bottom and had nothing to lose."

This year marks a decade since Prozac, the antidepressant that's achieved a celebrity normally associated with movie stars and rock groups, first hit the market. Since then, it's been glorified as a miracle cure and vilified in a backlash centering on claims that Prozac makes some users violent. It's also been attacked as a "happy pill," a quick fix that allows users to ignore the psychological issues at the root of their depression.

Yet even with its luster tarnished, Prozac prospers. With 1995 sales topping $2 billion, up 24% from 1994, it's the second biggest moneymaking drug in the U.S., after the ulcer medicine Zantac. According to the manufacturer, Eli Lilly, more than 14 million Americans have joined the Prozac generation.

The drug has touched the lives of women in particular, primarily because they're twice as likely as men to suffer from major depression—a partly genetic disorder marked by persistent symptoms including sadness, fatigue, sleep or appetite problems and suicidal thoughts. Women also tend to have higher rates of other disorders for which Prozac is now prescribed, such as dysthmyia (chronic mild depression), some forms of anxiety (panic attacks and obsessive-compulsive disorder), severe PMS and bulimia.

Has the advent of Prozac been a boon for women, or will it come to be seen as the 1990s equivalent of "Mother's Little Helper"? Has the drug transformed the treatment of mental illness, or will it cause as yet unknown health problems down the line? Such questions are all the more pressing in this era of managed care, when there's a growing tendency to treat psychological disorders with medication rather than prolonged (read: pricey) talk therapy. And with a host of newer antidepressant clones such as Zoloft, Paxil and Serzone flooding the market, should Prozac still reign as the drug of choice? Ten years into the Prozac phenomenon, we're starting to get some answers.

A Revolution in Treatment

Antidepressants work by altering balances of mood-regulating chemicals, such as serotonin, in the brain. The most popular antidepressants used to be a class of drug known as tricyclics, which were developed in the 1950s and are still in use. But tricyclics affect not only the brain chemicals they're supposed to but also some they aren't. This can lead to side effects ranging from constipation, dizziness and weight gain to more dangerous problems such as heart rhythm abnormalities.

In contrast, Prozac, Paxil and Zoloft, which belong to a class of drugs known as selective serotonin reuptake inhibitors, or SSRI's, affect serotonin regulation much more directly, which means users tolerate them better. "It doesn't matter how well a drug works if, because of the side effects, people don't take it regularly," says Michael Norden, M.D., a psychiatrist at the University of Washington in Seattle and author of *Beyond Prozac*. "So Prozac was a tremendous step forward."

Women in particular seem to find Prozac and the other SSRI's easy to tolerate. In an ongoing multicenter study of people with chronic depression, women and men were randomly assigned to tricyclic or SSRI treatment. More than 25% of the women on tricyclics stopped taking them, largely because of the side effects, while less than 15% of women on SSRI's quit. They also reported better moods while using SSRI's. (Men, on the other hand, tended to do better on tricyclics.)

With findings such as these, it comes as no surprise that antidepressants are now prescribed more liberally than ever. Some 60% are given out by family doctors, rather than mental health specialists. They're also prescribed for a far greater range of ailments and for less serious disorders: Whereas tricyclics were once reserved only for those with severe depression, these days it's not uncommon for physicians to prescribe Prozac for a case of the blues.

Happy All the Time?

Prozac's easy accessibility has also raised fears that doctors are handing out the drug like M&M's and people are popping it for "personality face-lifts." The real story is more complicated. Plenty of experts agree that the drugs are too readily available. "Their popularity has led to some inappropriate use," says Sidney Zisook, M.D., a professor of psychiatry at the University of California at San Diego. "There are a lot of sloppy diagnoses, cases where they're given for the wrong reasons or for too long. There are also patients who just want to be perfect, to always enjoy themselves, and they think they can do it the easy way, with Prozac. But it' wrong to use these medicines to try to solve all of life's problems."

Others point to a tendency, encouraged by managed care, for doctors to prescribe a pill instead of steering patients toward psychotherapy. "There are maybe 20% to 30% of depressed patients who can just take a drug and get well," says New York University psychiatrist Eric Peselow, M.D. "But the majority need psychotherapy as part of treatment. Racing to Prozac isn't the only answer." Unfortunately people who pop a pill without doing the hard work of self examination may find themselves back where they started when they quit taking the medication.

Yet with only one in three depressed people today getting treatment, cries of "Prozac abuse!" can be misleading. "There are far more people who could benefit from these drugs and aren't taking them than there are people taking them inappropriately," says Dr. Zisook. Prozac's trendiness shouldn't obscure the fact that the drug and its progeny help many people dramatically.

Despite her initial skepticism, for instance, Thompson found the drug "life transforming. I felt like myself again." Prozac also pulled Isabel Leigh up from despair. Leigh, 41, a New York City editor who has struggled with depression on and off for years, was reluctant to try the drug. "I didn't want to be just one more trendy Prozac taker," she says. "I told myself it was a crutch I could do without." But about a year ago she found herself feeling lethargic, hopeless and unable to concentrate; she withdrew from friends and let work slide. Finally Leigh went to a doctor and got a Prozac prescription. "It took a few weeks, but the difference was incredible." she says. "I realized I'd been trying to overcome a biochemical problem with willpower alone."

Prozac Pitfalls

Glowing testimonials aside, Prozac isn't perfect. Like any currently available antidepressant, it works in only 60% to 70% of cases. There's often a lag of up to eight weeks before the drug starts working. And Prozac isn't free of side effects either: potential problems include agitation, insomnia, headache and weight gain or loss. What's more perhaps a third of those who stay on Prozac for nine months or more find that its uplifting effects fade away, a problem ingloriously known as "Prozac poopout." (Increasing the dose once or twice often helps.)

A growing number of studies also show that up to half of all Prozac users experience decreased libido and delayed or no orgasm. Sharon Keene, 39, a writer in Laguna Hills, CA, took Prozac for three months and "it seemed to help in just about every way," she says. "But I ended up stopping, because I couldn't achieve orgasm. If I wasn't married, maybe I wouldn't have cared so much, but it was affecting my relationship with my husband."

Though other SSRI's can impair sexual function too, Zoloft and Paxil leave the bloodstream faster than Prozac, so users may be able to circumvent trouble in bed by taking drug "holidays" a day or two before the act (so much for spontaneity). Serzone, on the market since 1995, is kinder to users' sex lives. So is Wellbutrin, a medication with a slightly different mechanism of action than Serzone and the SSRI's. It does add a very slight risk of seizures, though....

The bottom line: None of the new antidepressants is clearly superior. "They all have advantages and disadvantages," says Dr. Zisook. "We never know with certainty which drug will work best. There's always some trial and error involved."

The Price of Fame

As the leader of the pack, Prozac is often the drug of choice by benefit of name recognition alone. But its fame works against it too. Even today Prozac's reputation is clouded by rumors it can't quite shake. Within two years of its introduction in the U.S., headlines and lawsuits began claiming that Prozac drives some users to bizarre, violent behavior. One notorious 1989 incident, the subject of a new book called *The Power to Harm* by John Cornwell, involved a 47-year-old printing plant worker who shot 20 coworkers and then committed suicide after being on Prozac. Survivors and relatives of the victims sued Eli Lilly and lost, but the damage to Prozac's reputation was done.

Today you can surf the Net and still find horror stories from disgruntled folks in "Prozac survivor" support groups. Mary Beth Mrozek, a 33-year-old Buffalo, NY, mother of three who has bipolar illness, says that while on the drug she hallucinated, became convinced people were plotting against her and violently attacked loved ones. "I was a totally different person," she says.

Should the average Prozac user worry about having a Jekyll and Hyde reaction? Bipolar patients who take Prozac may be at slightly higher risk for an episode of mania. But that's a risk associated with any antidepressant (though possibly less so with Wellbutrin). Based on a substantial body of research, experts agree that Prozac users overall aren't at greater risk for violent or suicidal behavior. In fact, says Dr. Norden, "Depressed people who avoid Prozac are probably placing themselves in greater danger. Nothing increases suicide risk as much as depression itself."

A Cancer Connection?

Perhaps a more realistic worry involves unknowns about the long-term effects of Prozac and the other SSRI's, especially since some users of these drugs are now staying on the drugs indefinitely. A slender body of evidence, based mostly on animal and very preliminary human studies, suggests that antidepressants, including Prozac, could accelerate tumor growth in some people who have a predisposition to cancer or preexisting tumors. Not surprisingly, Eli Lilly disputes these findings. "Lilly's long-term animal studies have been extensively reviewed by the FDA," says Freda Lewis-Hall, M.D., a psychiatrist who heads the Lilly Center for Women's Health in Indianapolis. "There is absolutely no scientifically credible evidence that it either causes or promotes cancer."

Not everyone agrees. Oncologist Lorne Brandes, M.D., of the Manitoba Cancer Treatment and Research Foundation in Winnipeg, Canada, questions how carefully Lilly interpreted some of its data. But at the same time, he says that antidepressants are "absolutely warranted to treat depression. I'd just suggest trying to get off them as soon as you comfortably can."

Ultimately, however, we may remember Prozac not for its side effects, trendiness or even its effectiveness, but for the attention it has focused on depression-and that can only benefit women in the end. "Once, to be depressed was to be morally and spiritually weak," says Dr. Zisook. "Now people in line at the grocery store are talking about being on Prozac. The drug has brought depression out of the closet."

Leigh, for one, is grateful that it did. "It's not like I have a perfect life with Prozac," she says. "I still have ups and downs. But now I know that if I do get down, I'll come back up. Before Prozac, I was never sure."

Debate Presenter Form

Follow the guidelines for debate presenters contained in the introduction of this text and those given to you by your instructor. Use the format below to organize the material for your debate. Remember to include all relevant citation information and to present the related information in your own words. Give credit to authors when you cite a quote and be as thorough as possible when writing about your points so you will be prepared for your debate.

Reference citation #1:

Author: _____

Title: _____

Date: _____

Source: _____

_____

Content from reference citation #1: _____

_____

_____

_____

_____

_____

_____

_____

_____

_____

_____

_____

_____

_____

Reference citation #2:

Author: _____

Title: _____

Date: _____

Source: _____

_____

Content from reference citation #2: _____

_____

_____

_____

_____

_____

Reference citation #3:

Author: _____

Title: _____

Date: _____

Source: _____

_____

Content from reference citation #3: _____

_____

_____

_____

_____

Name _____

Section _____

Audience Preparation Form

Follow the guidelines for preparing to be an informed audience member on the day of the debate included in the introduction to this text. After reading both sides of the debate from this chapter, answer the following questions. Be as thorough as possible so that you will be able to make a contribution to the debate by asking informed questions or making provocative comments. This form is usually due on the day of the debate.

State the issue in your own words. Do not plagiarize the text. Demonstrate that you understand the topic and it's relevant arguments.

_____

_____

_____

_____

_____

Discuss two points on the "yes" side of the debate.

Point #1: _____

_____

Point #2: _____

_____

Discuss two points on the "no" side of the debate.

Point #1: _____

_____

Point #2: _____

_____

What is your opinion on this topic?

_____

_____

_____

_____

_____

_____

_____

What has contributed to the development of your views about this topic?

_____

_____

_____

_____

_____

_____

_____

_____

What information would be necessary to cause you to change your thinking about this topic?

_____

_____

_____

_____

_____

Debate Response Form

Follow the guidelines for responding to the debates in the introductory chapter of this text. Complete this form and submit your answers at the class following the debate. Try to be thorough and convince your instructor that you were an active listener during the debate.

List a quote from a debate presenter that you think was important and explain why you think this comment was significant.

_____

_____

_____

_____

Which side of the debate do you think made the most convincing arguments, why?

_____

_____

_____

_____

_____

After hearing the debate, in what way has your thinking been affected?

_____

_____

_____

_____

_____

_____

ISSUE 5

Can You Trust the Consumer Reports Conclusion That Psychotherapy Is Effective?

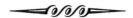

YES Martin E.P. Seligman, *The Effectiveness of Psychotherapy: The Consumer Reports Study*

NO Neil S. Jacobson and Andrew Christensen, *Studying the Effectiveness of Psychotherapy: How Well Can Clinical Trials Do the Job?*

In the applied arena of psychology, where countless hours of psychotherapy are delivered to mental health consumers, the central question is, "Does psychotherapy really help?" In a daring departure from their usual evaluation of products, *Consumer Reports* took on this question using a reader survey.

Twenty two thousand readers responded by rating how they felt prior to and after therapy. Overwhelmingly, people reported significant improvement with therapy. Martin Seligman suggests that this type of "effectiveness" study be considered seriously as a method of evaluating therapy outcomes.

Jacobsen and Christensen argue that significant methodological flaws exist in the Consumer Reports study and they reject this type of "effectiveness" study as invalid. These authors cite six major design flaws in the survey and they emphasize that the conclusions reached have been previously substantiated by empirical studies of the value psychotherapy. Jacobsen and Christensen support "efficacy" studies as demonstrating the true effectiveness of counseling.

Applications

1. Which type of study, effectiveness or efficacy, do you think is more convincing in terms of psychotherapy outcomes, why?

2. Do you think the results of this type of survey are convincing to a *Consumer Reports* reader who is considering whether or not to seek psychotherapy? Why or why not?

3. What would you change about the methodology of the *Consumer Reports* study to obtain results that would persuade you to seek counseling if you needed it?

The Effectiveness of Psychotherapy
The Consumer Reports Study

Martin E.P. Seligman

How do we find out whether psychotherapy works? To answer this, two methods have arisen: the *efficacy study* and the *effectiveness study*. An efficacy study is the more popular method. It contrasts some kind of therapy to a comparison group under well-controlled conditions....

The high praise "empirically validated" is now virtually synonymous with positive results in efficacy studies, and many investigators have come to think that an efficacy study is the "gold standard" for measuring whether a treatment works...

But my belief has changed about what counts as a "gold standard." And it was a study by *Consumer Reports* (1995, November) that singlehandedly shook my belief. I came to see that deciding whether one treatment, under highly controlled conditions, works better that another treatment or a control group is a different question from deciding what works in the field (Munoz, Hollon, McGrath, Rehm, & VandenBos, 1994). I no longer believe that efficacy studies are the only, or even the best, way of finding out what treatments actually work in the field. I have come to believe that the "effectiveness" study of how patients fare under the actual conditions of treatment in the field, can yield useful and credible "empirical validation" of psychotherapy and medication. This is the method that Consumer Reports pioneered...

Consumer Reports Survey

Consumer Reports (CR) included a supplementary survey about psychotherapy and drugs in one version of its 1994 annual questionnaire, along with its customary inquiries drugs in one version of its 1994 annual questionnaire, along with its customary inquiries about appliances and services. CR's 180,000 readers received this version, which included approximately 100 questions about automobiles and about mental health. CR asked readers to fill out the mental health section "if at any time over the past three years you experienced stress or other emotional problems for which you sought help from any of the following: friends, relatives, or a member of the clergy; a mental health professional like a psychologist or a psychiatrist; your family doctor; or a support group." Twenty-two thousand readers responded. Of these, approximately 7,000 subscribers responded to the mental health questions. Of these 7,000 about 3,000 had just talked to friends, relatives, or clergy, and 4,100 went to some combination of mental health professionals, family doctors, and support groups. Of these 4,100, 2,900 saw a mental health professional: Psychologists (37%) were the most frequently seen mental health professional, followed by psychiatrists (22%), social workers (14%), and marriage counselors (9%). Other mental health professionals made up 18%. In addition, 1,300 joined self-help groups, and about 1,000 saw family physicians. The respondents as a whole were highly educated, predominantly middle class; about half were women, and the median age was 46....

There were a number of clear-cut results, among them:

- Treatment by a mental health professional usually worked. Most respondents got a lot better. Averaged over all mental health professionals, of the 426 people who were feeling *very poor* when they began therapy, 87% were feeling *very good, good,* or at least so-so by the time of the survey. Of the 786 people who were feeling *fairly poor* at the outset, 92% were feeling *very good, good,* or at least so-so by the time of the survey. These findings converge with meta-analyses of efficacy (Lipsey & Wilson, 1993; Shapiro & Shapiro, 1982, Smith, Miller, & Glass, 1980).

- Long-term therapy produced more improvement than short-term therapy. This result was very robust, and held up over all statistical models....

- There was no difference between psychotherapy alone and psychotherapy plus medication for any disorder (very few respondents reported that they had medication with no psychotherapy at all).

- While all mental health professionals appeared to help their patients, psychologists, psychiatrists, and social workers did equally well and better than marriage counselors. Their patients' overall improvement scores (0–300 scale) were 220, 226, 225 (not significantly different from each other), and 208 (significantly worse than the first three), respectively.

- Family doctors did just as well as mental health professionals in the short term, but worse in the long term. Some patients saw both family doctors and mental health professionals, and those who saw both had more severe problems. For patients who relied solely on family doctors, their overall improvement scores when treated for up to six months was 213, and it remained at that level (212) for those treated longer than six months. In contrast, the overall improvement scores for patients of mental health professionals was 211 up to six months, but climbed to 232 when treatment went on for more than six months. The advantage of long-term treatment by a mental health professional held not only for the specific problems that led to treatment, but for a variety of general functioning scores as well: ability to relate to others, coping with everyday stress, enjoying life more, personal growth and understanding, self-esteem and confidence.

- Alcoholics Anonymous (AA) did especially well, with an average improvement score of 251, significantly bettering mental health professionals. People who went to non-AA groups had less severe problems and did not do as well as those who went to AA (average score=215).

- Active shoppers and active clients did better in treatment than passive recipients (determined by responses to "Was it mostly your idea to seek therapy? When choosing this therapist, did you discuss qualifications, therapist's experience, discuss frequency, duration, and cost, speak to someone who was treated by this therapist, check out other therapists? During therapy, did you try to be as open as possible, ask for explanation of diagnosis and unclear terms, do homework, not cancel sessions often, discuss negative feelings toward therapist?").

- No specific modality of psychotherapy did any better than any other for any problem. These results confirm the "dodo bird" hypothesis, that all forms of psychotherapies do about equally well (Luborsky, Singer, & Luborsky, 1975). They come as a rude shock to efficacy researchers, since the main theme of efficacy studies has been the demonstration of the usefulness of specific techniques for specific disorders.

- Respondents whose choice of therapist or duration of care was limited by their insurance coverage did worse,...(determined by responses to "Did limitations on your insurance coverage affect any of the following choices you made? Type of therapist I chose; How often I met with my therapist; How long I stayed in therapy").

These findings are obviously important, and some of them could not be included in the original CR article because of space limitations. Some of these findings were quite contrary to what I expected, but it is not my intention to discuss their substance here. Rather, I want to explore the methodological adequacy of this survey. My underlying questions are "Should we believe the findings?" and "Can the method be improved to give more authoritative answers?"

Consumer Reports Survey: Methodological Virtues

Sampling. This survey is, as far as I have been able to determine, the most extensive study of psychotherapy effectiveness on record. The sample is not representative of the United

States as a whole, but my guess is that it is roughly representative of the middle class and educated population who make up the bulk of psychotherapy patients. It is important that the sample represents people who choose to go to treatment for their problems, not people who do not "believe in" psychotherapy or drugs. The CR sample, moreover, is probably weighted toward "problem solvers," people who actively try to do something about what troubles them.

Treatment duration.   CR sampled all treatment durations from one month or less through two years or more. Because the study was naturalistic, treatment, it can be supposed, continued until the patient (a) was better, (b) gave up unimproved, or (c) had his or her coverage run out. This, by definition, mirrors what actually happens in the field. In contrast to all efficacy studies, which are of fixed conferences of the National Institute of Mental Health, or even from the halls of academe...

The Ideal Study

The *CR* study, then, is to be taken seriously—not only for its results and its credible source, but for its method. It is large-scale; it samples treatment as it is actually delivered in the field; it samples without obvious bias those who seek out treatment; it measures multiple outcomes including specific improvement and more global gains such as growth, insight, productivity, mood, enjoyment of life, and interpersonal relations; it is statistically stringent and finds clinically meaningful results. Furthermore, it is highly cost-effective.

Its major advantage over the efficacy method for studying the effectiveness of psychotherapy and medications is that it captures how and to whom treatment is actually delivered and toward what end. At the very least, the *CR* study and its underlying survey method provides a powerful addition to what we know about the effectiveness of psychotherapy and a pioneering way of finding out more.

The study is not without flaws, the chief one being the limited meaning of its answer to the question "Can psychotherapy help?" This question has three possible kinds of answers. The first is that psychotherapy does better than something else, such as talking to friends, going to church, or doing nothing at all. Because it lacks comparison groups. The *CR* study only answers this question indirectly. The second possible answer is that psychotherapy returns people to normality or more liberally to within, say, two standard deviations of the average. The *CR* study, lacking an untroubled group and lacking measures of how people were before they became troubled, does not answer this question. The third answer is "Do people have fewer symptoms and a better life after therapy than they did before?" This is the question that the *CR* study answers with a clear "yes."

Issue 5
NO

Studying the Effectiveness of Psychotherapy

Neil S. Jacobson
Andrew Christensen

[T]here is considerable debate about the merits of a recent *Consumer Reports (CR)* survey (1995)....This survey has received a great deal of attention within psychology and has been publicized in the popular press. Seligman (1995) suggested that this is the best study ever conducted on the effectiveness of psychotherapy.

Much like Freud's case studies, the report by *CR* (1995) is very persuasive and will probably have a great deal of influence on the public perception of psychotherapy. However, the purpose of this article is to show that most of what the *CR* study says has already been proven to the satisfaction of both practitioners and psychotherapy researchers. Moreover, those findings from the *CR* study that have not been previously established are highly questionable because of the study's methodological shortcomings. Finally, controlled experiments that avoid the methodological pitfalls of the *CR* study can answer virtually all of the questions considered by Seligman (1995) to be beyond the scope of clinical trials. In fact, it would be unfortunate if the field of psychotherapy research abandoned the controlled experiment when attempting to answer questions regarding the effectiveness of psychotherapy. Although clinical trials have their limitations and may need to be supplemented by other types of methodologies, they are far superior to the type of design reflected in the *CR* study, a design that has already been debated and rejected by both practitioners and researchers...

Adapted from *American Psychologist*, October 1996 Vol. 51, pp. 1031–1039 by Neil S. Jacobson and Andrew Christensen. Copyright © 1996 by The American Psychological Association. Reprinted by permission.

A Critique of the New Findings from the Consumer Reports Survey

The methodological shortcomings of the *CR* (1995) survey greatly limit their evidentiary value. Seligman (1995) mentioned some of these shortcomings but not others; the ones he did mention tended to be minimized. Here are a sample of these shortcomings.

A Retrospective Survey Is Not an Ideal Prototype for Effectiveness Research

Seligman (1995) suggested that the *CR* (1995) study is a well-done effectiveness study and was careful to distinguish this study from an efficacy study—a randomized clinical trial. However, in fact, the CR survey is not necessarily a good model for an effectiveness study as that term is typically used. The main virtue of the *CR* survey, according to Seligman, is its "realism"; that is, it is a report about real therapy, conducted by real therapists, with real clients, in the real world. The retrospective biases that are impossible to rule out are not seen as fatal flaws but simply as aspects of the design that need to be refined.

There are two fundamental problems with retrospective surveys. The first is that, because they are retrospective, there is no opportunity to corroborate respondents' reports. When participants are reporting on their own previous experiences, whether in therapy or otherwise, there is no way of assessing their accuracy. Various biases may contaminate their responses, ranging from demand characteristics to memory distortion. With a prospective study, some of these biases can be minimized, whereas others can be evaluated, using corroborative measures coming from different modalities. For example, self-report data can be supplemented with observational data. With retrospective surveys, such validation is impossible, and thus the responses are hard to interpret.

The second problem with retrospective surveys is the possibility that an unrepresentative subsample of those surveyed returned their questionnaires. Although it cannot be proven that those who benefited from psychotherapy were more likely to complete the survey than were those who did not, neither can that possibility be disproven. With a prospective study, one doesn't have to guess. This additional problem makes the improvement rates reported in the *CR* (1995) survey hard to interpret.

The most striking example of this selectivity problem is in the findings pertaining to Alcoholics Anonymous (AA), which had the highest mean improvement rate of any treatment category reported by Seligman (1995). In fact, as a treatment, AA significantly outperformed other mental health professionals. This finding can be contrasted with the lack of evidence supporting the efficacy of AA in prospective studies (McCrady & Delaney, 1995). Seligman acknowledged the strong possibility of sampling bias in AA and offered some speculations on why one might expect AA to be particularly susceptible to such biases. However, he then inexplicably minimized the likelihood of similarly extensive biases operating in the sample as a whole, suggesting that a similar kind of sampling bias, *to a lesser degree* (italics added) cannot be overlooked for other kinds of treatment failures. At any rate, it is quite possible that there was a *large* (italics added) oversampling of successful AA cases and a *smaller* (italics added) oversampling of successful treatment for problems other than alcoholism. (p.971)

Is it not possible that the oversampling of successful cases was as large for other problems as it was for AA? Is there any evidence to the contrary?

In addition to contaminating the overall estimates of treatment gains, sampling bias could easily explain the apparent superiority of long-term therapy reported by the respondents in the *CR* (1995) study. Unlike Howard et al. (1986), who found a negatively accelerated dose—response relationship, the *CR* survey found a linear relationship: the more therapy, the better the outcome. This would indeed be an important finding if it were interpretable; unfortunately, it is not interpretable. Seligman (1995) argued against the possibility of sampling bias by focusing on one potential source. He suggested that, if early dropouts are treatment failures and those who remain in treatment are beneficiaries, then earlier dropouts should have lower rates of "problem resolution" than later dropouts. In fact, the rates are uniform: About two thirds of dropouts quit because the problem is resolved, whether they quit therapy one month or two years after they started.

The problem with Seligman's (1995) refutation is that it fails to rule out the primary source of interpretive ambiguity—spontaneous remission. The longer people stay in therapy, the greater the opportunity for factors other than therapy to produce improvement. There is no way of knowing whether the superiority of long-term therapy is due to the treatment itself or simply to increased opportunities for other factors to produce improvements.

Seligman (1995) argued that the main virtue of the *CR* (1995) study is its realism. If one thinks of realism using the metaphor of a snapshot, the implication is that the *CR* survey provides a snapshot of what psychotherapy is really like. But, because the study is retrospective, the snapshot may be out of focus. With a prospective study, one can take a snapshot of psychotherapy whose focus is indisputable. But, with a retrospective survey, the negatives are gone forever.

The Absence of Control Groups of Any Kind Constitutes an Additional Fatal Flaw

Seligman (1995) fully acknowledged the problems introduced by the uncontrolled nature of the study but suggested that there are "internal controls" that can be used as surrogates. Unfortunately, none of Seligman's internal controls can be considered adequate substitutes for control groups.

First, he suggested that the inferior performance of marriage counselors allowed them to serve as a reference group because they controlled for various non-specific factors such as the presence of an attentive listener. However, because marriage counselors may have differed systematically from other professionals in the client population with whom they worked, their performance cannot be compared with that of other mental health professionals who may have treated more mental health problems that were not primarily related to marital distress. In other words, there may have been a systematic confounding between type of problem treated and profession, which rendered marriage counselors useless as an internal control.

Second, Seligman (1995) noted that long-term treatment worked better than short-term treatment, thus allowing the use of the first point in the dose—response curve as a control group. As we have already suggested, this internal control is useless because of the confound with greater opportunity for spontaneous remission in long-term therapy.

Third, according to Seligman (1995), because it is known that drugs outperform placebos, and because psychotherapy did as well as psychotherapy plus drugs in the *CR* (1995) study, one can infer that psychotherapy would have outperformed an adequate placebo if one had been included in the *CR* study. This argument is specious for a number of reasons: It is not known what drugs were used for which problems in the *CR* study; it is not known whether the pharmacotherapy performed was adequate (compliance, dosage, etc.); and most importantly, it is not known whether the sample of patients in the *CR* study was similar to those in which drugs typically outperform placebos.

Fourth, family doctors did not perform as well as mental health professionals when treatment continued beyond six months, thus suggesting family doctors as an internal control. However, family doctors saw clients for a fewer number of sessions than did mental health professionals, creating a confound that Seligman (1995) himself acknowledged.

Seligman (1995) concluded that spontaneous remission is an unlikely explanation for the high improvement rates reported by respondents in the *CR* (1995) study. We come to a different conclusion, because none of the proposed internal controls are adequate. We conclude that factors other than psychotherapy might very well have accounted for the improvement rates reported by the respondents. We come to this conclusion for several reasons. First, there is no adequate control to rule it out, thus no compelling reason to reject the null hypothesis. Second, because the 4,000 respondents in the *CR* study were, to use Seligman's (1995) terminology, "middle class and educated" (p.969) and "a good-sized fraction were 'subclinical'...and would not meet *DSM-IV (Diagnostic and Statistical Manual of Mental Disorders, 4th Edition;* American Psychiatric Association, 1994) criteria for any disorder" (p. 970), we have the kind of sample that is most likely to spontaneously remit, or to benefit from any treatment, specific or non-specific (Jacobson & Hollon, 1996). As Seligman noted, in most clinical trials, the single largest basis for exclusion is that the client is not sufficiently distressed or dysfunctional to be included.

For example, in research on depression, by far the most common basis for exclusion is that not enough symptoms are present for the patient to meet criteria for major depressive disorder; even if *DSM-IV* criteria are met, participants are often excluded because the major depressive disorder is not severe enough (Jacobson et al., 1996). In efficacy studies, there is a good reason to exclude these participants: They seem to get better no matter what they receive. Even the less severe patients who make it into these trials tend to respond as well to placebos as they do to active treatments (cf. Jacobson & Hollon, 1996). Thus, it is a fair assumption that many of the respondents to the *CR* (1995) survey who improved would have improved without therapy.

The Measures in the *Consumer Reports* Survey Were Not Only Unreliable but Unrevealing

The *CR* (1995) survey measured little more than consumer satisfaction. Consumer satisfaction is far from trivial. However, consumer satisfaction ratings are uncorrelated with symptomatic outcome and general functioning. In the *CR* survey, three questions were asked in the assessment of improvement, one pertaining to "satisfaction with therapist", a second pertaining to "improvement in the presenting problem." and a third pertaining to "improvement in overall functioning." The latter measure was a change score, derived by subtracting posttest scores from pretest scores (both obtained retrospectively); the other two measures were simply posttest scores. Seligman (1995) seized on these three questions to argue that three different constructs are being measured: consumer satisfaction, symptom relief, and general functioning. However, since all three questions are global and retrospective and have method variance in common, they cannot be considered independent assessments of functioning or to be measuring different constructs. Furthermore, the three questions were combined into a multi-variate composite for the calculation of improvement rates, thus making it impossible to separate out consumer satisfaction from the other items.

The Specificity Question Revisited:

The *Consumer Reports* Survey Did Not Assess Which Therapies Led to Improvement in Which Problems

Researchers are long past the stage of referring to psychotherapy as if it were uniform, without specifying the nature of the problem being treated or the treatment used. Yet, the *CR* (1995) study failed to inform the public about any particular treatment for any particular problem and thus provides little information that advances knowledge about psychotherapy. The data may be available to answer more specific questions. But even if they were available, and were released, they would be based on respondent reports: Respondents would be reporting what their presenting problem was and the kind of treatment they received (we have already seen some data on this latter question), and they would be defining both the profession and the theoretical orientation of the therapist. How reliable are survey respondents at describing the theoretical orientation of their therapist or at fitting their presenting problem into one of a series of choices on a survey, especially in retrospect? Both of us have small private practices, and a large proportion of our clients are couples. We have heard ourselves referred to as marriage counselors, psychologists, and even, on occasion, psychiatrists. We doubt whether the number of our clients who could correctly identify our theoretical orientation would much exceed chance.

Even Assuming Methodological Adequacy, the Results as Reported by *Consumer Reports* and by Seligman Are Misleading

Although the sound bite coming out of both the *CR* (1995) report and Seligman's (1995) article says that 90% of the respondents found psychotherapy beneficial, it is worth noting that this figure comes from combining those who were helped "a great deal," "a lot," and "somehat." Only 54% reported that they were helped "a great deal." This is not a very impressive figure from the standpoint of clinical significance, especially when one takes into account the number of subclinical respondents in the sample and the possibility that the respondents may be overrepresented by those who found treatment to be helpful.

The Eysenck Evaluation Revisited

The *CR* (1995) survey bears remarkable resemblance to the controversial evaluation of psychotherapy reported by Eysenck (1952). In this report, Eysenck summarized the results of 24 reports of psychoanalytic and eclectic psychotherapy with more than 7,000 neurotic patients treated in naturalistic settings. Using therapist ratings of improvement, Eysenck reported a 44% improvement rate for psychoanalytic therapy and a 64% improvement rate for eclectic psychotherapy. Unlike the *CR* survey, however, these reports were prospective in that the therapist evaluations occurred at the time of termination. Also unlike the *CR* survey, Eysenck used control groups: One consisted of all improved patients who had been discharged from hospitals in New York between 1917 and 1934 for "neurotic" conditions, receiving nothing but custodial care; the other consisted of 500 disability claimants who were periodically evaluated by general practitioners without receiving psychotherapy, so it could be determined whether they were improved enough to go back to work. Improvement for this latter control group was defined as their ability to return to work, which was decided by the general practitioner. Eysenck reported, on the basis of these two control groups, that the spontaneous remission rate for these minimally treated patients was 72% and that psychotherapy was therefore ineffective.

The merits of these findings and the methodology supporting them were debated vigorously for 20 years. Initially, Luborsky (1954) criticized the study on the grounds that the measures of improvement were flawed, the control groups were inadequate, and the treatments were lacking on both uniformity and representativeness. Similar critiques were registered by Rosenzweig (1954) and De Charrus, Levy, and Wertheimer (1954). These and more recent critiques (e.g., Bergin, 1971) argued, with considerable merit, the Eysenck (1952) had underestimated the success of therapy and overestimated the spontaneous remission rate. As recently as the mid-1970s, Eysenck's study was subject to refutation by more optimistic appraisals and interpretations of psychotherapy's impact (Luborsky et al., 1975; Meltzoff & Kornreich, 1970). Now, the controversy has largely subsided, and Eysenck's study has been rejected by clinical scientists. In fact, in the most recent edition of Bergin and Garfield's (1994) *Handbook of Psychotherapy and Behavioral Change* the study is not even cited.

When it is referenced nowadays, it is primarily for its historical impact and its heuristic value.

What is interesting about examining Eysenck's (1952) study in light of the *CR* (1995) survey is that virtually all of the criticisms leveled at Eysenck's evaluation also apply to the *CR* survey, even though Eysenck's evaluation was more sophisticated from a methodological perspective. Eysenck had a sample that was almost twice as large as the sample reported in the CR survey; he did at least include control groups, however inadequate they might have been; the measures of improvement were concurrent rather than retrospective; and the measures were obtained from trained therapists rather than from the clients themselves. Given Seligman's (1995) assumptions that therapists are able to self-correct their therapeutic work and cannily select which clients need drugs and psychotherapy, therapists should also be better judges of when clients have made genuine improvement versus transitory symptom change. However, the field was correct in rejecting Eysenck's evaluation: The control groups and the measures of outcome were inadequate. We don't see any reason to revert to a methodology that was rejected for its methodological inadequacies 20 years ago.

Debate Presenter Form

Follow the guidelines for debate presenters contained in the introduction of this text and those given to you by your instructor. Use the format below to organize the material for your debate. Remember to include all relevant citation information and to present the related information in your own words. Give credit to authors when you cite a quote and be as thorough as possible when writing about your points so you will be prepared for your debate.

Reference citation #1:

Author: _____

Title: _____

Date: _____

Source: _____

_____

Content from reference citation #1: _____

_____

_____

_____

_____

_____

_____

_____

_____

_____

_____

_____

_____

Reference citation #2:

Author: _____

Title: _____

Date: _____

Source: _____

_____

Content from reference citation #2: _____

_____

_____

_____

_____

_____

_____

Reference citation #3:

Author: _____

Title: _____

Date: _____

Source: _____

_____

Content from reference citation #3: _____

_____

_____

_____

_____

Audience Preparation Form

Follow the guidelines for preparing to be an informed audience member on the day of the debate included in the introduction to this text. After reading both sides of the debate from this chapter, answer the following questions. Be as thorough as possible so that you will be able to make a contribution to the debate by asking informed questions or making provocative comments. This form is usually due on the day of the debate.

State the issue in your own words. Do not plagiarize the text. Demonstrate that you understand the topic and it's relevant arguments.

_____

_____

_____

_____

_____

Discuss two points on the "yes" side of the debate.

Point #1: _____

_____

Point #2: _____

_____

Discuss two points on the "no" side of the debate.

Point #1: _____

_____

Point #2: _____

_____

What is your opinion on this topic?

_____

_____

_____

_____

_____

_____

_____

_____

What has contributed to the development of your views about this topic?

_____

_____

_____

_____

_____

_____

_____

_____

What information would be necessary to cause you to change your thinking about this topic?

_____

_____

_____

_____

_____

Debate Response Form

Follow the guidelines for responding to the debates in the introductory chapter of this text. Complete this form and submit your answers at the class following the debate. Try to be thorough and convince your instructor that you were an active listener during the debate.

List a quote from a debate presenter that you think was important and explain why you think this comment was significant.

_____

_____

_____

_____

Which side of the debate do you think made the most convincing arguments, why?

_____

_____

_____

_____

_____

After hearing the debate, in what way has your thinking been affected?

_____

_____

_____

_____

_____

_____

Psychological Treatment

I S S U E 6

Do Religiously Committed Individuals Enjoy Greater Mental Health?

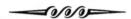

YES David B. Larson, *Have Faith: Religion Can Heal Mental Ills*

NO Albert Ellis, *Dogmatic Devotion Doesn't Help, It Hurts*

David B. Larson supports the assertion that spirituality can have a positive effect on mental illness. He cites research demonstrating the benefits of religion and spirituality on psychological disorders ranging from depression to suicide. Marital satisfaction, recovery from illness and surgery, and personal sense of well-being are also cited by Larson as being enhanced by religious commitment.

Larson concludes with an explanation for the rejection of religiosity as an asset to mental well being. He explains that mental health professionals have a significantly lower rate of belief in God than the general population. For this reason, these professionals are quick to see problems in patients as caused by what may be deemed as religious "delusions."

Albert Ellis takes a strong opposing viewpoint. He not only negates the benefits of religion, but attributes mental illness to the practice of religion. Ellis' concerns with the research regarding the relationship between religion and mental health include flaws in scientific method, experimenter bias, and participant bias in self-report.

Ellis also presents research to contradict studies reviewed by Larson. He discusses cases of the devoutly religious and describes them as "often disturbed." In some specific cases religious belief and practice have been the direct cause of mental illness according to Ellis. These include antiabortion killers, Muslim extremists, the aggressive Ayatollah Komeine, religious wars, and cult-related multiple suicides.

Ellis distinguishes between devout and moderate religiosity and believes the later to be fairly emotionally healthy. It is the fanatically religious that Ellis predicts to be mentally ill. He concludes with a description of the religious beliefs held by people most likely to be mentally disturbed.

Applications

1. How do you think your views about religion affect your mental health?

2. Give examples of the benefits of religion to people you know.

3. Give examples of the detriments of religion to people you know.

YES

Have Faith
Religion Can Heal Mental Ills

David B. Larson

If a new health treatment were discovered that helped to reduce the rate of teenage suicide, prevent drug and alcohol abuse, improve treatment for depression, reduce recovery time from surgery, lower divorce rates and enhance a sense of well-being, one would think that every physician in the country would be scrambling to try it. Yet, what if critics denounced this treatment as harmful, despite research findings that showed it to be effective more than 80 percent of the time? Which would you be more ready to believe—the assertions of the critics based on their opinions or the results of the clinical trials based upon research?

As a research epidemiologist and board-certified psychiatrist, I have encountered this situation time and again during the last 15 years of my practice. The hypothetical medical treatment really does exist, but it is not a new drug: It is spirituality. While medical professionals have been privately assuming and publicly stating for years that religion is detrimental to mental health, when I actually looked at the available empirical research on the relationship between religion and health, the findings were overwhelmingly positive.

Just what are the correlations that exist between religion and mental health? First, religion has been found to be associated with a decrease in destructive behavior such as suicide. A 1991 review of the published research on the relationship between religious commitment and suicide rates conducted by my colleagues and I found that religious commitment produced lower rates of suicide in nearly every published study located. In fact, Stephen Stack, now of Wayne State University, showed that non-church attenders were four times more likely to kill themselves than were frequent attenders and that church attendance predicted suicide rates more effectively than any other factor including unemployment.

What scientific findings could explain these lower rates of suicide? First, several researchers have noted that the religiously committed report experiencing fewer suicidal impulses and have a more negative attitude toward suicidal behavior than do the nonreligious. In addition, suicide is a less-acceptable alternative for the religiously committed because of their belief in a moral accountability to God, thus making them less susceptible than the nonreligious to this life-ending alternative. Finally, the foundational religious beliefs in an afterlife, divine justice and the possibility of eternal condemnation all help to reduce the appeal of potentially self-destructive behavior.

If religion can reduce the appeal of potentially self-destructive behavior such as suicide, could it also play a role in decreasing other self-destructive behavior such as drug abuse? When this question has been examined empirically, the overwhelming response is yes. When Richard Gorsuch conducted a review of the relationship between religious commitment and drug abuse nearly 20 years ago, he noted that religious commitment "predicts those who have not used an illicit drug regardless of whether the religious variable is defined in terms of membership, active participation, religious upbringing or the meaningfulness of religion as viewed by the person himself."

More recent reviews have substantiated the earlier findings of Gorsuch, demonstrating that even when employing varying measures of religion, religious commitment predicted curtailed drug abuse. Interestingly, a national survey of 14,000 adolescents found the lowest rates of adolescent drug abuse in the most "politically incorrect" religious group—theologically conservative teens. The drug-abuse rates of teens from more liberal religious groups rose a little higher but still sank below rates of drug abuse among nonreligious teens. The correlations between the six measures of religion employed in the survey and the eight measures of substance abuse all were consistently negative. These findings lead the authors of the study to conclude that the amount of importance individuals place on religion in their lives is the best predictor of a lack of substance abuse, implying that "the (internal) controls operating here are a result of deeply internalized norms and values rather than fear...or peer pressure." For teens living in a society in which drug rates continue to spiral, religion may not be so bad after all.

Just as religious commitment seems to be negatively correlated with drug abuse, similar results are found when examining the relationship between religious commitment and alcohol abuse. When I investigated this area myself, I found that those who abuse alcohol rarely have a strong religious commitment. Indeed, when my colleagues and I surveyed a group of alcoholics, we found that almost 90 percent had lost interest in religion during their teenage years, whereas among the general population, nearly that same percentage reported no change or even a slight increase in their religious practices during adolescence. Furthermore, a relationship between religious commitment and the nonuse or moderate use of alcohol has been extensively documented in the research literature. Some of the most intriguing results have been obtained by Acheampong Amoateng and Stephen Bahr of Brigham Young University, who found that whether or not a religion specifically proscribed alcohol use, those who were active in a religious group consumed substantially less than those who were not active.

Not only does religion protect against clinical problems such as suicide and drug and alcohol abuse, but religious commitment also has been shown to enhance positive life experiences such as marital satisfaction and personal well-being. When I reviewed the published studies on divorce and religious commitment, I found a negative relationship between church attendance and divorce in nearly every study that I located.

To what can these lower rates of divorce be attributed? Some critics argue that the religiously committed stay in unsatisfactory marriages due to religious prohibitions against divorce. However research has found little if any support for this view. In my review I found that, as a group, the religiously committed report a higher rate of marital satisfaction than the nonreligious. In fact, people from long-lasting marriages rank religion as one of the most important components of a happy marriage, with church attendance being strongly associated with the hypothetical willingness to remarry a spouse—a very strong indicator of marital satisfaction. Could these findings be skewed because, as is believed by some in the mental-health field, religious people falsify their response to such questions to make themselves look better? When the studies were controlled for such a factor the researchers found that the religiously committed were not falsifying their responses or answering in a socially acceptable manner and truly were more satisfied in their marriages.

Although the religiously committed are satisfied with their marriages, is this level of satisfaction also found in the sexual fulfillment of married couples? Though the prevailing public opinion is that religious individuals are prudish or even sexually repressed, empirical evidence has shown otherwise. Using data from *Redbook* magazine's survey of 100,000 women in 1975, Carole Tavris and Susan Sadd contradicted the longstanding assumption that religious commitment fosters sexual dysfunction. Tavris and Sadd found that it is the most religious women who report the greatest happiness and satisfaction with marital sex—more so than either moderately religious or nonreligious women. Religious women also report reaching orgasm more frequently than nonreligious women and are more satisfied with the frequency of their sexual activity than the less pious. Thus, while surprising to many, research suggests that religious commitment may play a role in improving rather than hindering sexual expression and satisfaction in marriage.

Not only has religious commitment been found to enhance sexual satisfaction, but overall life satisfaction as well. For example, David Myers of Hope College reviewed well-being literature and found that the religiously committed have a greater sense of overall life satisfaction than the nonreligious. Religion not only seems to foster a sense of well-being and life satisfaction but also may play a role in protecting against stress, with religiously committed respondents reporting much lower stress levels than the less committed. Even when the religiously committed have stress levels that are similar to the nonreligious, the more committed report experiencing fewer mental-illness problems than do the less committed.

Mental-health status has been found to improve for those attending religious services on a regular basis. Indeed, several studies have found a significant reduction in diverse psychiatric symptomatology following increased religious involvement. Chung-Chou Chu and colleagues at the Nebraska Psychiatric Institute in Omaha found lower rates of rehospitalization among schizophrenics who attended church or were given supportive aftercare by religious homemakers and ministers. One of my own studies confirmed that religious commitment can improve recovery rates as well. When my colleagues and I examined elderly women recovering from hip fractures, we found that those women with stronger religious beliefs suffered less from depression and thus were more likely to walk sooner and farther than their nonreligious counterparts.

***

Yet, despite the abundance of studies demonstrating the beneficial effects of religious commitment on physical and mental health, many members of the medical community seem immune to this evidence. This resistance to empirical findings on the mental-health benefits of religious commitment may stem from the anti-religious views espoused by significant mental-health theorists. For example, Sigmund Freud called religion a "universal obsessional neurosis" and regarded mystical experience as "infantile helplessness" and a "regression to primary narcissism." More recently, Albert Ellis, the originator of rational-emotive therapy, has argued that "unbelief, humanism, skepticism and even thorough-going atheism not only abet but are practically synonymous with mental health; and that devout belief, dogmatism and religiosity distinctly contribute to, and in some ways are equal to, mental or emotional disturbance." Other clinicians have continued to perpetuate the misconception that religion is associated with psychopathology by labeling spiritual experiences as, among other things, borderline psychosis, a psychotic episode or the result of temporal-lobe dysfunction. Even the consensus report, "Mysticism: Spiritual Quest or Psychological Disturbance," by the Group for the Advancement of Psychiatry supported the long-standing view of religion as psychopathology; calling religious and mystical experiences "a regression, an escape, a projection upon the world of a primitive infantile state."

What is perhaps most surprising about these negative opinions of religion's effect on mental health is the startling absence of empirical evidence to support these views. Indeed, the same scientists who were trained to accept or reject a hypothesis based on hard data seem to rely solely on their own opinions and biases when assessing the effect of religion on health. When I conducted a systematic review of all articles published in the two leading journals of psychiatry, the *American Journal of Psychiatry* and the *Archives of General Psychiatry*, which assessed the association between religious commitment and mental health, I found that more than 80 percent of the religious-mental health associations located were clinically beneficial while only 15 percent of the associations were harmful—findings that run counter to the heavily publicized opinion of mental-health professionals. Thus, even though the vast majority of published research studies show religion as having a positive influence on mental health, religious commitment remains at best ignored or at worst, maligned by the professional community.

The question then begs to be asked: Why do medical professionals seem to ignore such positive evidence about religion's beneficial effect on mental health? One possible source of this tension could lie in clinicians' unfamiliarity with or rejection of traditional religious expression. For example, not only do mental-health professionals generally hold levels of religious commitment that diverge significantly from the general population, but they have much higher rates of atheism and agnosticism as well. The most recent survey of the belief systems of mental-health professionals found that less than 45 percent of the members of the American Psychiatric Association and the American Psychological Association believed in God—a percentage less than half that of the general population. When asked whether they agreed with the statement, "My whole approach to life is based on my religion," only one-third of clinical psychologists and two-fifths of psychiatrists agreed with that statement—again, a percentage that is nearly half that of the U.S. population. Indeed, more than 25 percent of psychiatrists and clinical psychologists and more than 40 percent of psychoanalysts claimed that they had abandoned a theistic belief system, compared with just less than 5 percent of the general population reporting the same feelings.

Science is assumed to be a domain that progresses through the gradual accumulation of new data or study findings, yet the mental-health community seems to be stalled in its understanding of the interface between religion and mental health. If a field is to progress in its knowledge and understanding of a controversial issue such as religion, empirical data and research must be relied upon more than personal opinions and biases. At a time when the rising cost of health care is causing so much discussion in our country, no factor that may be so beneficial to health can be ignored. The continuing neglect of published research on religion prevents clinicians and policymakers from fully understanding the important role of religion in health care and deprives patients as well as themselves of improved skills and methods in clinical prevention, coping with illness and quality of care. The mental health establishment needs to begin to recognize that it is treating a whole person—mind, body and, yes, even spirits.

Dogmatic Devotion Doesn't Help, It Hurts

Albert Ellis

According to the psychological studies cited by David Larson, religious believers have more satisfying marriages, more enjoyable sex lives, less psychological stress, less depression and less drug and alcohol abuse than nonreligious people. Do these studies present a "true" picture of the mental health benefits of being religious? Probably not, for several reasons. First, the scientific method itself has been shown by many postmodernists to be far from "objective" and unassailable because it is created and used by highly subjective, often biased individuals. Scientists are never purely dispassionate observers of "reality" but frequently bring their own biases to their experiments and conclusions.

Second, practically all the studies that Larson cites were conducted by religious believers; some were published in religious journals. Many of the researchers were motivated to structure studies to "prove" that religionists are "healthier" than nonreligionists and only to publish studies that "proved" this.

None of the studies cited—as I noted when I read many of them myself—eliminated the almost inevitable bias of the subjects they used. I showed, in two comprehensive reviews of personality questionnaires that were published in the *Psychological Bulletin* in 1946 and 1948 and in several other psychological papers, that people often can figure out the "right" and "wrong" answers to these questionnaires and consequently "show" that they are "healthy" when they actually are not. I also showed, in an article in the *American Sociological Review* in 1948, that conservative and religious subjects probably more often were claiming falsely to have "happier" marriages on the Burgess-Locke Marriage Prediction Test than were liberal and nonreligious subjects.

This tendency of conservative, religious, job-seeking and otherwise motivated individuals to overemphasize their "good" and deemphasize their "poor" behavior on questionnaires has been pointed out by a number of other reviewers of psychological studies. Because all these studies included a number of strongly religious subjects, I would guess that many of these religionists had a distinct tendency to claim to be happier, less stressful and less addictive personalities than a good clinician would find them to be. I believe that this is a common finding of psychologists and was confirmed by my reviews mentioned previously.

Although Larson has spent a number of years locating studies that demonstrated that religious believers are healthier than nonreligious subjects, a large number of researchers have demonstrated the opposite. Several other studies have found that people who rigidly and dogmatically maintain religious views are more disturbed than less-rigid religious followers. But all these studies, once again, are suspect because none of them seem to have eliminated the problem of the biased answers of some of their subjects who consciously or unconsciously want to show how healthy they are.

Larson points out that many psychologists are sure that religionists are more disturbed than nonreligionists in spite of their having no real scientific evidence to substantiate their opinions. He is largely right about this, in view of what I have already said. Nonetheless, some reasonably good data back up the views of these psychologists that devout religionists often are disturbed.

Antiabortion killers such as Paul Hill have demonstrated that fanatical beliefs can have deadly consequences. But lesser-known fanatical religious believers have used ruthless tactics to oppose such "enlightened" views as birth control, women's liberation and even separation of church and state. Some religious zealots have jailed, maimed or even killed liberal proponents of their own religions. Nobel laureate Naguib Mahfouz is still recovering from stab wounds inflicted by Muslim extremists last October near his home in Cairo. (Mahfouz, considered by many to be a devout Muslim, frequently has ridiculed religious hypocrisy in his work.) Indian-born author Salman Rushdie has lived for seven years under a death sentence pronounced by the late Ayatollah Khomeini. Rushdie explained to the *New York Times* that dissidents within the Muslim world become "persons whose blood is unclean and therefore deserves to be spilled."

Religious persecution and wars against members of other religions have involved millions of casualties throughout human history Islamic fundamentalists from North Africa to Pakistan have established, or done their best to establish, state religions that force all the citizens of a country or other political group to strictly obey the rules of a specific religious group.

People diagnosed as being psychotic and of having severe personality disorders frequently have been obsessed with religious ideas and practices and compulsively and scrupulously follow religious teachings.

The tragic, multiple suicides of members of the Switzerland-based Order of the Solar Temple last October is only the most recent illustration of an extremist religious cult which manipulated its adherents and induced some of them to harm and kill themselves.

Do these manifestations of religious-oriented fanaticism, despotism, cultism and psychosis prove that religious-minded people generally are more disturbed than nonreligious individuals? Of course not. Many—probably most—religionists oppose the extreme views and practices I have just listed, and some actually make efforts to counteract them. One should not conclude, then, that pious religiosity in and of itself equals emotional disturbance.

However, as a psychotherapist and the founder of a school of psychotherapy called rational emotive behavior therapy, I have for many years distinguished between people who hold moderate religious views and those who espouse devout, dogmatic, rigid religious attitudes. In my judgment, most intelligent and educated people are in the former group and temperately believe God (such as Jehovah) exists, that He or She created the universe and the creatures in it, and that we preferably should follow religious, ethical laws but that a Supreme Being forgives us fallible humans when we do not follow His or Her rules. These "moderate" religionists prefer to be "religious" but do not insist that the rest of us absolutely and completely always must obey God's and the church's precepts. Therefore, they still mainly run their own lives and rarely damn themselves (and others) for religious nonobservance. In regard to God and His or Her Commandments, they live and let live.

The second kind of religious adherents—those who are devout, absolutistic and dogmatic—are decidedly different. They differ among themselves but most of them tend to believe that there absolutely has to be a Supreme Being, that He or She specifically runs the universe, must be completely obeyed and will eternally damn all believers and nonbelievers who deviate from His or Her sacred commands.

Another devout and absolutistic group of people do not believe in anything supernatural, but do rigidly subscribe to a dogmatic, secular belief system—such as Nazism, Fascism or Communism—which vests complete authority in the state or in some other organization and which insists that nonallegiance or opposition to this Great Power must be ruthlessly fought, overthrown, punished and annihilated.

As an advocate of mental and emotional health, I have always seen "moderate" religious believers as reasonably sound individuals who usually are no more neurotic (or otherwise disturbed) than are skeptical, nonreligious people. Like nonbelievers, they are relatively open-minded, democratic and unbigoted. They allow themselves to follow and experience "religious" and "secular" values, enjoyment and commitment. Therefore, they infrequently get into serious emotional trouble with themselves or with others because of their religious beliefs and actions.

This is not the case with fanatical, pietistic religionists. Whether they are righteously devoted to God and the church or to secular organizations and cults (some of which may be atheistic) these extreme religionists are not open-minded, tolerant and undamning. Like nonreligious neurotics and individuals with severe personality disorders, they do not merely wish that other religionists and nonbelievers agree with them and worship their own Supreme Being and their churchly values. They insist, demand and command that their God's and their church's will be done.

Since the age of 12, I have been skeptical of anything supernatural or god-like. But I always believed that undogmatic religionists can get along well in the world and be helpful to others, and I relate nicely to them. Many, if not most, of the mental-health professionals with whom I have worked in the field of rational emotive behavior therapy are religious. A surprisingly large number of them have been ordained as Protestant ministers, Catholic priests or nuns or Jewish rabbis. A few have even been fundamentalists! So some forms of psychotherapy and moderate religious belief hardly are incompatible.

The important question remains: Is there a high degree of correlation between devout, one-sided, dogmatic religiosity and neurosis (and other personality disorders)? My experience as a clinical psychologist leads me to conclude that there well may be. Some of the disturbed traits and behaviors that pietistic religionists tend to have (but, of course, not always have) include these:

A dearth of enlightened self-interest and self-direction. Pietistic religionists tend to be overdevoted, instead, to unduly sacrificing themselves for God, the church (or the state) and to ritualistic self-deprivation that they feel "bound" to follow for "sacred" reasons. They often give masochistic and self-abasing allegiance to ecclesiastical (and/or secular) lords and leaders. Instead of largely planning and directing their own lives, they often are mindlessly overdependent on religious-directed (or state-directed) creeds, rules and commandments.

Reduced social and human interest. Dogmatic religionists are overly focused on godly, spiritual and monastic interests. They often give greater service to God than to humanity and frequently start holy wars against dissidents to their deity and their church. Witness the recent murders by allegedly devout antiabortionists.

Refusal to accept ambiguity and uncertainty. In an obsessive-compulsive fashion, they hold to absolute necessity and complete certainty, even though our universe only seems to include probability and chance. They deny pliancy, alternative-seeking and pluralism in their own and other people's lives. They negate the scientific view that no hypothesis is proved indisputably "true" under all conditions at all times.

Allergy to unconditional self-acceptance. Emotionally healthy people accept themselves (and other humans) unconditionally—that is, whether they achieve success and whether all significant others approve of them. Dogmatic religionists unhealthily and conditionally accept themselves (and others) only when their God, their church (or state) and similar religionists approve of their thoughts, feelings and behaviors. Therefore, they steadily remain prone to, and often are in the throes of, severe anxiety guilt and self-condemnation.

In rational-emotive therapy we show people that they "get" emotionally disturbed not only by early or later traumas in their lives but mainly by choosing goals and values that they strongly prefer and by unrealistically, illogically and defeatingly making them into one, two or three grandiose demands: (1) "I absolutely must succeed at important projects or I am an utterly worthless person"; (2) Other people must treat me nicely or they are totally damnable"; (3) "Life conditions are utterly obligated to give me everything that I think I need or my existence is valueless."

When people clearly see that they are largely upsetting themselves with these godlike commandments, and when they convert them to reasonable—but often still compulsive—desires, they are able to reconstruct their disturbed thoughts, feelings and actions and make themselves much less anxious, depressed, enraged and self-hating and much more self-actualizing and happy.

Being a philosophical system of psychotherapy, rational emotive behavior therapy has much to learn from theological and secular religions. But individuals who choose to be religious also may learn something important from it, namely: Believe whatever you wish about God, the church, people and the universe. But see if you can choose a moderate instead of a fanatical form of religion. Try to avoid a doctrinal system through which you are dogmatically convinced that you absolutely must devote yourself to the one, only, right and unerring deity and to the one, true and infallible church. And try to avoid the certitude that you are God. Otherwise, in my view as a psychotherapist, you most probably are headed for emotional trouble.

Name _____

Section _____

Debate Presenter Form

Follow the guidelines for debate presenters contained in the introduction of this text and those given to you by your instructor. Use the format below to organize the material for your debate. Remember to include all relevant citation information and to present the related information in your own words. Give credit to authors when you cite a quote and be as thorough as possible when writing about your points so you will be prepared for your debate.

Reference citation #1:

Author: _____

Title: _____

Date: _____

Source: _____

_____

Content from reference citation #1: _____

_____

_____

_____

_____

_____

_____

_____

_____

_____

_____

_____

_____

Reference citation #2:

Author: _____

Title: _____

Date: _____

Source: _____

_____

Content from reference citation #2: _____

_____

_____

_____

_____

_____

_____

Reference citation #3:

Author: _____

Title: _____

Date: _____

Source: _____

_____

Content from reference citation #3: _____

_____

_____

_____

_____

Audience Preparation Form

Follow the guidelines for preparing to be an informed audience member on the day of the debate included in the introduction to this text. After reading both sides of the debate from this chapter, answer the following questions. Be as thorough as possible so that you will be able to make a contribution to the debate by asking informed questions or making provocative comments. This form is usually due on the day of the debate.

State the issue in your own words. Do not plagiarize the text. Demonstrate that you understand the topic and it's relevant arguments.

_____

_____

_____

_____

_____

Discuss two points on the "yes" side of the debate.

Point #1: _____

_____

Point #2: _____

_____

Discuss two points on the "no" side of the debate.

Point #1: _____

_____

Point #2: _____

_____

What is your opinion on this topic?

_____

_____

_____

_____

_____

_____

_____

_____

What has contributed to the development of your views about this topic?

_____

_____

_____

_____

_____

_____

_____

_____

What information would be necessary to cause you to change your thinking about this topic?

_____

_____

_____

_____

_____

Debate Response Form

Follow the guidelines for responding to the debates in the introductory chapter of this text. Complete this form and submit your answers at the class following the debate. Try to be thorough and convince your instructor that you were an active listener during the debate.

List a quote from a debate presenter that you think was important and explain why you think this comment was significant.

_____

_____

_____

_____

Which side of the debate do you think made the most convincing arguments, why?

_____

_____

_____

_____

_____

After hearing the debate, in what way has your thinking been affected?

_____

_____

_____

_____

_____

_____

Human Sexual Behavior

ISSUE 7

Is Our Sexual Behavior Based in Our Genetics?

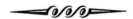

YES Robert Wright, *Our Cheating Hearts*

NO Richard N. Williams, *Science or Story Telling? Evolutionary Explanations of Human Sexuality*

In his article "Our Cheating Hearts" Robert Wright describes compelling explanations for what most of us know to be true: it is difficult for us to be monogamous. Although we may be evolutionarily designed to fall in love, we are not designed to stay in love according to Wright.

He also suggests that the objective of the human mind is to transmit genes. He offers multiple reasons for differences in males and females as they make an attempt to distribute their genes. Evolutionary patterns are offered as explanation for promiscuity, jealousy, weight of testes, polygyny, child abuse, romantic love, infanticide, paternal love, divorce, the spoils of status and male monopolization of female fertility.

Richard Williams, focusing directly on the content of Wright's article, describes Wright's assertions as an example of creative story telling. He cites the importance of distinguishing between evolutionary theory and genetic biology. Whereas genetic biology presents verifiable fact, evolutionary theory is just that: theory.

William's position against Wright's explanations rests on two points: that there is no proof that genetics produce mental events or that evolution controls these psychological phenomena. He urges us to be cautious about accepting evolutionary theory just because it makes sense. It may not contain any scientific proof.

Evolutionary explanations are popular at present although they rest on philosophical tenet rather than fact according to Williams. He applies the rules of logical argumentation to Wright's evolutionary explanations to demonstrate the fallacy of his approach.

Applications

1. Do you think your own sexual behavior is a result of genetic influences or cultural influences? Explain your answer.

2. Do you think it is legitimate to explain our behavior with theory or do you believe we must only rely on what we can prove as explanations for behavior? Why?

3. Give your thoughts about Wright's explanations of promiscuity, jealousy, and romantic love.

Our Cheating Hearts

Robert Wright

The language of zoology used to be so reassuring. Human beings were called a "pair-bonding" species. Lasting monogamy, it seemed, was natural for us, just as it was for geese, swans and the other winged creatures that have filled our lexicon with such labels as "love-birds" and "lovey-dovey." Family values, some experts said, were in our genes. In the 1967 best seller *The Naked Ape*, zoologist Desmond Morris wrote with comforting authority that the evolutionary purpose of human sexuality is "to strengthen the pair-bond and maintain the family unit."

This picture has lately acquired some blemishes. To begin with, birds are no longer such uplifting role models. Using DNA fingerprinting, ornithologists can now check to see if a mother bird's mate really is the father of her offspring. It turns out that some female chickadees (as in "my little chickadee") indulge in extramarital trysts with males that out-rank their mates in the social hierarchy. For female barn swallows, it's a male with a long tail that makes extracurriculars irresistible. The innocent-looking indigo bunting has a cuckoldry rate of 40%. And so on. The idea that most bird species are truly monogamous has gone from conventional wisdom to punctured myth in a few short years. As a result, the fidelity of other pair-bonding species has fallen under suspicion.

Which brings us to the other problem with the idea that humans are by nature endur-ingly monogamous: humans. Of course, you don't need a Ph.D. to see that 'till-death-do-we-part fidelity doesn't come as naturally to people as, say, eating. But an emerging field known as evolutionary psychology can now put a finer point on the matter. By studying how the process of natural selection shaped the mind, evolutionary psychologists are painting a new portrait of human nature, with fresh detail about the feelings and thoughts that draw us into marriage—or push us out.

The good news is that human beings are designed to fall in love. The bad news is that they aren't designed to stay there. According to evolutionary psychology, it is "natural" for both men and women—at some times, under some circumstances—to commit adultery or to sour on a mate, to suddenly find a spouse unattractive, irritating, wholly unreasonable. (It may even be *natural* to become irritating and wholly unreasonable, and thus hasten the departure of a mate you've soured on.) It is similarly natural to find some attractive colleague superior on all counts to the sorry wreck of a spouse you're saddled with. When we see a couple celebrate a golden anniversary, one apt reaction is the famous remark about a dog walking on two legs: the point is not that the feat was done well but that it was done at all.

All of this may sound like cause for grim resignation to the further decline of the American family. But what's "natural" isn't necessarily unchangeable. Evolutionary psychology, unlike past gene-centered views of human nature, illuminates the tremendous flexibility of the human mind and the powerful role of environment in shaping behavior. In particular, evolutionary psychology shows how inhospitable the current social environment is to monogamy. And while the science offers no easy cures, it does suggest avenues for change.

***

The premise of evolutionary psychology is simple. The human mind, like any other organ, was designed for the purpose of transmitting genes to the next generation; the feelings and thoughts it creates are best understood in these terms. Thus the feeling of hunger, no less than the stomach, is here because it helped keep our ancestors alive long enough to reproduce and rear their young. Feelings of lust, no less than the sex organs, are here because they aided reproduction directly. Any ancestors who lacked stomachs or hunger or sex organs or lust—well, they wouldn't have become ancestors, would they? Their traits would have been discarded by natural selection.

This logic goes beyond such obviously Darwinian feelings as hunger and lust. According to evolutionary psychologists, our everyday, ever shifting attitudes toward a mate or prospective mate—trust, suspicion, rhapsody, revulsion, warmth, iciness—are the handiwork of natural selection that remain with us today because in the past they led to behaviors that helped spread genes.

How can evolutionary psychologists be so sure? In part, their faith rests on the whole data base of evolutionary biology. In all sorts of species, and in organs ranging from brains to bladders, nature's attention to the subtlest aspects of genetic transmission is evident. Consider the crafting of primate testicles—specifically, their custom tailoring to the monogamy or lack thereof, of females. If you take a series of male apes and weigh their testicles (not recommended, actually), you will find a pattern. Chimpanzees and other species with high "relative testes weight" (testes weight is comparison to body weight) feature quite promiscuous females. Species with low relative testes weight are either fairly monogamous (gibbons, for example) or systematically polygynous (gorillas), with one male monopolizing a harem of females. The explanation is simple. When females breed with many males, male genes can profit by producing lots of semen for their own transportation. Which male succeeds in getting his genes into a given egg may be a question of sheer volume, as competing hordes of sperm do battle.

The Trouble with Women

Patterns like these, in addition to showcasing nature's ingenuity, allow a kind of detective work. If testicles evolved to match female behavior, then they are clues to the natural behavior of females. Via men's testicles, we can peer through the mists of prehistory and see how women behaved in the social environment of our evolution, free from the influence of modern culture; we can glimpse part of a pristine female mind.

The relative testes weight of humans falls between that of the chimpanzee and the gorilla. This suggests that women, while not nearly so wild as chimpanzee females (who can be veritable sex machines), are by nature somewhat adventurous. If they were not, why would natural selection divert precious resources to the construction and maintenance of weighty testicles?

There is finer evidence, as well, of natural female infidelity. You might think that the number of sperm cells in a husband's ejaculate would depend only on how long it has been since he last had sex. Wrong. What matters more, according to a recent study, is how long his mate has been out of sight. A man who hasn't had sex for, say, a week will have a higher sperm count if his wife was away on a business trip than is she's been home with the flu. In short, what really counts is whether the woman has had the opportunity to stray. The more chances she has had to collect sperm from other males, the more profusely her mate sends in his own troops. Again: that natural selection designed such an elaborate weapon is evidence of something for the weapon to combat—female faithlessness.

So here is problem No. 1 with the pair-bond thesis: women are not by nature paragons of fidelity. Wanderlust is an innate part of their minds, ready to surface under propitious circumstances. Here's problem No. 2: if you think women are bad, you should see men.

The Trouble with Men

With men too, clues from physiology help uncover the mind. Consider "sexual dimorphism"—the difference between average male and female body size. Extreme sexual dimorphism is typical of a polygynous species, in which one male may impregnate several females, leaving other males without offspring. Since the winning males usually secure their trophies by fighting or intimidating other males, the genes of brawny, aggressive males get passed on while the genes of less formidable males are deposited in the dust-bin of history. Thus male gorillas who get a whole haremful of mates if they win lots of fights and no mates if they win none, are twice as big as females. With humans, males are about 15% bigger—sufficient to suggest that male departures from monogamy, like female departures, are not just a recent cultural invention.

Anthropology offers further evidence. Nearly 1,000 of the 1,154 past or present human societies ever studied—and these include most of the world's "hunter-gatherer" societies—have permitted a man to have more than one wife. These are the closest things we have to living examples of the "ancestral environment"—the social context of human evolution, the setting for which the mind was designed. The presumption is that people reared in such societies—the!Kung San of southern Africa, the Ache of Paraguay, the 19th century Eskimo—behave fairly "naturally." More so, at least, than people reared amid influences that weren't part of the ancestral environment: TVs, cars, jail time for bigamy.

There are vanishingly few anthropological examples of systematic female polygamy, or polyandry—women monopolizing sexual access to more than one man at once. So, while both sexes are prone under the right circumstances to infidelity, men seem much more deeply inclined to actually acquire a second or third mate—to keep a harem.

They are also more inclined toward the casual fling. Men are less finicky about sex partners. Prostitution—sex with someone you don't know and don't care to know—is a service sought overwhelmingly by males the world round. And almost all pornography that relies sheerly on visual stimulation—images of anonymous people, spiritless flesh—is consumed by males.

Many studies confirm the more discriminating nature of women. One evolutionary psychologist surveyed men and women about the minimal level of intelligence they would accept in a person they were "dating." The average response for both male and female: average intelligence. And how smart would the potential date have to be before they would consent to sex? Said the women: Oh, in that case, markedly above average. Said the men: Oh, in that case, markedly below average.

There is no dispute among evolutionary psychologists over the basic source of this male open-mindedness. A woman, regardless of how many sex partners she has, can generally have only one offspring a year. For a man, each new mate offers a real chance for pumping genes into the future. According to the *Guiness Book of Records*, the most prolific human parent in world history was Moulay ("The Bloodthirsty") Ismail, the last Sharifian Emperor of Morocco, who died in 1727. He fathered more than 1,000 children.

The logic behind undiscerning male lust seems obvious now, but it wasn't always. Darwin had noted that in species after species the female is "less eager than the male," but he never figured out why. Only in the late 1960s and early 1970s did biologists George Williams and Robert Trivers attribute the raging libido of males to their nearly infinite potential rate of reproduction.

Why Do Women Cheat?

Even then the female capacity for promiscuity remained puzzling. For women, more sex doesn't mean more offspring. Shouldn't they focus on quality rather than quantity—look for a robust, clever mate whose genes may bode well for the offspring's robustness and cleverness? There's ample evidence that women are drawn to such traits, but in our species genes are not all a male has to offer. Unlike our nearest ape relatives, we are a species of "high male-parental investment." In every known hunter-gatherer culture, marriage is the norm—not necessarily monogamous marriage, and not always lasting marriage, but marriage of some sort; and via this institution, fathers help provide for their children.

In our species, then, a female's genetic legacy is best amplified by a mate with two things: good genes and much to invest. But what if she can't find one man who has both? One solution would be to trick a devoted, generous and perhaps wealthy but not especially brawny or brainy mate into raising the offspring of another male. The woman need not be aware of this strategy, but at some level, conscious or unconscious, deft timing is in order. One study found that women who cheat on mates tend to do so around ovulation, when they are most likely to get pregnant.

For that matter, cheating during the infertile part of the monthly cycle might have its own logic, as a way (unconsciously) to turn the paramour into a dupe; the woman extracts goods or services from him in exchange for his fruitless conquest. Of course the flowers he buys may not help her genes, but in the ancestral environment, less frivolous gifts—notably food— would have. Nisa, a woman in a !Kung San hunter-gatherer village, told an anthropologist that "when you have lovers, one brings you something and another brings you something else. One comes at night with meat, another with money, another with beads. Your husband also does things and gives them to you."

Multiple lovers have other uses too. The anthropologist Sarah Blaffer Hrdy has theorized that women copulate with more than one man to leave several men under the impression that they might be the father of particular offspring. Then, presumably, they will treat the offspring kindly. Her theory was inspired by langur monkeys. Male langurs sometimes kill infants sired by others as a kind of sexual icebreaker, a prelude to pairing up with the (former) mother. What better way to return her to ovulation—by putting an emphatic end to her breast-feeding—and to focus her energies on the offspring to come?

Anyone tempted to launch into a sweeping indictment of langur morality should first note that infanticide on grounds of infidelity has been acceptable in a number of human societies. Among the Yanomamö of South America and the Tikopia of the Solomon Islands, men have been known to demand, upon marrying women with a past, that their babies be killed. And Ache men sometimes collectively decide to kill a newly fatherless child. For a woman in the ancestral environment, then, the benefits of multiple sex partners could have ranged from their sparing her child's life to their defending or otherwise investing in her youngster.

Again, this logic does not depend on a conscious understanding of it. Male langurs presumably do not grasp the concept of paternity. Still, genes that make males sensitive to cues that certain infants may or may not carry their genes have survived. A gene that says, "Be nice to children if you've had lots of sex with their mothers," will prosper over the long haul.

The Invention and Corruption of Love

Genes don't talk, of course. They affect behavior by creating feelings and thoughts—by building and maintaining the brain. Whenever evolutionary psychologists talk about some evolved behavioral tendency—a polygamous or monogamous bent, say, or male parental investment—they are also talking about an underlying mental infrastructure.

The advent of male parental investment, for example, required the invention of a compelling emotion: parental love. At some point in our past, genes that inclined a man to love his offspring began to flourish at the expense of genes that promoted remoteness. The reason, presumably, is that changes in circumstance—an upsurge in predators, say—made it more likely that the offspring of undevoted, unprotective fathers would perish.

Crossing this threshold meant love not only for the child; the first step toward becoming devoted parents consists of the man and woman developing a mutual attraction. The genetic payoff of having two parents committed to a child's welfare seems to be the central reason men and women can fall into swoons over one another.

Until recently, this claim was heresy. "Romantic love" was thought to be the unnatural invention of Western culture. The Mangaians of Polynesia, for instance, were said to be "puzzled" by references to marital affection. But lately anthropologists have taken a second look at purportedly loveless cultures, including the Mangaians, and have discovered what nonanthropologists already knew: love between man and woman is a human universal.

In this sense the pair-bonding label is apt. Still, that term—and for that matter the term love—conveys a sense of permanence and symmetry that is wildly misleading. Evolution not only invented romantic love but from the beginning also corrupted it. The corruption lies in conflicts of interest inherent in male parental investment. It is the goal of maximizing male investment, remember, that sometimes leads a woman to infidelity. Yet it is the preciousness of this investment that makes her infidelity lethal to her mate's interests. Not long for this world are the genes of a man who showers time and energy on children who are not his.

Meanwhile, male parental investment also makes the man's naturally polygynous bent inimical to his wife's reproductive interests. His quest for a new wife could lead him to withdram, or at least dilute, investment in his first wife's children. This reallocation of resources may on balance help his genes but certainly not hers.

The living legacy of these long-running genetic conflicts is human jealousy—or, rather, human jealousies. In theory, there should be two kinds of jealousy—one male and one female. A man's jealousy should focus on sexual infidelity, since cuckoldry is the greatest genetic threat he faces. A woman, though she'll hardly applaud a partner's strictly sexual infidelity (it does consume time and divert some resources), should be more concerned with emotional infidelity—the sort of magnetic commitment to another woman that could lead to a much larger shift in resources.

David Buss, an evolutionary psychologist at the University of Michigan, has confirmed this prediction vividly. He placed electrodes on men and women and had them envision their mates doing various disturbing things. When men imagined sexual infidelity, their heart rates took leaps of a magnitude typically induced by three cups of coffee. They sweated. Their brows wrinkled. When they imagined a budding emotional attachment, they calmed down, though not quite to their normal level. For women, things were reversed: envisioning emotional infidelity—redirected love, not supplementary sex—brought the deeper distress.

That jealousy is so finely tuned to these forms of treachery is yet more evidence that they have a long evolutionary history. Still, the modern environment has carried them to new heights, making marriage dicier than ever. Men and women have always, in a sense, been designed to make each other miserable, but these days they are especially good at it.

Modern Obstacles to Monogamy

To begin with, infidelity is easier in an anonymous city than in a small hunter-gatherer village. Whereas paternity studies show that 2% of the children in a !Kung San village result from cuckoldry, the rate runs higher than 20% in some modern neighborhoods.

Contraceptive technology may also complicate marriage. During human evolution, there were no condoms or birth-control pills. If an adult couple slept together for a year or two and produced no baby, the chances were good that one of them was not fertile. No way of telling which one, but from their genes' point of view, there was little to lose and much to gain by ending the partnership and finding a new mate. Perhaps, some have speculated, natural selection favored genes inclining men and women to sour on a mate after long periods of sex without issue. And it is true that barren marriages are especially likely to break up.

Another possible challenge to monogamy in the modern world lies in movies, billboards and magazines. There was no photography in the long-ago world that shaped the human male mind. So at some deep level, that mind may respond to glossy images of pinups and fashion models as if they were viable mates—alluring alternatives to dull, monogamous devotion. Evolutionary psychologist Douglas Kenrick has suggested as much. According to his research, men who are shown pictures of *Playboy* models later describe themselves as less in love with their wives than do men shown other images. (Women shown pictures from *Playgirl* felt no such attitude adjustment toward spouses.)

Perhaps the largest modern obstacle to lasting monogamy is economic inequality. To see why, it helps to grasp a subtle point made by Donald Symons, author of the 1979 classic *The Evolution of Human Sexuality*. Though men who leave their wives may be driven by "natural" impulses, that does not mean men have a natural impulse designed expressly to make them leave their wives. After all, in the ancestral environment, gaining a second wife didn't mean leaving the first. So why leave her? Why not stay near existing offspring and keep giving some support? Symons believes men are designed less for opportune desertion than for opportune polygyny. It's just that when polygyny is illegal, a polygynous impulse will find other outlets, such as divorce.

If Symons is right, the question of what makes a man feel the restlessness that leads to divorce can be rephrased: What circumstances, in the ancestral environment, would have permitted the acquisition of a second wife? Answer: possessing markedly more resources, power or social status than the average Joe.

Even in some "egalitarian" hunter-gatherer societies, men with slightly more status or power than average are slightly more likely to have multiple wives. In less egalitarian pre-industrial societies, the anthropologist Laura Betzig has shown, the pattern is dramatic. In Incan society, the four political offices from petty chief to chief were allotted ceilings of seven, eight, 15 and 30 women. Polygyny reaches its zenith under the most despotic regimes. Among the Zulu, where coughing or sneezing at the king's dinner table was punishable by death, his highness might monopolize more than 100 women.

To an evolutionary psychologist, such numbers are just extreme examples of a simple fact: the ultimate purpose of the wealth and power that men seek so ardently is genetic proliferation. It is only natural that the exquisitely flexible human mind should be designed to capitalize on this power once it is obtained. Thus it is natural that a rising corporate star, upon getting a big promotion, should feel a strong attraction to women other than his wife. Testosterone—which expands a male's sexual appetites—has shown to rise in nonhuman primates following social triumphs, and there are hints that it does so in human males too. Certainly the world is full of triumphant men—Johnny Carson, Donald Trump—who trade in aging wives for younger, more fertile models. (The multi-wived J. Paul Getty said, "A lasting relationship with a woman is only possible if you are a business failure.")

A man's exalted social status can give his offspring a leg up in life, so it's natural that women should lust after the high-status men who lust after them. Among the Ache, the best hunters also have more extramarital affairs and more illegitimate children than lesser hunters. In modern societies, contraception keeps much of this sex appeal from translating into offspring. But last year a study by Canadian anthropologist Daniel Pérusse found that single men of high socioeconomic status have sex with more partners than lower-status men.

One might think that the appeal of rich or powerful men is losing its strength. After all, as more women enter the work force, they can better afford to premise their marital decisions on something other than a man's income. But we're dealing here with deep romantic attractions, not just conscious calculation, and these feelings were forged in a different environment. Evolutionary psychologists have shown that the tendency of women to place greater emphasis than men on a mate's financial prospects remains strong regardless of the income or expected income of the women in question.

The upshot of all this is that economic inequality is monogamy's worst enemy. Affluent men are inclined to leave their aging wives, and young women—including some wives of less affluent men—are inclined to offer themselves as replacements.

Objections to this sort of analysis are predictable: "But people leave marriages for emotional reasons. They don't add up their offspring and pull out their calculators." True. But emotions are just evolution's executioners. Beneath the thoughts and feelings and temperamental differences marriage counselors spend their time sensitively assessing are the stratagems of the genes—cold, hard equations composed of simple variables: social status, age of spouse, number of children, their ages, outside romantic opportunities and so on. Is the wife really duller and more nagging than she was 20 years ago? Maybe, but maybe the husband's tolerance for nagging has dropped now that she is 45 and has no reproductive future. And the promotion he just got, which has already drawn some admiring glances from a young woman at work, has not helped.

Similarly, we might ask the young, childless wife who finds her husband intolerably insensitive why the insensitivity wasn't so oppressive a year ago, before he lost his job and she met the kindly, affluent bachelor who seems to be flirting with her. Of course, maybe her husband's abuses are quite real, in which case they signal his disaffection and perhaps his impending departure—and merit just the sort of pre-emptive strike the wife is now mustering.

The Fallout from Monogamy's Demise

Not only does male social inequality favor divorce. Divorce can also reinforce male social inequality; it is a tool of class exploitation. Consider Johnny Carson. Like many wealthy, high-status males, he spent his career dominating the reproductive years of a series of women. Somewhere out there is a man who wanted a family and a pretty wife and, if it hadn't been for Johnny Carson, would have married one of these women. And if this man has managed to find another woman, she was similarly snatched from the clutches of some other man. And so on—a domino effect: a scarcity of fertile females trickles down the social scale.

As theoretical as this sounds, it cannot help happening. There are only about 25 years of fertility per woman. When some men dominate more than 25 years' worth, some man somewhere must do with less. And when, in addition to all the serial husbands, you count the men who live with a woman for five years before deciding not to marry her, and then do it again (perhaps finally at 35 marrying a 28-year-old), the net effect is not trivial. As some Darwinians have put it, serial monogamy is tantamount to polygyny. Like polygyny, it lets powerful men grab extra sexual resources (a.k.a. women), leaving less fortunate men with-out mates—or at least without mates young enough to bear children. Thus rampant divorce not only ends the marriages of some men but also prevents the marriage of others. In 1960, when the divorce rate was around 25%, the portion of the never married population age 40 or older was about the same for men and women. By 1990, with the divorce rate running at 50%, the portion for men was larger by 20% than for women.

Viewing serial monogamy as polygyny by another name throws a kink into the family-values debate. So far, conservatives have got the most political mileage out of decrying divorce. Yet life-long monogamy—one woman per man for rich and poor alike—would seem to be a natural rallying cry for liberals.

One other kind of fallout from serial monogamy comes plainly into focus through the lens of evolutionary psychology: the toll taken on children. Martin Daly and Margo Wilson of McMaster University in Ontario, two of the field's seminal thinkers, have written that one of the "most obvious" Darwinian predictions is that stepparents will "tend to care less profoundly for children than natural parents." After all, parental investment is a precious resource. So natural selection should "favor those parental psyches that do not squander it on non-relatives"—who, after all, do not carry the parent's genes.

Indeed, in combing through 1976 crime data, Daly and Wilson found that an American child living with one or more substitute parents was about 100 times as likely to be fatally abused as a child living with biological parents. In a Canadian city in the 1980s, a child age two or younger was 70 times as likely to be killed by a parent if living with a stepparent and a natural parent than if living with two natural parents.

Of course, murdered children are a tiny fraction of all children living with stepparents; divorce and remarriage hardly amount to a child's death warrant. But consider the more common problem of nonfatal abuse. Children under 10 were, depending on their age and the study in question, three to 40 times as likely to suffer parental abuse if living with a stepparent and a biological parent instead of two biological parents.

There are ways to fool Mother Nature, to induce parents to love children who are not theirs. (Hence cuckoldry.) After all, people cannot telepathically sense that a child is carrying their genes. Instead they rely on cues that in the ancestral environment would have signaled as much. If a woman feeds and cuddles an infant day after day, she may grow to love the child, and so may the woman's mate. This sort of bonding is what makes adopted children lovable (and is one reason relationships between stepparent and child are often harmonious). But the older a child is when first seen, the less profound the attachment will probably be. Most children who acquire stepfathers are past infancy.

Polygynous cultures, such as the 19th century Mormons, are routinely dismissed as cruelty sexist. But they do have at least one virtue: they do not submit children to the indifference or hostility of a surrogate father. What we have now—serial monogamy, quasi-polygyny— is in this sense worse than true polygyny. It massively wastes the most precious evolutionary resource: love.

Is There Hope?

Given the toll of divorce—on children, on low income men, and for that matter on mothers and fathers—it would be nice to come up with a magic monogamy-restoration plan. Alas, the importance of this task seems rivaled only by its difficulty. Lifelong monogamous devotion just isn't natural, and the modern environment makes it harder than ever. What to do?

As Laura Netzig has noted, some income redistribution might help. One standard conservative argument against antipoverty policies is their cost: taxes burden the affluent and thus, by lowering work incentive, reduce economic output. But if one goal of the policy is to bolster monogamy, then making the affluent less so would help. Monogamy is threatened not just by poverty in an absolute sense but also by the relative wealth of the rich. This is what lures a young woman to a wealthy married man or formerly married man. It is also what makes the man who attracts her feel too good for just one wife.

As for the economic consequences, the costs of soaking the rich might well be outweighed by the benefits, financial and otherwise, of more stable marriages, fewer divorces, fewer abused children and less loneliness and depression.

There are other levers for bolstering monogamy, such as divorce law. In the short run, divorce brings the average man a marked rise in standard of living, while his wife, along with her children, suffers the opposite. Maybe we should not lock people into unhappy marriages with financial disincentives to divorce, but surely we should not reward men for leaving their wives either.

A Moral Animal

The problem of divorce is by no means one of public policy alone. Progress will also depend on people using the explosive insight of evolutionary psychology in a morally responsible way. Ideally this insight would lead people to subject their own feelings to more acute scrutiny. Maybe for starters, men and women will realize that their constantly fluctuating perceptions of a mate are essentially illusions, created for the (rather absurd, really) purpose of genetic proliferation, and that these illusions can do harm. Thus men might beware the restlessness designed by natural selection to encourage polygyny. Now that it brings divorce, it can inflict great emotional and even physical damage on their children.

And men and women alike might bear in mind that impulses of wanderlust, or marital discontent, are not always a sign that you married the "wrong person." They may just signify that you are a member of our species who married another member of our species. Nor, as evolutionary psychiatrist Randolph L. Nesse has noted, should we believe such impulses are a sign of psychopathology. Rather, he writes, they are "expected impulses that must, for the most part, be inhibited for the sake of marriage."

The danger is that people will take the opposite tack: react to the new knowledge by surrendering to "natural" impulses, as if what's "in our genes" were beyond reach of self-control. They may even conveniently assume that what is "natural" is good.

This notion was common earlier in this century. Natural selection was thought of almost as a benign deity, constantly "improving" our species for the greater good. But evolutionary psychology rests on a quite different world view: recognition that natural selection does not work toward overall social welfare, that much of human nature boils down to ruthless genetic self-interest, that people are naturally oblivious to their ruthlessness.

George Williams, whose 1966 book *Adaptation and Natural Selection* helped dispel the once popular idea that evolution often works for "the good of the group," has even taken to calling natural selection "evil" and "the enemy." The moral life, in his view, consists largely of battling human nature.

Darwin himself believed the human species to be a moral one—in fact, the only moral animal species. "A moral being is one who is capable of comparing his past and future actions or motives, and of approving or disapproving of them," he wrote.

In this sense, yes, we are moral. We have at least the technical capacity to lead an examined life: self-awareness, memory, foresight and judgment. Still, chronically subjecting ourselves to moral scrutiny and adjusting our behavior accordingly is hardly a reflex. We are potentially moral animals—which is more than any other animal can say—but we are not naturally moral animals. The first step to being moral is to realize how thoroughly we aren't.

Science or Story Telling? Evolutionary Explanations of Human Sexuality

Richard N. Williams

Robert Wright's article, "Our Cheating Hearts," provides a good example of how genetic explanations of behavior (derived from evolutionary theory) have become popular in the social sciences, and thus, how they have found their way into the mainstream of our culture. Wright introduces his audience to the new field of environmental psychology, which attempts to explain some of our most important and meaningful human behaviors, like sexuality and marital fidelity, in terms of evolutionary and genetic processes. However, a careful analysis of Wright's article illuminates the problems and conceptual gaps found in attempts to explain human behavior as being caused by evolutionary forces or genes.

On the surface of his article, Wright seems to be simply reporting scientific facts that have been discovered about how and why animals engage in sexual behaviors, and how they have evolved in ways that facilitate such behaviors. Wright's article is similar to a great many other articles and books all trying to make the point that human behaviors are governed by genes, and by evolutionary processes, and, therefore, humans are essentially like animals in their sexual and other behaviors. However, the kind of data used to support this kind of explanation is not scientific in the usual sense. It is composed mostly of stories and analogies. On the surface, Wright seems to be merely pointing out the truths of the similarities of animal to human behavior, and then offering the obvious explanation for these similarities—that evolution, through the workings of our genes, has guided, and continues to control our behaviors. A closer look at the so-called evidence that evolutionary psychology uses to explain our sexual behaviors reveals that it is not at all convincing. It is more story telling than it is science.

Is There Compelling Evidence That Our Intimate or Sexual Behaviors Are Determined by Evolution or Genes?

The idea that human sexual behaviors and intimate relationships are governed by biological structures or evolutionary forces is not scientific in the sense in which we usually use that term. We usually consider scientific facts to be those that are discovered through careful experimentation giving rise to unambiguous results. Scientific work on which evolutionary psychology bases its explanations of human behavior is of quite a different sort. To make this point clear, it is important to distinguish between what we might call "evolutionary theory," and genetic biology.

Scientific studies in the field of genetic biology are very sophisticated and careful. They have provided us a convincing picture of what genes are and how they work. Studies in genetics have resulted in hybrid strains of plants and animals, and in new, and even patented, life forms. However, all this work demonstrates only that genetic material is responsible for a number of *physical* structures and attributes. There is little argument that our genetic material plays a major role in such things as eye color, physical stature, and certain diseases. These are physical characteristics and have a recognizably physical and/or chemical foundation. However, the claims of evolutionary psychology are quite different.

There are several important ideas that Wright and the evolutionary psychologists take for granted that are not established by hard scientific evidence. What is not established by careful scientific work is: (a) that psychological or mental events and behaviors (such as human intimacy and sexual attraction) can be produced by genetic material; and (b) that *evolution* controls these events and governs their development and their manifestation.[1] Wright, and the evolutionary psychologists, assume that these two points are true. However, before we are willing to accept them, and Wright's explanations for our sexual behavior, these two points need to be clarified and examined more carefully. Because Wright simply accepts these two claims as true, he is able to tell an evolutionary story about us and our sexual behavior. I argue that Wright's account is a creative story about human sexuality and not a report of scientific facts of human sexuality.

Evolution Explanation as Story

Evolutionary theory is convincing to many people chiefly because the living world we experience seems to be like evolutionary theory would predict it should be. In other words, evolutionary theory seems to be true because it fits the data. Evolutionary theorists have offered an account or story of the origin of life, how it developed, and how it regulates itself that makes sense. It seems reasonable, and we can think of very few examples of phenomena that evolutionary theory could not explain. However, it should be kept in mind that because a theory or story can be shown to fit the world and explain it reasonably well, it is not necessarily the case that the story is true. Certainly this is not enough to establish the story as scientific fact. To see why this is the case, we need only ask ourselves what people used to think about the world before evolutionary theories became popular. Did they live in a world they could not explain? Did the world not make sense to them? Certainly a study of history reveals that before evolutionary theories as we know them came into vogue as explanations, people had other stories that made sense of the living world, its origins, and its development. The truth or falsity of evolutionary explanations is not a scientific question because it would be impossible to formulate a properly scientific test of these explanations in contrast to other nonevolutionary explanations. Instead, evidence for evolutionary theory is philosophical and conceptual. Evolutionary theorists observe the world and the nature and behavior of various species and then offer a story of what might be the case. Wright's notion of evolutionary psychology thus rests on conceptual and philosophical rather than scientific grounds.

For example, evolutionary theory suggests that humans are motivated above all to insure the survival of their own genes in succeeding generations. This, in turn, suggests that the best way to do this would be to make sure our offspring survive. And this, in turn, suggests that humans will take better care of their own biological children than stepchildren who do not share their genes. Statistics are reported in Wright's article that show that children who live with one or more stepparents are much more likely to be abused than are children who live with both of their biological parents. Evolutionary theorists will claim that this statistic supports evolutionary theory because it is consistent with what an evolutionary story would predict. However, it seems clear that there are more obvious and immediate factors that might explain why children living with stepparents are more likely to be abused. It seems obvious that children living with stepparents are doing so because of some trouble in their birth family. The factors that contributed to the breakup of the birth family in the first place are likely to continue with both parents and children into subsequent family arrangements. These factors include unsatisfactory relationships between parents, stresses from the breakup of the original family, economic troubles, and any number of other social and cultural factors. It seems that the evolutionary account of the abuse of these children is quite far removed from the immediate and compelling circumstances of the case. Evolutionary forces do not seem—even by common sense—to be the most direct or obvious source of the problem of abused stepchildren. There does not seem to be anything obvious that would argue that the evolutionary explanation of the statistics of abuse is the best, or most sensible one. Rather, the evolutionary account of this tragedy seems rather contrived. It should also be noted that there is no scientific test that could possibly separate evolutionary causes from the host of social and personal causes of this sort of child abuse.

Wright's account of the evolutionary origins of human intimacy provides many good illustrations of this sort of story telling. For example, he points out that the size of the testicles (relative to body weight) in various primate species is correlated with the extent to which the species tend to be monogamous or polygynous. The story of evolutionary biology is consistent with this bit of data, however, there is nothing about these data that suggest in the least that some evolutionary process is the *cause* of the correlation. Similarly, Wright reports that nearly 1,000 of 1,154 past or present human societies have at one time or another permitted the practice or polygamy. This is also consistent with evolutionary theory—or, rather, evolutionary theory can fit this bit of information into its story. However, there are many other reasons for which cultures might practice polygamy besides evolutionary forces. Some societies practice it for religious reasons, some for seemingly pragmatic reasons, and some, perhaps, for purely social reasons. The point is that these alternative stories can also "make sense" of this bit of data. The datum itself (i.e., the practice of polygamy) does not demand an evolutionary explanation. Which story we prefer is not based on scientific evidence but on our historical prejudices, and current preferences for some kinds of explanations over others. Evolutionary explanations are currently very popular.

In summary then, evolutionary explanations of our behavior rest not on sound scientific demonstration but on our perceptions that evolutionary accounts, like the one Wright gives, makes sense, and fit the data. Support for the story of evolution is grounded in how well the story can be used to make sense of the data of the world.

The Logical Fallacy of Affirming the Consequent

We will leave the specifics of Wright's evolutionary analysis in order to make an important but more general point and then show how this general point applies to Wright's argument. From the analysis of evolutionary theories just given, it can be concluded that the truth or falsity of evolutionary theory as an explanation of human behavior is not a genuinely scientific question because it depends for support not on hard scientific data but on reason and argument and a certain degree of cleverness in making the story fit. Since evolutionary accounts of our behavior stand or fall on the basis of reason and argument, we should be very careful about the kind of reasoning and arguments that are used to support the evolutionary explanation of our actions. From the very beginnings of our Western intellectual tradition, scholars have spent much effort detailing what kinds of reasoning and arguments were valid and trustworthy and what kinds were not. Rules have been established for logical analysis so that we can be confident of the conclusions we reach from our arguments. Likewise, certain kinds of errors have been identified which make our arguments and conclusions invalid—or illogical. This is not the forum to fully discuss the nature of human reason itself, and the power of logic. We need only point out that by the rules scholars have traditionally accepted certain forms of argument are considered invalid, and do not bring us to valid necessary conclusions.[2]

One of the most common and well known logical fallacies is *affirming the consequent*. To see what this fallacy looks like, let us consider one common type of logical argument. It has the following form:

1. *If* Socrates is a man, *then* he is mortal.

2. Socrates is a man.

3. Therefore, he is mortal.

Note that this whole argument hangs on the validity of a very important assumption that is not even stated in the argument—that *all men really are mortal*. If this is not true, then the argument, while still valid according to the rules of logic, is not sensible. Many theoretical arguments, including many of those supporting evolutionary explanations of human behavior, have assumptions that are presumed to be true but are almost never stated, much less examined.

Whenever an argument is presented in the form just presented, it is considered, by the rules of logic, to be valid. That is, the conclusion is reasonable, and we should agree with it and comprehend that it is true. The part of the argument (in statement 1) that follows the word *if* is called the antecedent of the argument. The part following the word *then* is the consequent. In statement 2 the antecedent is restated. That is, it is shown to be true—Socrates really is a man. Whenever we can show that the antecedent is true, then, as we see in statement 3, the consequent follows—it is taken to be true. If he *is* a man—we can show or accept that he is—then he *is* mortal. This classical type of arguing is called affirming the antecedent.

What would have happened, however, if the argument had been made in the following form?

1. *If* Socrates is a man, *then* he is mortal.

2. Socrates *is* mortal.

3. Therefore, he is (must be) a man.

Notice that in this argument we have stated that the consequent is true in statement 2, rather than the antecedent. Then we try to conclude that the antecedent must also be true in statement 3. A moment's reflection is sufficient to show that our conclusion is not valid. Socrates could be a dog—since dogs are mortal. Just because he is mortal, we do not know that he is a man. The conclusion is not valid because the form of the argument is not valid. This is an illustration of a classical logical fallacy called affirming the consequent. Even though this is a commonly understood logical fallacy, it is a commonly employed strategy in arguing for the validity of theories.

In Wright's exposition of the evolutionary basis of human sexuality, there are numerous examples of this fallacy of affirming the consequent. For example, as I noted above, Wright uses evidence of sexual dimorphism—the difference in the average size of human males and females—to argue for the validity of his evolutionary account. The argument has the following form:

1. *If* evolution makes humans prone to polygyny, *then* we will find sexual dimorphism in humans (because there is dimorphism in polygynous animals).

2. We do find sexual dimorphism in humans. (The consequent is true.)

3. Therefore, evolution makes humans prone to polygyny. (The antecedent supposedly follows.)

This is, of course, a classic example of affirming the consequent.

Wright's article offers a long string of similar but unsound arguments. In its general form the foundational argument for evolutionary explanations of human behavior is:

1. *If* evolutionary theory is true, *then* we should observe that humans do X (some phenomenon).

2. We observe that humans do X (this phenomenon).

3. Therefore, evolutionary theory is true.

In summary, it should be noted that this style of reasoning by affirming the consequent is not sound scientific practice. Thus, the evidence generally marshalled in favor of evolutionary accounts of human behavior, such as evolutionary psychology, is not genuinely scientific. Rather, it is argument and deduction. And, as has been shown, most often it is not sound argument.

The Criterion of Falsifiability

At least since the publication of the influential work of Karl Popper (1959), a philosopher of science, it has been accepted in most scientific circles that a good theory—a genuinely scientific theory—must be of the type that can be proven false. That is, sound scientific practice demands that a theory must be capable of being tested in such a way that if the results don't turn out to be consistent with the predictions of the theory, then it can be concluded that the theory is false. Theories that cannot be shown to be false are not to be considered genuinely scientific theories. I have already argued in the previous sections of this essay that evolutionary explanations of human behavior are not falsifiable in this sense. There is no experimental test that can settle the question of the validity of these explanations.

However, most proponents of evolutionary theories of human behavior do not even attempt to formulate or explain their theories in a way that can be falsified.[3] While it should be acknowledged that Wright's article is written more for a popular audience than for a professional audience, it nonetheless is illustrative of the approach taken even in more technical and scientific presentations of evolutionary theory. Thus it provides a good example of how the theories are generally presented in unfalsifiable form.

In order to see how evolutionary theories are presented in unfalsifiable form let us pay attention to the way in which Wright reassures his readers that the new evolutionary psychology does not subscribe to the strict and fatalistic theories of previous evolutionary and genetic explanations. He points out that "what's 'natural' isn't necessarily unchangeable." This is because of the "tremendous flexibility of the human mind and the powerful role of the environment in shaping behavior." Two important points are illustrated in this quotation. The first is that most proponents of evolutionary or genetic explanations of human behavior allow for some determining influence from the environment. However, being caused to behave by our environment does not make for a much better image of our humanity than does being caused by our biology. Acknowledging the causal role of the environment is not much of a corrective to the strict fatalism of biological explanations of our behavior.

The other point, more relevant to the present discussion, is that Wright suggests that the flexibility of the human mind is a source of power to counteract some of the natural process-es that might otherwise control us. The problem, however, is that according to Wright's own account of the evolutionary perspective, the human mind is "built and maintained" by genes to serve their (reproductive) purposes. For example, evolutionary theory might predict that since our overriding concern is to get our genes into the next generation, we (especially males) would not care much for one another, especially, for reproductive rivals. We would expect males to be aggressive with all other males. However, as we study societies through-out history, we notice that humans, even males, have tended to be rather civilized and caring, even altruistic. On the surface, this seems to counter evolutionary explanations. However, many evolutionary accounts would claim that our minds (or brains) evolved the capacity to care for others and be kind because being kind and caring had survival value, and actually would help us make sure our genes survived into the next generation, because if we care for others, they are likely to care for us and our children. So, no matter what we observe about the behavior of human males—aggression or cooperation—evolutionary theory can claim the observation as evidence that it is true.

If we take this kind of argument seriously, then, when we see people behaving in accor-dance with the predictions of evolutionary theory, it is evidence that evolutionary theory is true. And when we see people behaving in a way that seems not to be consistent with evolu-tionary theory, it is because of the influence of a "tremendously flexible" mind—which, in turn, has evolved according to the dictates of evolutionary theory to serve the ends of evolu-tion itself. So when evolutionary theory seems to work as an explanation we can assume it is true. When it does not seem to work so well it is still true because it is merely *appearing* to work against itself via the evolved human mind. Evolutionary theory is thus unfalsifiable because both observations that confirm predictions, and observations that do not, are count-ed as evidence for the validity of evolution as an explanation.

Myths of Magic Genes

There is one aspect of evolutionary theory that has a firm foundation of scientific research. This is the structure and function of genes and their role in determining important characteristics of organisms. These are, for the most part, physical characteristics. Very sophisticated research assures us that many important characteristics of organisms have their origins in genetic codes contained in the chromosomes of the tissues of the organism. However, even though we know much about the structure and function of genes, the picture is not at all clear when we turn attention to the relationship between genes and psychologi-cal—rather than strictly physical—characteristics and behaviors of organisms, especially humans.[4]

We find in Wright's essay the following:

> Genes don't talk, of course. They affect behavior by creating feelings and thoughts—by building and maintaining...an underlying mental infrastructure.

The claim here is quite clear: genes create mental phenomena. Wright also speaks of "genes that inclined a man to love his offspring," and suggests that the purposes of the genes required "the invention of a compelling emotion: parental love." Not only are genes sophisticated enough to invent emotions, but, according to Wright, also to contradict them. "Evolution not only invented romantic love but from the beginning also corrupted it."

According to evolutionary theory, not only are genes capable of producing particular emotions, they are also capable of predicting and monitoring behavioral outcomes. This portrayal of genes and their activities is problematic for a number of reasons. The description of genes as intelligent and possessing "stratagems" is problematic in that it seems to overlook what genes really are. We need to remind ourselves as we read evolutionary and genetic accounts of our behavior that genes are simply molecules—chemicals—locked away in the nuclei of the cells of our bodies. How, we might ask, could genes as molecules of chemicals be aware of such things as "outside romantic opportunities" in order to motivate us to take advantage of them? The orthodox evolutionary answer, of course, is that the genes are not aware of such things (that would be silly). Rather, the genes give rise to minds, thoughts, feelings, and sophisticated mental capacities for monitoring all of these social factors and deciding what should be done. But here we run headlong into the fundamental and perpetually vexing question of evolutionary and genetic theories of our behavior. The response to this question determines the adequacy and believability of the accounts of our behavior these theories offer. The question is this: How do chemical compounds locked within the nuclei of the cells of the tissues of our bodies give rise to nonchemical and intelligent things like particular ideas, feelings, emotions, and stratagems? Ideas, feelings, emotions, and stratagems are not simply and strictly chemical or physical. "Stratagems," and "romantic opportunities" are not chemical substances, nor substances at all. It is not at all clear how they might arise from molecules of chemicals that compose our genes. There seems to be no answer to this essential question in all the literature on evolutionary and genetic accounts of human behavior. It is simply assumed that it can happen and does happen because then the theory "fits."

Conclusion

This response to "evolutionary psychology" and Wright's treatment of it has centered on the argument that evolutionary and genetic explanations of human behaviors are not based on hard scientific data and that they are really more like story telling than science. However, much more is at stake than a mere disagreement about how certain observations should be interpreted. Simply making the case that there are other and simpler explanations for our behaviors than the evolutionary explanation, or that such evolutionary explanations are not truly scientific, is not in itself a strong refutation and is hardly sufficient grounds for rejecting them. The larger issues need to be made clear.

Evolutionary and genetic explanations of human behavior are not just stories about us; they are stories that pretend not to be stories. Furthermore, they ask us to reduce our most human and most meaningful behaviors to the level of simple animal behaviors. They ask us to accept that the same fundamental processes are at work to determine our intimate relationships as determine "mating behaviors" in animal species. Evolutionary psychologists accomplish this reduction subtly by using the same terms to describe both animal and human behaviors. This reduction of the human to the animal and the application of a common vocabulary destroys the meaning of human behavior. If, as evolutionary psychology declares, human and animal sexuality have the same roots, then human intimacy is no more meaningful than the copulatory acts of common breeding stock. Proponents of evolution claim that we are recompensed for the loss of meaning in our lives by scientific credibility. But if, as I argue, there is no convincing scientific base for the evolutionary account of our behaviors, then we are being asked to sacrifice the meaning of human intimacy for nothing.

The end result of evolutionary and genetic accounts of human behavior is a moral vacuum in which we do not engage one another as moral agents at all but as organisms controlled by biological forces beyond our control. Until such time as there is overwhelming scientific evidence that chemicals in our cells can produce morality and human affections, we are morally obligated to resist explanations that destroy the meaning and morality of our lives. The evolutionary story exacts too great a price both in credulity and in humanity.

Notes

1.   Some evolutionary theorists might argue that at some future date when technology has advanced and when they are given permission to manipulate human genes, genuine scientific validation will be available. It is axiomatic in science, however, that one does not rely on nor claim credibility from what might someday be done. To argue in this way moves one from science to science fiction.

2.   The interested reader is referred to Slife & Williams (1995) for a fuller account of how logic plays a role in scientific and theoretical work, and how both scientists and theorists too easily fall into the practice of affirming the consequent.

3.   The work of most experimental geneticists is sophisticated and scientifically sound. Their experiments are routinely set up so that their *predictions can* be falsified. However, to falsify a prediction derived from a theory such as evolution is not at all the same thing as to falsify the theory itself. Even though it has generated much credible scientific work, evolutionary theory as a world view has never been at risk. Because of the way it is formulated and promulgated it is unfalsifiable.

4.   Some would argue that some behavioral characteristics can also be shown to be genetically determined. Whether this is the case depends in large part on how the term "behavior" is defined. For example, is a plant's "growing" a behavior?

References

James, W. (1897/1956). The dilemma of determinism. In W. James, *The will to believe and other essays in popular philosophy* (pp. 145–184). New York: Dover.

Popper, K. (1959). *The logic of scientific discovery*. New York: Basic Books.

Slife, B. D., & Williams, R.N. (1995). *What's behind the research? Discovering hidden assumptions in the behavioral sciences*. Newbury Park, CA: Sage Publications.

Debate Presenter Form

Follow the guidelines for debate presenters contained in the introduction of this text and those given to you by your instructor. Use the format below to organize the material for your debate. Remember to include all relevant citation information and to present the related information in your own words. Give credit to authors when you cite a quote and be as thorough as possible when writing about your points so you will be prepared for your debate.

Reference citation #1:

Author: _____

Title: _____

Date: _____

Source: _____

_____

Content from reference citation #1: _____

_____

_____

_____

_____

_____

_____

_____

_____

_____

_____

_____

_____

_____

Reference citation #2:

Author: _____

Title: _____

Date: _____

Source: _____

_____

Content from reference citation #2: _____

_____

_____

_____

_____

_____

Reference citation #3:

Author: _____

Title: _____

Date: _____

Source: _____

_____

Content from reference citation #3: _____

_____

_____

_____

_____

Audience Preparation Form

Follow the guidelines for preparing to be an informed audience member on the day of the debate included in the introduction to this text. After reading both sides of the debate from this chapter, answer the following questions. Be as thorough as possible so that you will be able to make a contribution to the debate by asking informed questions or making provocative comments. This form is usually due on the day of the debate.

State the issue in your own words. Do not plagiarize the text. Demonstrate that you understand the topic and it's relevant arguments.

_____

_____

_____

_____

_____

Discuss two points on the "yes" side of the debate.

Point #1: _____

_____

Point #2: _____

_____

Discuss two points on the "no" side of the debate.

Point #1: _____

_____

Point #2: _____

_____

What is your opinion on this topic?

_____
_____
_____
_____
_____
_____
_____
_____

What has contributed to the development of your views about this topic?

_____
_____
_____
_____
_____
_____
_____
_____

What information would be necessary to cause you to change your thinking about this topic?

_____
_____
_____
_____
_____
_____

Debate Response Form

Follow the guidelines for responding to the debates in the introductory chapter of this text. Complete this form and submit your answers at the class following the debate. Try to be thorough and convince your instructor that you were an active listener during the debate.

List a quote from a debate presenter that you think was important and explain why you think this comment was significant.

_____

_____

_____

_____

Which side of the debate do you think made the most convincing arguments, why?

_____

_____

_____

_____

_____

After hearing the debate, in what way has your thinking been affected?

_____

_____

_____

_____

_____

_____

ISSUE 8

Is the Use of Pornography between Consenting Adults Harmful?

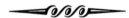

YES Victor Cline, *A Psychologist's View of Pornography*

NO F. M. Christensen, *Pornography: The Other Side*

Victor Cline begins his argument against pornography by laying a foundation for the general impact of cinematic violence on criminal violence. Within this media context, Cline asserts that sexual aggression too is the result of viewing television and movie pictorials of sexual contact that is predominantly illicit.

Cline holds pornography in the United States accountable for increases in rate of rape, degradation of women, male conditioning toward sexual deviation and violence. He goes as far as suggesting that we have made a spectator sport of man's inhumanity to women and men. He describes a sizable body of research demonstrating that this sanctioned voyeurism results in disastrous criminal consequences.

F. M. Christensen proclaims that there is nothing inherently evil about pornography. He rejects the notion that one is a victim of pornography and reminds readers of the concept of free will. Rather than identifying pornography as the culprit, Christensen suggests that members of our society who have rebelled against the sanctions set forth in other arenas are likely to also have less constraint on their sexual behavior. He describes the idea that gratification of sexual feelings leads to moral corruption and lack of self-discipline as "superstitious".

Christensen concludes his argument with the suggestion that pornography can be a benefit to couples seeking to enhance their sex lives. This improvement in sexual satisfaction can be an asset to the longevity of a marriage. In this sense, pornography can be a benefit to prevention of divorce, the stability of the family structure and ultimately to the children who are parented in intact families.

Applications

1. Examine your history and discuss the various influences you have experienced regarding the formation of your own opinion on pornography.

2. Do you think there should be some controls in place regarding pornography and if so, what would these be?

3. Do you believe criminals when they blame pornography for their crimes? Explain.

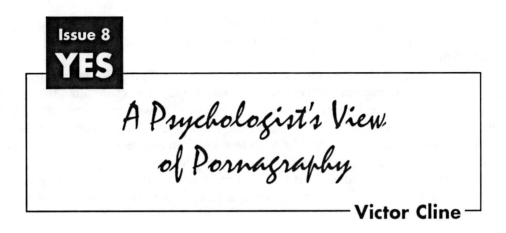

Issue 8
YES

A Psychologist's View of Pornography

Victor Cline

Violent Crime on Increase

The United States is by far the most violent country in the world compared with all of the other advanced societies. For example, the U.S. rape rate is many times higher than that of the United Kingdom. We have more homicides annually on just the island of Manhattan than those reported in all of England, Scotland, and troubled Ireland combined. Our homicide rate is ten times that of the Scandinavian countries. At the present time crimes of violence in the U.S. are increasing at four to five times the rate of population growth.

Behavioral scientists recognize that there are many causes for any violent act, and it behooves us to investigate and understand those key triggers or contributors—if we care at all about the kind of society we want for ourselves and our children. Many lines of evidence have pointed to media influences such as commercial cinema and television as being especially suspect; as presenting inappropriate models and instigations of violent and antisocial behavior, especially for our young.

Mental Health Study Blames TV Violence

In reviewing all of the scientific evidence relating to the effect TV violence has on our behavior, the National Institute of Mental Health in 1984 issued a ten-year-report that concluded that there is indeed "overwhelming evidence of a casual relationship between violence on television and later aggressive behavior."

Some long-term studies and cross national studies also indicate that this learned aggressive behavior is stable over time—the victims stay aggressive. It is by no means just a transient kind of effect.

The reviewers of the research at the National Institute of Mental Health also note the role that TV (and by implication, commercial cinema) play as sex educators for our children. TV contributes significantly to sex role socialization as well as shaping attitudes and values about human sexuality. Various studies suggest that in TV presentations sex is commonly linked with violence. Erotic relationships are seldom seen as warm, loving, or stable. When sex is depicted it is almost always illicit. It is rather rare to suggest or depict sexual relations between a man and a woman married and who love each other. This agrees with similar results from my own research on the content of commercial cinema conducted several years ago.

Rape Rate Grows 700 Percent

Aggression against women is increasingly becoming a serious social problem. This can be seen in the escalation of wife battering, sexual molestation of female children, and sexual assaults on adult females.

Examining empirical data on the incidence of this type of thing is risky. This is because nearly all statistics on rape, for example, tend to underreport its actual occurrence. Many women for reasons of shame, humiliation, embarrassment, or seeking to avoid further trauma do not report these experiences. Data from many sources indicates that police get reports on one in four attempted or actual rapes. And of those reported less than 5 percent result in prosecution and conviction. Since 1933 the increase in the rape rate in the U.S. is in excess of 700 percent (this is in relation to population growth—in actual numbers the increase is much greater).

This means that the chances of a woman being sexually attacked are seven times greater now than in 1933. This clearly indicates major changes in male attitudes about sexual aggressiveness toward women. Obviously, more men today have a lower esteem of women. Why should this be in an age such as ours when women are being heard and winning rights?

Pornography Degrades Women

Feminists such as Susan Brownmiller, Diana Russell, Laura Lederer, and Kathleen Barry point to the fact that our culture influences men to regard women as things—to be used. They note, for example, that nearly all pornography is created by males for a primarily male audience. Most of it is hostile to women. There is much woman hatred in it. It is devoid of foreplay, tenderness, caring, to say nothing of love and romance. They see its main purpose to humiliate and degrade the female body for the purpose of commercial entertainment, erotic stimulation, and pleasure for the male viewer. This is perceived as creating a cultural climate in which a rapist feels he is merely giving in to a normal urge and a woman is encouraged to believe that sexual masochism is healthy liberated fun.

Susan Brownmiller states, "Pornography, like rape, is a male invention designed to dehumanize women."

Many of the men's magazines such as *Hustler* are filled with antifemale messages both overt and covert. The victims in most "hard R" slasher movies are women—it is they who are most often sexually assaulted, tortured, and degraded. The feminist's concern is that these films sexually stimulate men while at the same time pairing this erotic arousal with images of violent assaults on women. The possibility of conditioning a potential male viewer into deviancy certainly has to be considered here.

Men Conditioned to Sexual Deviation

In a laboratory experiment using classical conditioning procedures at the Naudsley Hospital in London, England, Dr. Stanley Rachman conditioned a number of young males into being fetishists—a mild form of sexual deviation. A number of studies by such investigators as Davison, Bandura, Evans, Hackson, and McGuire suggest that deviant sexual fantasies through a process of masturbatory conditioning are related in many instances to later acted-out deviant sexual behavior. What happens here is that deviant sexual fantasies in the man's mind are paired with direct sexual stimulation and orgasm via masturbation. In this way the deviant fantasies acquire strong sexually arousing properties—which help sustain the sexual interest in the deviant behavior. Thus reinforced sexual imagery and thoughts (accompanied via masturbation) are a link in the acquisition and maintenance of new deviant sexual arousal and behavior. In the light of this, media portrayals of sex modeling male aggression against women logically can have a harmful effect on certain viewers. These portrayals, it would be concluded, facilitate deviant conditioning by providing new malignant fantasy material as well as increased motivation for masturbatory experiences—leading to changes in the man's sexual attitudes, appetites, and behavior.

For example: A Los Angeles firm is currently marketing an 8mm motion picture film, available through the mails to anybody wishing it, which depicts two girl scouts in their uniforms selling cookies from door to door. At one residence they are invited in by a mature, sexually aggressive male who proceeds to subject them to a variety of unusual and extremely explicit sexual acts—all shown in great detail. This film is what is usually referred to as "hard-core" pornography. If the research of Rachman, McGuire, and others has any meaning at all, it suggests that such a film could potentially condition some male viewers, via masturbatory conditioning, into fantasies and later behavior involving aggressive sex with female minors.

Also, we might mention, that sex therapists have for years used carefully selected erotic material to recondition men with sexual deviations and help them out of their problems. In other words, the conditioning can go both ways using erotic materials. If all sexual deviations are learned, as psychologist Albert Bandura suggests, then one would assume that most deviations occur through "accidental conditioning"—which is exactly what many feminists have concerns about—especially as they see how they are treated in male-oriented media presentations.

At the present time in most urban areas of the U.S., there have arisen groups of women with concerns about what the media are doing to them—and especially about the social/sexual enculturation of males. Women Against Violence in Pornography and Media, based in San Francisco, is one example of this kind of group. Initially, their concerns were intuitive, moralistic, and emotional. They picketed various establishments—movie houses, adult bookstores, etc., selling or marketing highly sexist and antifemale materials—material that might tend to engender hate toward women. This includes the so-called "snuff films" in which women were supposedly murdered on-camera for the voyeuristic entertainment of male viewers.

However, in the last five years there has been a flood of well-done behavioral studies by researchers that appear to scientifically legitimize the concerns of these groups. These studies have repeatedly given documentation of potential harms to viewers of aggressive erotic materials, especially males.

These findings have been given very little attention by the popular press and are known only to a few scientists who are privy to the journals that these articles are showing up in. Thus, most ordinary citizens, journalists, as well as professionals in other disciplines, are not aware of these studies. For example, one of the editors of the *Utah Daily Chronicle* on March 1, 1985, in an editorial column discussing the cable TV bills before our state legislature, wrote, "Research has shown there is no demonstrable relationship between watching TV and increased aggressiveness...[and] regardless of what Utah legislators may believe, there is no scientific correlation between obscenity and antisocial conduct."

Both of these statements are totally incorrect. I am sure they were written as a result of ignorance, not as a conscious attempt at deception. In fact, quite ironically, on the day this editorial appeared, the Department of Psychology was sponsoring a widely publicized seminar featuring one of the nation's leading authorities on television effects, Dr. Raoul Huesmann, who discussed a pioneering 22-year study on the long-term negative effects of TV violence viewing.

World's Most Violent Advanced Society

I will not further belabor the issue of media violence and its potential negative effects on viewers. The evidence is really quite overwhelming on this issue. But let me briefly summarize what the literature suggests:

1. We are the most violent advanced society in the world.

2. We have the highest rates of media violence (in our entertainments) of any nation.

3. There are something like 20 years of behavioral studies linking exposure to media vio-

lence with violent behavior. These include both laboratory and field studies. And while there are many contributions to any particular violent act, I do not think that any fair reviewer of the literature can deny that the media are one important contributor to the violence problems in our society.

In my judgment repeated violence viewing also desensitizes the observer to the pathology in the film or material witnessed. It becomes with repeated viewing more acceptable and tolerable. We lose the capacity to empathize with the victim. Man's inhumanity to man (or woman) becomes a spectator sport. We develop and cultivate an appetite for it, no different than in early Rome, where people watched gladiatorial contests in which men fought to their deaths, dismembering their opponents' bodies. In other contests, others fought wild animals barehanded, eventually to be eaten alive. Again, a spectator sport. We become to some extent debased, even dehumanized, if you wish, by participating in these kinds of experiences. And, of course, approximations of what happened in the Roman arena nightly occur in some movie houses and on some TV screens—especially the cable variety where explicit violence is broadcast unedited. And usually—women are the victims.

Increasing Assaults in Marriage

Let us now move to the issue of linking aggressive pornography to increased aggressive behavior in marriage. It can be physical abuse, psychological abuse, or both. I see many couples in marital counseling. Violence between spouses is a common problem. Of course many women have learned to fight back. And this leads to an ever-escalating exchange of anger and hostility. Divorce usually doesn't solve the problem. If you don't know how to handle anger and aggressive feelings in one relationship, switching partners doesn't necessarily solve the problem for you in the next relationship.

There have been many experiments on aggressive pornography and its effects on consumers conducted by such capable investigators as Edward Donnerstein and Leonard Berkowitz at the University of Wisconsin; Nell Malamuth and James Check at the University of Manitoba; Dolf Zillman and Jennings Bryant at Indiana University; and Seymour Feshbach and his associates at UCLA.

Sexual Arousal, Aggression Linked

There has been a convergence of evidence from many sources suggesting that sexual arousal and aggression are linked or are mutually enhancing. Thus materials that are sexually exciting can stimulate aggressive behavior and, contrariwise, portrayals of aggression in books, magazines, and films can raise some people's levels of sexual arousal.

Thus it is not by accident that some four-letter words are frequently used in the context of an epithet or as part of a verbal attack on another.

Many theorists have noted the intimate relationship between sex and aggression—including Sigmund Freud, or more recently, Robert Stoler at UCLA who suggest that frequently it is hostility that generates and enhances sexual excitement.

A large number of research studies consistently and repetitiously keep coming to one conclusion—those subjects who are sexually aroused by strong erotic stimuli show significantly greater aggression than nonaroused controls.

The typical experiment will sexually arouse with pornographic stimuli a group of experimental subjects who will then be given an opportunity to punish a confederate with electric shock. Their aggressiveness will be compared to a neutral group who will have seen only a bland nonsexual film or reading material.

If the film combines both erotic *and* aggressive elements, this usually produces even higher levels of aggressiveness (as measured by the subjects' willingness to shock their partners at even higher and apparently more painful levels of shock intensity). If the erotic material is very mild—like pin-ups and cheesecake type photos—then it appears to have reverse effect on aggression—tending to dampen it.

In the situation of reading about or witnessing a filmed presentation of rape, if the female victim is seen as in great pain this can also have a dampening effect on aggressive arousal. It serves as an inhibitor. But if the portrayal showing the woman as finally succumbing to and enjoying the act (as is typical of most pornography), then the situation is reversed for males (but not females). It becomes very arousing. For men, the fantasy of a woman becoming sexually excited as a result of a sexual assault reverses any inhibitions that might have been initially mobilized by the coercive nature of the act and seeing the woman initially in pain.

This message—that pain and humiliation can be "fun"—encourages in men the relaxation of inhibitions against rape.

Doctors Gager and Schurr in their studies on the causes of rape note that a common theme in pornography is that women enjoy being raped and sexually violated. Sexual sadism is presented as a source of sexual pleasure for women. The Gager and Schurr studies note: "The pattern rarely changes in the porno culture....After a few preliminary skirmishes, women invite or demand further violation, begging male masters to rape them into submission, torture, and violence. In this fantasy land, females wallow in physical abuse and degradation. It is a pattern of horror which we have seen in our examination of sex cases translated again and again into actual assaults."

University Study Shows Effects of Movies

Going outside the laboratory, Neal Malamuth at the University of Manitoba sent hundreds of students to movies playing in the community. He wanted to see what the effects would be of their being exposed to films portraying sexual violence as having positive consequences. The movies they went to see were not pornography, but everyday "sex and violence" of the R-rated variety. The films includes *Swept Away* (about a violent male aggressor and a woman who learns to crave sexual sadism; they find love on a deserted island). A second film, *The Getaway*, tells about a woman who falls in love with the man who raped her in front of her husband, then both taunt the husband until he commits suicide.

A second group of students was assigned to see two control films, *A Man and a Woman*, and *Hooper*, both showing tender romance and nonexplicit sex. Within a week of seeing the films, Malamuth administered an attitude survey to all students who had participated in the experiment. The students did not know that the survey had anything to do with the films which they seen. Embedded within the survey were questions relating to acceptance of interpersonal violence and acceptance of such rape myths as "women enjoy being raped." Examples of questions asked also included: "Many women have an unconscious wish to be raped and may unconsciously set up a situation in which they are likely to be attacked."

The results of the survey indicated that exposure to the films portraying sexual violence significantly increased male subjects' acceptance of interpersonal violence against women. For females, the trend was in the opposite direction.

Dr. Malamuth concluded: "The present findings constitute the first demonstration in a nonlaboratory setting... of relatively long-term effects of movies that fuse sexuality and violence." And, of course, these were not hard-core pornography but rather R-rated type, edited films that have appeared on national commercial TV and unedited films shown on cable TV.

As I review the literature on media effects, it appears that in the areas of both sex and violence materials depicting these kinds of behaviors do several things: (1) they stimulate and arouse aggressive and sexual feeling—especially in males; (2) they show or instruct in detail *how* to do the acts—much of it antisocial; (3) when seen frequently enough have a desensitization effect which reduces feelings of conscience, guilt, inhibitions, or inner controls, the act is in a sense legitimized by its repetitious exposure; and finally, (4) there is increased likelihood that the individual will act out what he has witnessed.

Seymour Feshbach's research at UCLA has a direct bearing on this issue. After exposing a group of male college students to a sadomasochistic rape story taken from *Penthouse* magazine—telling of a woman's pleasure at being sexually mistreated—he asked these men if they would like to emulate what the rapist did to the woman. Seventeen percent said they would. When asked the same question but with the added assurance they would not get caught—51 percent indicated a likelihood of raping. This finding has been replicated in a number of other studies—though the percentages vary somewhat from research to research.

Doctors Edward Donnerstein and Neil Malamuth, in reviewing a large number of both field and laboratory experiments, found that exposure to media materials that mix both sex and violence causes six things to happen: (1) it sexually excites and arouses (especially) the male viewer; (2) it increases both his aggressive *attitudes* and *behavior*; (3) it stimulates the production of aggressive rape fantasies; (4) it increases men's acceptance of so-called rape myths (such as: "women ask for it"); (5) it produces a lessened sensitivity about rape (and increased callousness); and (6) it leads to men admitting an increased possibility of themselves raping someone—especially if they think they can get away with it.

Pornography Reduces Compassion

What about exposure to nonaggressive erotic materials? Do these have any kind of effects on the consumer? Doctors Dolf Zillman and Jennings Bryant at Indiana University studied 160 male and female undergraduates who were divided into groups where they were exposed to : (1) massive amounts of pornography over a period of six weeks; (2) a moderate amount of pornography over that time period; and (3) no exposure over the same time period. Among their many findings were that being exposed to a lot of pornography led to a desensitization effect. The more they saw, the less offensive and objectionable it became to them. They also tended to see rape as a more trivial offense. They had an increasing loss of compassion for women as rape victims (even though no aggressive pornography was shown them).

Massive exposure to nonaggressive pornography clearly promoted sexual callousness in males toward women generally. This was measured by a scale where men agreed with such items as: "Pickups should expect to put out." Or, "If they are old enough to bleed, they are old enough to butcher" (referring to women).

The thrust of this presentation is to suggest that there is an abundance of scientific evidence suggesting social harms from some types of media exposure as has been previously discussed. The studies we have discussed are only illustrative. Many others have not been mentioned due to time limitations. Extensive documentation and lengthy bibliographies on this subject matter are available from the speaker on request.

Can We Control Pornography?

We now come to the really hot issue—the bottom line. Does a community have a constitutional right through democratically enacted laws to censor or limit the public broadcast of these kinds of materials—because of their malignant nature? The recent controversy about the First Amendment of the Constitution? Where does or where can one draw the line? How bad or pathological does material have to be before it can be limited? Or should our position be: anything goes regardless of the consequences? Free speech is free speech.

Seymour Feshbach, the UCLA psychologist, states: "As psychologists, we would support community efforts to restrict violence in erotica to adults who are fully cognizant of the nature of the material and who choose knowingly to buy it. We are opposed to advertisements that have appeared in some popular magazines depicting sadomasochism; a recent fashion layout in *Vogue*, for instance, featured a man brutally slapping an attractive woman. We also oppose the practice of some therapists who try to help their patients overcome sexual inhibitions by showing them films of rape or by encouraging them to indulge in rape fantasies. Psychologists, in our judgment, ought not to support, implicitly or explicitly, the use and dissemination of violent erotic materials."

In reference to the First Amendment to our Constitution, we must recognize that today there are many kinds of democratically enacted prohibitions of speech and expression. These, of course, can be amended or repealed anytime we wish. Examples include libel, slander, perjury, conspiracy, false advertising, excitement to violence or speech that might create a "clear and present danger" such as yelling "Fire" in a crowded theater. Still other examples include TV cigarette advertisements and also obscenity. In fact most of the people who went to jail in the Watergate scandal did so because of what they said—or for words they spoke (e.g., perjury and conspiracy).

In certain public broadcast mediums such as TV and radio, even obscene language can be proscribed without running afoul of the First Amendment.

At present, cable TV is the most controversial area about what is appropriate or inappropriate for broadcast. Currently there are virtually no restrictions on what can be aired. There are some channels in the U.S. broadcasting the roughest kind of hard-core pornography. There are others, including some in Utah, that are regularly broadcasting soft-core pornography mixed with violence. Last spring one of the local cable networks broadcast some 15 times *Eyes of a Stranger*. This film shows in explicit detail a young woman and her boyfriend being attacked by a sadist. He chops the boyfriend's head off, then proceeds to tear the girl's clothes off, strangles her, then rapes the dead body. The film continues with a series of attacks, rapes, and killings of other females. In my judgment this kind of programming, some of it in primetime, represents antisocial and irresponsible behavior on the part of the cable station owners.

Of course, there are many other similar type films which are being regularly broadcast. This is not an isolated incident. But along with this are films of great merit and quality which represent a major contribution to our cultural life as well as entertainment.

At present close to 30 percent of homes in the U.S. have cable. Industry analysts project that by 1985 this will be up to 50 percent and by the end of the decade 80-90 percent. This means that within a few years most of all of us will have cable. This is not hard to understand when you consider that very shortly the cable networks will be able to outbid the regular networks for choice sporting events, fights, new Broadway musicals, etc. Even now all the latest movies come to cable before they reach regular commercial TV.

At present there is a double standard in television. The FCC (Federal Communications Commission) has control over the broadcast of appropriate materials by the regular commercial TV channels. They cannot air obscene or other objectionable material without threat of losing their licenses. Cable TV has no restrictions whatever. And, of course, cable firms are taking advantage of this. And there are some adults in our community who are delighted. Others are appalled and have concerns, especially about exposing their children to this kind of programming.

As with most controversial issues, there are no simple solutions which will please everybody. But somewhere a line must be drawn—if we care about the quality of life in our community. We have a right to protect ourselves in our own self-interest.

Media Savagery Grows

George Elliot has commented: "If one is for civilization, for being civilized..., then one must be willing to take a middle way and pay the price for responsibility. To be civilized, to accept authority, to rule with order, costs deep in the soul, and not the least of what it costs is likely to be some of the sensuality of the irresponsible." Some have argued, as Elliott notes, that since guilt reduces pleasure in sex, the obvious solution is to abolish all sexual taboos and liberate pornography, which in turn would supposedly free the human spirit—and the body.

This is a cheery optimistic view, not unlike the sweet hopefulness of the old-fashioned anarchist who thought that all we had to do in order to attain happiness was to get rid of governments so that we might all express our essentially good nature unrestrained. But sexual anarchism, or the aggressive impulse turned loose, like political anarchism before it, is a "lovely" but fraudulent daydream. Perhaps, before civilization, savages were noble, but if there is anything we have learned in this century, it is that those who regress from civilization become ignoble beyond all toleration. They may aspire to innocent savagery, but what they achieve too often is brutality and loss of their essential humanity.

The issue of how we should deal with the savagery which continues to escalate in our media presentations is just as much your problem as mine. I have shared with you some of the consequences of its presence on our culture. But the solution has to be a shared one—if we really believe in democracy.

Alleged Ill Effects from Use

F.M. Christensen

[T]he belief that pornography is evil in itself is simply wrong. This leaves open the important question of whether it has effects on the user's attitudes or behavior that are harmful to anyone. Charges that this is so are continually being made, so...we will explore [a few aspects of] that issue [here]...

One particularly profound problem involves the issue of human agency. Now, some people are logically inconsistent in regard to this issue. In response to the suggestion that a violent criminal was made that way by a traumatic childhood, they invoke a notion of absolute free will: "His circumstances are not to blame; he *chose* to let them affect him!" But let the subject be something as comparatively minor as exposure to words and pictures, and suddenly the same people insist on a causal influence. The perennial debate over freedom of the will can hardly be discussed here. But one thing is perfectly clear from all the evidence: heredity and environment have a powerful influence on human behavior. The only room for rational debate is over whether that influence is total (deterministic) or not—and, once more, over just how much effect different types of causal factor exert...

The Domino Theory of Character

The first of the claims we will discuss is usually expressed in vague generalities; it is basically the charge that use of pornography tends to produce all sorts of wrongful behavior. From the rhetoric some of its proponents employ, one would swear they believe sexual thoughts that are not strictly confined will create a desire to rush out and break windows and steal cars. It is as if they retained the primitive belief that individuals are motivated by only two basic desires—to do good or to do evil—rather than by a complex panoply of needs and emotions. In the minds of some, this idea seems to rest on the conviction that one sort of corruption just naturally leads to others. Few, if any, scientists take such ideas seriously today; "degeneracy theory," with its concept that physical, psychological, and moral defects are all bound together, was popular in the last century but died with the rise of psychology and scientific medicine. In the rest of the population, unfortunately, notions like this one linger on.

The more specific suggestion is sometimes made that "losing self-control" in regard to sex—as allegedly might be precipitated by the use of pornography—produces a general lack of self-discipline, hence a tendency toward selfish libertinism or worse. This sort of thinking has a long history. In Victorian times, married couples were advised to limit the frequency of their sexual activities strictly lest they lead to a weakening of the will and of general character. And the myth that sexual excess brought about the decline and fall of Rome has been around for centuries, having come down to us with those old suspicions about bodily pleasure. (Never mind the gladiators and slavery and brutal imperialism; sexual pleasure was Rome's real failing.) Part of what is involved in the thinking, evidently, is an inability to distinguish between the very specific matter of sexual "permissiveness" and the rejection of *all* restraints on behavior. Alternatively, it is a confusion between a strong interest in sex and a failure to care about any other sources of happiness, or else a tendency to be concerned only with one's own happiness or with the pleasures of the moment. Such tendencies are certainly bad; for example, a person or nation fixated on momentary satisfactions will lack the discipline to plan for and protect future happiness. But there is no reason to suppose that sexual desires are any more apt to have such consequences than are other strong desires.

...[I]t is revealing to point out the inconsistency between these concerns and the lack of fears associated with other needs and pleasures, say, those involving food, love, religious devotion, or the arts. How many are alarmed that our lack of eating taboos—so common in other cultures—will lead to a general obsession with the happiness of the moment? Perhaps we should ban the Wednesday food section in the newspaper, with its seductive pictures and emphasis on the pleasure of eating over its utilitarian function. How many suppose that getting great enjoyment from music or dance will lead to a general lack of self-discipline, or to a disregard for the welfare of others (say, of those who perform them)? The rhetoric about the perils of "pleasure-seeking" is remarkably selective in regard to which pleasures it notices. The real source of this belief, it seems clear, is the sexual anxiety with which so many are raised; it produces the fear that something terrible will happen if one should ever "let go."

The most important response to such charges, however, is that those who make them do not have a shred of genuine evidence. They have been accepted and repeated endlessly, like so many other cultural beliefs, without critical examination. In earlier times, when racism was more socially acceptable than it is now, mixing of the races was often alleged to have brought about the decline of Rome and other civilizations—on the basis of the same worthless *post hoc* reasoning....Certain commentators have claimed to have evidence from one or two studies that reported finding a statistical association between exposure to sexual materials and juvenile delinquency in the United States. It could well be true that in this society, there has been a tendency for those who lack the traditional sexual attitudes to reject other social standards as well. The former is easily explained as a result of the latter, however: those who have been less well socialized into or have rebelled against the system as a whole will naturally be among the ones whose sexual behavior is less constrained. Alternatively, those whose needs have led them to break one social taboo will feel less threatened by other societal rules....

Of course, that a belief is held for bad reasons does not mean there are no good reasons for it. Nonetheless, it can be said without hesitation that the evidence available is strongly against the "domino theory" of character. One has only to consider the cross-cultural picture to begin to realize this, say, the promiscuous children and youth of Mangaia or the Trobriand Islands or the Muria villages, who grow up into hard-working adults who have internalized all of their society's moral standards. More generally, there is no indication that sexually positive cultures have greater amounts of antisocial behavior. In fact, one cross-cultural survey found significantly more personal crime in groups where premarital sex is strongly punished than in others. (The fact that the crime rate in permissive northern Europe is much lower than that in the United States may already be known to the reader—but beware of *post hoc* thinking.) The belief that gratifying sexual feelings tends somehow to turn into a general state of moral corruption, or even to damage one's capacity for self-discipline, is sheer superstition....

Personal Relationships

A second variety of claim that pornography has ill effects is that its use tends to damage personal relationships between men and women. This charge takes several different forms, including some that are bizarre (e.g., the idea that many men prefer it to real women and hence will avoid relationships with them if given that option). The simplest of these allegations, however, just points out that numerous women are upset by their partners' interest in pornography, so that it becomes a source of conflict. Part of the problem here is jealousy: the mere biologically normal fact that the partner is attracted to other persons is threatening to some, even when it is all fantasy. But that is evidently not the main difficulty. Few men feel upset over their partners' interest in love stories, say, in soap operas, with their romantic hunks and adulterous love affairs. The real problem seems to be the woman's aversion to nudity and sexual openness.

That being so, this argument presupposes that pornography is hurtful rather than proving it. For it could equally well be said that it is the woman's prudishness, rather than the man's interest in pornography, that is "the real" source of the trouble; which it is would have to be argued for rather than just assumed. Mention to the feminists and religionists who employ this objection that women's liberation or religious devotion has broken up many relationships, and they will make the same basic point....[M]oreover, it seems clear which one is the real culprit. In earlier years, the attitude that explicit sex is offensive to women led men to go off by themselves to watch "stag films"; what could have been an enjoyable shared experience became a source of alienation. Although female interest in such things might never approach that of males, the ones who divide the sexes are those who say, "My desires are noble and yours are nasty," not those who believe in the equal worth and dignity of the needs of both.

One special argument of this kind alleges that pornography harms relationships by its overemphasis on sex, and also by its underemphasis on companionship or romantic love. It is said to "teach men" to value the former too much and the latter too little. With its culture-bound and egocentric notions of how much emphasis is too much or too little, this claim ignores the possibility of keeping the sexes in harmony by teaching women to want sex in the same way. Its biggest error, however, lies in assigning to media depictions far more power to influence basic desires that is at all justified. As usual, those who make this claim express no similar beliefs about the persuasive power of the constant barrage of love songs and love stories in all the entertainment media. If such exposure were really so effective, one would think, we would all be incurable love-junkies by now. In any case, there is certainly no lack of publicity promoting love and companionship in our society. Moreover, male sexuality is not detectably different in cultures without appreciable amounts of pornography; indeed, it is evidently very much the same the world over.

What really underlies this claim is an old problem: the unfortunate fact that, on average, men's and women's needs in regard to love/commitment and sex are not well matched. Unable—or perhaps just unwilling—to believe men could ultimately have such different needs than they themselves do, some women suppose it must be in the different amount of stress on sex or love among men that does it. One common response is simply to deny that men are really different. For example, these women say men just *think* they have a strong need for sex because advertisers keep telling them they do. Others grant the reality of male sexual responses but do not want to believe they are natural. (Among feminists, this is just part of the wider conviction that there are *no* innate differences between the sexes except anatomical ones.) Yet those who make both claims insist it is men who have been most affected by culture in this regard. Over and again, without offering any argument as to which is cause and which effect, they assert that men would not be so interested in sex, or so attracted to female bodies, if only there were not so much emphasis on those things in this society. Besides projecting their own responses onto male nature—responses that are themselves largely culture-conditioned—the women (and sometimes men) who make such claims are somehow blind to all the societal efforts to suppress male sexuality and promote female needs.

What is true is that a double standard is still taught to adolescents in our culture. But it is glaringly false to say that it encourages males to be sexual; it merely discourages them less. Consider the common charge that "this society" teaches young males they have to "score" to be real men, for example. In fact, you will not find this preached by any of the major socializing institutions, not by church, government, school, family, *or* the media. Even that small segment of the latter that celebrates sex overtly cannot really be said to do this—and it is standardly maligned and even banned by the society at large. The one place where such a thing is taught is in the peer groups of some young men as they themselves rebel against society's teaching on the subject, trying to justify their own needs and feelings. However all this may be, the point remains that pornography is not the cause of male sexuality. It has again become a scapegoat in connection with male-female conflicts whose real causes lie in biology, or at least much deeper in the socialization of men—or of women....

Some have claimed there is scientific evidence that standard pornography causes misperception of other people's sexual desires. In a certain type of experiment, volunteers are exposed to a presentation of some kind and then asked questions about their beliefs or attitudes.(A subterfuge is used to keep them from realizing the true purpose of the test.) In one version of this test, subjects who have been shown sexual materials indicated they regarded women (as well as men) as somewhat more sexually liberal than did subjects who had not been shown the materials. In itself, this is no evidence of misperception; the former might have been closer to the truth than the latter. In any case, the result is not in the least remarkable. A recent or extended experience of *any* kind looms large in one's consciousness. Hence just about any book or movie, *or* real person that one has recently met, would have a similar influence on one's other judgments, temporarily. For a more striking example, one who has just seen a scary movie is much more likely to look under the bed before retiring at night. The effect soon fades, however, it is swamped by that of subsequently encountered books or movies or real people. And most of the latter tend to promote the culture's current party line on sex, just as they do on other subjects. Except in unusual circumstances, the conclusion remains: sexual entertainment will have little effect on perceptions of reality.

A variant of this objection says the ecstatic pleasure often portrayed in pornography will tend to make the readers or viewers disappointed with their own sexual experience and, hence, with their partners or their partners' performance. (Although it is women who standardly complain about the latter, this new claim is usually framed in terms of male dissatisfaction.) It is not always clear whether those who present the argument believe ordinary tepid sex is really all that is possible—the half-hour orgasms of Mangaian women argue otherwise—or whether for some reason they just think it unwise to aspire to greater enjoyment. In any case, few people would be misled even by genuine exaggeration, which is an extremely common part of life. Does the hysterical euphoria of the consumers in commercials for hamburgers and soft drinks make anyone seriously expect them to taste different? Once again, the only reason for possibly being misled in the special case of sex is societally imposed ignorance. And it is people who use arguments like this one who often want to keep young people in that vulnerable state....

Most of the...claims about pornography's "effects" assume that too much stress on sex is dangerous to an intimate relationship. This can certainly be true, but the proper balance of emphasis between sex and other needs in that context is one that requires sensitive exploration, not dogma. In fact, those who give these fallacious arguments typically overlook the opposite problem. Surveys and clinical experience have long revealed that a high percentage of couples have unsatisfying sex lives. That is a major destroyer of relationships in itself. There are many reasons for this, but a serious one continues to be the sexual inhibition this society inculcates, with its *negative* stress on sex. Conversely,...countless women have discovered that sex could be a joy rather than a burden, and they have done so precisely by learning to become more sexually assertive and more adventurous in bed.

What is especially relevant to our purposes about the latter fact is that pornography has often aided in the process. Large numbers of people have reported that it has helped their sex lives and hence their relationships. In one survey of couples who went to sex movies together, for example, 42 percent made that claim. In her beautiful little book on female sexuality, *For Yourself*, Dr. Lonnie Barbach tells how women have overcome difficulty in getting sexually aroused, or in having orgasms, by learning to use fantasy and pornography. Indeed, it has become standard practice for therapists to use sex films to treat the sexual disabilities of individuals and couples. The ways in which they help are very revealing in light of what has just been discussed: they aid in overcoming inhibition, enhance arousal in preparation for sex, and introduce ideas and techniques that bring freshness to a stale routine. So far from harming intimate personal relationships, pornography can have the very opposite effect.

Marriage and the Family

A third general charge of social harm from pornography has been put forth, mostly by traditionalists. Its use is seen as a threat, not to love and personal relationships as such, but to marriage and the family. The basic claim is that by celebrating sex for its own sake, pornography entices people to leave or refrain from entering committed relationships— "Why be married if you can get sex without it?"—or else leads to their breakup by encouraging extramarital adventures that result in jealous conflicts. This is a serious charge indeed. The legalistic concern some have with marriage ceremonies is highly questionable; but the family, in its role of raising children, is of crucial importance. And divorce, with its adverse effects on children, has become increasingly common in recent decades. Such a large and complex topic can hardly be explored adequately here, but we can address two relevant questions: Is a positive attitude toward sex for its own sake necessarily a threat to marriage? And is pornography an appreciable factor in promoting that sort of attitude, hence itself such a threat?

The answer to the first question seems to be negative. For one thing, there have been many cultures with a stable family life and also an accepting attitude toward nonmarital sex. In fact, prior to the rise of the world religions and the empires that spread them, socially sanctioned premarital sex may well have been the cross-cultural norm. It has even been suggested that such behavior contributes to later marital stability by providing young people with experience on which to base a wiser choice of mate. In any case, it does not speak very well of marriage to suggest that, given a choice, people will reject it. As a matter of fact, most do have a strong inclination toward pair-bonding. Since they do not marry just for sex in the first place (and *shouldn't* do so), liberal sexual attitudes are not likely to dissuade them; only the timing is apt to be affected. In addition, there are many good reasons for not forcing young people to rush into marriage by making it the only way they can get sex.

As for the case of *extra*marital sex, where it has been socially sanctioned and controlled, it too has not been a serious threat to the stability of the family. It is true that jealousy is a powerful emotion. But it is also true that humans are far from being strictly monogamous in their feelings. Although our culture has traditionally taken jealousy as morally justified and condemned extramarital desires, others have done just the reverse: they have sought to mitigate the conflict between the two emotions by controlling the former more than the latter. And the anthropological reports indicate that they succeed rather well. It just may be, for all we know, that their system works better than ours in this respect. In fact, it can be argued that our unbending attitude toward sexual exclusivity contributes to marital breakup by creating unrealistic expectations. The offending party may not want such a break but feel it is necessary to satisfy other desires; and the offended one may fear loss of face in not avenging the act, or else think there must be something wrong with one of them or with the marriage for such a thing to have happened.

However all this may be, it is not the immediate question here. For us the issue is whether pornography is, in any of the ways suggested, a threat to the family in our culture. In spite of what many assume, it is far from obvious that it is. Indeed, it may be more likely to act as a "safety valve" for preventing marital breakup by providing a substitute way to satisfy nonmonogamous desires. Many cultures of the world have had special festival times and special locations in which the usual sexual taboos could be broken. (For just one example, consider the temple "prostitution" of the ancient Near East, in which all men and women took part.) The seeming value of such institutions in maintaining both monogamy and mental health has been noted by many students of the subject. The fact that such large numbers of strictly monogamous couples in the present time have come to use sexual entertainment together hints that it can serve the same purpose. Given the strong biological urge to have more than one sex partner, this may be an extremely important consideration.

Furthermore, pornography can help to preserve marriages by means of the positive effects listed earlier. As for the chance that it can also have the opposite effect, it might be suggested that romantic love stories present more of a danger to long-term pairing by awakening desires that many a marriage gone stale cannot satisfy. After all, falling in love with someone else is more likely to produce the wish for divorce than is a one-night stand. In any case, factors other than sexual fantasies have been vastly more influential in creating marital instability. The data indicate that such things as the following have been responsible for increasing divorce rates: greater independence for women (most female advocates of long-term commitment do not assail *this* casual factor), changes in laws and attitudes regarding divorce, unemployment and other financial troubles, and the greater mobility of the population, which has led to loss of controls by the extended family and the community.

To really answer the question before us, however, we must consider the possible dynamics. Exactly how might pornography produce the allegedly destabilizing desires? Those who make the charge sometimes talk as if it is just a matter of arousing feelings that would not otherwise exist. But that is *their* fantasy, for biology can quite adequately do so. It does not take "outside agitators" like pornography to produce lust and wandering eyes. There is one thing, however, that pornography certainly can do, and that is to thwart attempts to suppress such feelings. Efforts to promote one moral point of view are indeed apt to be hampered when people are allowed to become aware of others views as genuine alternatives. This is just to say, however, that freedom and knowledge are an obstacle to attempts at thought control. "How're you gonna keep 'em down on the farm, after they've seen Paris?" asks an old song. It was not only the pill, but the loosening of restraints on sexual content in the media, that launched the reassessment of traditional sexual attitudes that occurred in the 1960s.

So there is a much broader point here that is very important. It is clear that formal and informal education—learning more about the world—tend to make people more tolerant and liberal in their views. For just one apparent example, surveys have revealed that half the readers of sex magazines are college educated, in contrast to a third of the readers of magazines in general. Ideologues, however, do not like such tolerance; what they are opposed to at bottom is the right of other people to make up their own minds. (From Moscow to Washington, they answer, "Don't *let* 'em see Paris.") But it cannot easily be argued that keeping people in ignorance of different ideas is best for them. As Carl Sagan pointed out in *Cosmos*, science has flourished at those times and places in history where there have been the greatest social openness and freedom. So it is for good reasons that we have our tradition of freedom of expression: aside from the great value of liberty itself, we have a better chance of discovering truth in a "free marketplace of ideas" than in conditions where only certain beliefs and attitudes may be extolled.

In particular, our best hope of working out the most viable social arrangement concerning sex and the family is to allow an open dialogue in which all human needs are given consideration. It is just as wrong to censor portrayals of alternative sexual lifestyles as it is to suppress those of different political or religious systems. In all likelihood, given the large range of human differences that exists, the best system in the present regard is a pluralistic one that allows individuals to discover the different modes of living that maximize their fulfillment. To rigidly impose the same kinds of relationships upon everyone (on homosexual and heterosexual, pair-bonder and non-pair-bonder and so forth) surely does not serve the best interests of individual people. And the common assumption that what is best for society as a whole is the product, not of a careful study of alternatives, but of the very prejudice that censors consideration of alternatives. Socially enforced error is self-perpetuating.

Debate Presenter Form

Follow the guidelines for debate presenters contained in the introduction of this text and those given to you by your instructor. Use the format below to organize the material for your debate. Remember to include all relevant citation information and to present the related information in your own words. Give credit to authors when you cite a quote and be as thorough as possible when writing about your points so you will be prepared for your debate.

Reference citation #1:

Author: _____

Title: _____

Date: _____

Source: _____

_____

Content from reference citation #1: _____

_____

_____

_____

_____

_____

_____

_____

_____

_____

_____

_____

Reference citation #2:

Author: _____

Title: _____

Date: _____

Source: _____

_____

Content from reference citation #2: _____

_____

_____

_____

_____

_____

_____

Reference citation #3:

Author: _____

Title: _____

Date: _____

Source: _____

_____

Content from reference citation #3: _____

_____

_____

_____

_____

Audience Preparation Form

Follow the guidelines for preparing to be an informed audience member on the day of the debate included in the introduction to this text. After reading both sides of the debate from this chapter, answer the following questions. Be as thorough as possible so that you will be able to make a contribution to the debate by asking informed questions or making provocative comments. This form is usually due on the day of the debate.

State the issue in your own words. Do not plagiarize the text. Demonstrate that you understand the topic and it's relevant arguments.

_____

_____

_____

_____

_____

Discuss two points on the "yes" side of the debate.

Point #1: _____

_____

Point #2: _____

_____

Discuss two points on the "no" side of the debate.

Point #1: _____

_____

Point #2: _____

_____

What is your opinion on this topic?

_____

_____

_____

_____

_____

_____

_____

What has contributed to the development of your views about this topic?

_____

_____

_____

_____

_____

_____

_____

_____

What information would be necessary to cause you to change your thinking about this topic?

_____

_____

_____

_____

_____

Debate Response Form

Follow the guidelines for responding to the debates in the introductory chapter of this text. Complete this form and submit your answers at the class following the debate. Try to be thorough and convince your instructor that you were an active listener during the debate.

List a quote from a debate presenter that you think was important and explain why you think this comment was significant.

_____

_____

_____

_____

Which side of the debate do you think made the most convincing arguments, why?

_____

_____

_____

_____

_____

After hearing the debate, in what way has your thinking been affected?

_____

_____

_____

_____

_____

_____

Human Sexual Behavior

ISSUE 9

Should Prostitution Be Legal?

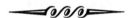

YES James Bovard, *Safeguard Public Health: Legalize Contractual Sex*

NO Anastasia Volkonsky, *Legalizing the 'Profession' Would Sanction the Abuse*

James Bovard says that legalization of contractual sex (prostitution) would be a step toward protecting the public from health hazards such as Aids. Elimination of prosecution of those who sell sex would reduce enormous financial resources and hours the police spend on "sting" operations aimed toward the apprehension of those involved in prostitution. Then we could spend these resources on dealing with more serious crimes.

Bovard also points out that, with an already over-crowded prison system, it makes no sense to fill space needed for violent criminals with prostitutes and their customers. He concludes by questioning whether police suppression of prostitution actually makes our society a safer place to be. He asks whether the consideration by some that prostitution is immoral should make it legal.

Anastasia Volkonsky ardently disagrees with the claim that legalization of prostitution would produce any type of benefit to women and society at large. She describes statistics showing that to be a prostitute is to be physically and emotionally abused.

In response to those who would say that these abusive aspects of prostitution are due to it's illegality, Volkonsky replies that regulated prostitution is accompanied by a black market promoting illegal sex for sale. Legalizing some forms of prostitution would not eliminate the problems faced by prostitutes.

Volkonsky describes the problem with the two main areas of supposed benefit of legalization of prostitution. First, the women are not free to choose prostitution. With the rules and regulations of brothels prostitutes can earn little and suffer a lot. Second, police resources go into the regulation of the brothels and the peripheral crime that occurs in association with this legal sex industry. This author concludes with the assertion that legalizing this profession will not remove the harmful effects on women or protect the public's health or welfare.

Applications

1 Do you know of anyone who has benefited from prostitution? Do you think these benefits outweigh the problems associated with prostitution? Explain your answer.

2. Would you favor legalization of prostitution or not? Why?

3. What do you think about the idea that just because sex for sale seems immoral to some, that it does not necessarily mean it should be illegal?

Safeguard Public Health
Legalize Contractual Sex

James Bovard

The call to legalize prostitution once again is becoming a hot issue. Columnists have been complaining about the conviction of Heide Fleiss, the "Hollywood madam," saying it is unfair that the law punishes her but not her clients. San Francisco has appointed a task force to analyze the issue of legalizing prostitution. (A similar task force in Atlanta recommended legalization in 1986, but the city has not changed its policies.)

As more people fear the spread of AIDS, the legalization of prostitution offers one of the easiest means of limiting the spread of the disease and of improving the quality of law enforcement in this country.

Prostitution long has been illegal in all but one state. Unfortunately, laws against it often bring out the worst among the nation's law-enforcement agencies. Since neither prostitutes nor their customers routinely run to the police to complain about the other's conduct, police rely on trickery and deceit to arrest people.

In 1983, for example, police in Albuquerque, N.M., placed a classified advertisement in a local paper for men to work as paid escorts—and then arrested 50 men who responded for violating laws against prostitution. In 1985, Honolulu police paid private citizens to pick up prostitutes in their cars, have sex with them and then drive them to nearby police cars for arrest. (One convicted prostitute's lawyer complained: "You can now serve your community by fornicating. Once the word gets out there will be no shortage of volunteers.") In San Francisco, the police have wired rooms in the city's leading hotels to make videotapes of prostitutes servicing their customers. But given the minimal control over the videotaping operation, there was little to stop local police from watching and videotaping other hotel guests in bed.

Many prostitution-related entrapment operations make doubtful contributions to preserving public safety. In 1985, eight Fairfax County, VA., police officers rented two $88-a-night Holiday Inn rooms, purchased an ample supply of liquor and then phoned across the Potomac River to Washington to hire a professional stripper for a bachelor party. The stripper came, stripped and was busted for indecent exposure. She faced fines up to $1,000 and 12 months in jail. Fairfax County police justified the sting operation by claiming it was necessary to fight prostitution. But the department had made only 11 arrests on prostitution charges in the previous year—all with similar sting operations.

In 1992, police in Des Moines, Wash., hired a convicted rapist to have sex with masseuses. The local police explained that they hired the felon after plainclothed police officers could not persuade women at the local Body Care Center to have intercourse. Martin Pratt, police chief in the Seattle suburb, claimed that the ex-rapist was uniquely qualified for the job and, when asked why the police instructed the felon to consummate the acts with the alleged prostitutes, Pratt explained that stopping short "wouldn't have been appropriate."

A New York sting operation [in 1994] indirectly could have helped out the New York Mets: Two San Diego Padres baseball players were arrested after speaking to a female undercover officer. A Seattle journalist who also was busted described the police procedure to *Newsday*: "He said that he was stuck in traffic when he discovered that a miniskirted woman in a low-cut blouse was causing the jam, approaching the cars that were stopped. 'She came up to the windows, kind of swaggering,' he said. He said that she offered him sex, he made a suggestive reply, and the next thing he knew he was surrounded by police officers who dragged him out of his car and arrested him."

Many police appear to prefer chasing naked women than pursuing dangerous felons. As Lt. Bill Young of the Las Vegas Metro Police told Canada's *Vancouver Sun*, "You get up in a penthouse at Caesar's Palace with six naked women frolicking in the room and then say: 'Hey, baby, you're busted!' That's fun." (Las Vegas arrests between 300 to 400 prostitutes a month.) In August 1993, Charles County, Md,. police were embarrassed by reports that an undercover officer visiting a strip joint had had intercourse while receiving a "personal lap dance."

In some cities, laws against prostitution are transforming local police officers into de facto car thieves. Female officers masquerade as prostitutes; when a customer stops to negotiate, other police rush out and confiscate the person's car under local asset-forfeiture laws. Such programs are operating in Detroit, Washington, New York and Portland, Ore. The female officers who masquerade as prostitutes are, in some ways, worse than the prostitutes—since, at least, the hookers will exchange services for payment, while the police simply intend to shake down would-be customers.

Shortly after the Washington police began their car-grabbing program in 1992, one driver sped off after a plainclothes officer tried to force his way into the car after the driver spoke to an undercover female officer. One officer's foot was slightly injured, and police fired six shots into the rear of the car. The police volley could have killed two or three people—but apparently the Washington police consider the possibility of killing citizens a small price to pay for slightly and temporarily decreasing the rate of prostitution in one selected neighborhood.

The same tired, failed antiprostitution tactics tend to be repeated ad nauseam around the country. Aurora, Colo., recently announced plans to buy newspaper ads showing pictures of accused johns. The plan hit a rough spot when the *Denver Post* refused to publish the ads, choosing not to be an arm of the criminal-justice system. One Aurora councilman told radio host Mike Rosen that the city wanted to publish the pictures of the accused (and not wait until after convictions) because some of them might be found not guilty "because of some legal technicality."

In recent years, the Washington police force has tried one trick after another to suppress prostitution—including passing out tens of thousands of tickets to drivers for making right turns onto selected streets known to be venues of solicitation. (Didn't they see the tiny print on the street sign saying that right turns are illegal between 5 p.m. and 2 a.m.?) Yet, at the same time, the murder rate in Washington has skyrocketed and the city's arrest and conviction rates for murders have fallen by more than 50 percent.

The futile fight against prostitution is a major drain on local law-enforcement resources. A study published in the *Hastings Law Journal* in 1987 is perhaps the most reliable estimate of the cost to major cities. Author Julie Pearl observed: "This study focuses on sixteen of the nation's largest cities, in which only 28 percent of reported violent crimes result in arrest. On average, police in these cities made as many arrests for prostitution as for all violent offenses.

Last year, police in Boston, Cleveland, and Houston arrested twice as many people for prostitution as they did for all homicides, rapes, robberies, and assaults combined, while perpetrators evaded arrest for 90 percent of these violent crimes. Cleveland officers spent eighteen hours—the equivalent of two workdays—on prostitution duty for every violent offense failing to yield an arrest." The average cost per bust was almost $2,000 and "the average big-city police department spent 213 man-hours a day enforcing prostitution laws." Pearl estimated that 16 large American cities spent more than $120 million to suppress prostitution in 1985. In 1993, one Los Angeles official estimated that prostitution enforcement was costing the city more than $100 million a year.

Locking up prostitutes and their customers is especially irrational at a time when more than 35 states are under court orders to reduce prison overcrowding. Gerald Arenberg, executive director of the National Association of the Chiefs of Police, has come out in favor of legalizing prostitution. Dennis Martin, president of the same association, declared that prostitution law enforcement is "much too time-consuming, and police forces are short-staffed." Maryland Judge Darryl Russell observed: "We have to explore other alternatives to solving this problem because this eats up a lot of manpower of the police. We're just putting out brush fires while the forest is blazing." National surveys have shown that 94 percent of citizens believe that police do not respond quickly enough to calls for help, and the endless pursuit of prostitution is one factor that slows down many police departments from responding to other crimes.

Another good reason for reforming prostitution laws is to safeguard public health: Regulated prostitutes tend to be cleaner prostitutes. HIV-infection rates tend to be stratospheric among the nation's streetwalkers. In Newark, 57 percent of prostitutes were found to be HIV positive, according to a *Congressional Quarterly* report. In New York City, 35 percent of prostitutes were HIV-positive; in Washington, almost half.

In contrast, brothels, which are legal in 12 rural Nevada counties, tend to be comparative paragons of public safety. The University of California at Berkeley School of Public Health studied the health of legal Nevada brothel workers compared with that of jailed Nevada streetwalkers. None of the brothel workers had AIDS, while 6 percent of the unregulated streetwalkers did. Brothel owners had a strong incentive to police the health of their employees, since they could face liability if an infection were passed to a customer.

Prostitution is legal in several countries in Western Europe. In Hamburg, Germany, which some believe has a model program of legalized prostitution, streetwalkers are sanctioned in certain well-defined areas and prostitutes must undergo frequent health checks. Women with contagious diseases are strictly prohibited from plying their trade. (While some consider Amsterdam a model for legalization, the system there actually has serious problems. A spokesman for the association of Dutch brothels recently told the Associated Press: "The prostitutes these days are not so professional any more. In the past, prostitutes had more skills and they offered better services. Most of them work only one or two evenings per week, and that's not enough time for them to become good.")

Bans of prostitution actually generate public disorder—streetwalkers, police chases, pervasive disrespect for the law and condoms littering lawns. As long as people have both money and sexual frustration, some will continue paying others to gratify their desires. The issue is not whether prostitution is immoral, but whether police suppression of prostitution will make society a safer place. The ultimate question to ask about a crackdown on prostitution is: "How many murders are occurring while police are chasing after people who only want to spend a few bucks for pleasure?

In 1858, San Francisco Police Chief Martin Burke complained: "It is impossible to suppress prostitution altogether, yet it can, and ought to be regulated so as to limit the injury done to society, as much as possible." Vices are not crimes. Despite centuries of attempts to suppress prostitution, the profession continues to flourish. Simply because prostitution may be immoral is no reason for police to waste their time in a futile effort to suppress the oldest profession.

Legalizing the 'Profession' Would Sanction the Abuse

— Anastasia Vilkonsky —

Prostitution commonly is referred to as "the world's oldest profession." It's an emblematic statement about the status of women, for whom being sexually available and submissive to men is the oldest form of survival.

As the "world's oldest," prostitution is presented as an accepted fact of history, something that will always be with us that we cannot eradicate. As a "profession," selling access to one's body is being promoted as a viable choice for women. In an era in which the human-rights movement is taking on some of history's most deeply rooted oppressions and an era in which women have made unprecedented strides in politics and the professions, this soft-selling of prostitution is especially intolerable.

Calls for legalization and decriminalization of prostitution put forth by civil libertarians are not forward-thinking reforms. They represent acceptance and normalization of the traffic in human beings. Moreover, the civil-libertarian portrayal of the prostitute as a sexually free, consenting adult hides the vast network of traffickers, organized-crime syndicates, pimps, procurers and brothel keepers, as well as the customer demand that ultimately controls the trade.

In studies replicated in major cities throughout the United States, the conditions of this "profession" are revealed to be extreme sexual, physical and psychological abuse. Approximately 70 percent of prostitutes are raped repeatedly by their customers—an average of 31 times per year, according to a study in a 1993 issue of the *Cardoza Women's Law Journal*. In addition, 65 percent are physically assaulted repeatedly by customers and more by pimps. A majority (65 percent and higher) are drug addicts. Increasingly, prostituted women are HIV positive. Survivors testify to severe violence, torture and attempted murder. The mortality rate for prostitutes, according to Justice Department statistics from 1982, is 40 times the national average.

What can be said of a "profession" with such a job description? How can it be said that women freely choose sexual assault, harassment, abuse and the risk of death as a profession? Such a term might be appealing for women who are trapped in the life, as a last-ditch effort to regain some self-respect and identify with the promises of excitement and glamour that may have lured them into prostitution in the first place. A substantial portion of street-walkers are homeless or living below the poverty line. Even most women who work in outcall or escort services have no control over their income because they are at the mercy of a pimp or pusher. Most will leave prostitution without savings.

Prostitution is not a profession selected from among other options by today's career women. It comes as no surprise that the ranks of prostitutes both in the United States and globally are filled with society's most vulnerable members, those least able to resist recruitment. They are those most displaced and disadvantaged in the job market: women, especially the poor; the working class; racial and ethnic minorities; mothers with young children to support; battered women fleeing abuse; refugees; and illegal immigrants. Women are brought to the United States from Asia and Eastern Europe for prostitution. In a foreign country, with no contacts or language skills and fearing arrest or deportation, they are at the mercy of pimps and crime syndicates.

Most tellingly, the largest group of recruits to prostitution are children. The average age of entry into prostitution in the United States is approximately 14, sociologists Mimi Silbert and Ayala Pines found in a study performed for the Delancey Foundation in San Francisco. More than 65 percent of these child prostitutes are runaways. Most have experienced a major trauma: incest, domestic violence, rape or parental abandonment. At an age widely considered too young to handle activities such as voting, drinking alcohol, driving or holding down a job, these children survive by selling their bodies to strangers. These formative years will leave them with deep scars—should they survive to adulthood.

***

Sensing this contradiction between the reality of prostitution and the rhetoric of sexual freedom and consensual crime, some proposals to decriminalize prostitution attempt to draw a distinction between "forced" prostitution and "free" prostitution. A June 1993 *Times* article about the international sex industry notes that "faced with the difficulty of sorting out which women are prostitutes by choice and which are coerced, many officials shrug off the problem," implying that when one enters prostitution, it is a free choice. The distinction between force and freedom ends in assigning blame to an already victimized woman for "choosing" to accept prostitution in her circumstances.

"People take acceptance of the money as her consent to be violated," says Susan Hunter, executive director of the Council for Prostitution Alternatives, a Portland, OR-based social-service agency that has helped hundreds of women from around the country recover from the effects of prostitution. She likens prostituted women to battered women. When battered women live with their batterer or repeatedly go back to the batterer, we do not take this as a legal consent to battering. A woman's acceptance of money in prostitution should not be taken as her agreement to prostitution. She may take the money because she must survive, because it is the only recompense she will get for the harm that has been done to her and because she has been socialized to believe that this is her role in life. Just as battered women's actions now are understood in light of the effects of trauma and battered woman syndrome, prostituted women suffer psychologically in the aftermath of repeated physical and sexual assaults.

To make an informed choice about prostitution, says Hunter, women need to recover their safety, sobriety and self-esteem and learn about their options. The women in her program leave prostitution, she asserts, "not because we offer them high salaries, but because we offer them hope....Woman are not voluntarily returning to prostitution."

Proponents of a "consensual crime" approach hold that the dangers associated with prostitution are a result of its illegality. Legal prostitution will be safe, clean and professional, they argue; the related crimes will disappear.

Yet wherever there is regulated prostitution, it is matched by a flourishing black market. Despite the fact that prostitution is legal in 12 Nevada counties, prostitutes continue to work illegally in casinos to avoid the isolation and controls of the legal brothels. Even the legal brothels maintain a business link with the illegal pimping circuit by paying a finder's fee to pimps for bringing in new women.

Ironically, legalization, which frequently is touted as an alternative to spending money on police vice squads, creates its own set of regulations to be monitored. To get prostitutes and pimps to comply with licensing rules, the penalties must be heightened and policing increased—adding to law-enforcement costs.

Behind the facade of a regulated industry, brothel prostitutes in Nevada are captive in conditions analogous to slavery. Women often are procured for the brothels from other areas by pimps who dump them at the house in order to collect the referral fee. Women report working in shifts commonly as long as 12 hours, even when ill, menstruating or pregnant, with no right to refuse a customer who has requested them or to refuse the sexual act for which he has paid. The dozen or so prostitutes I interviewed said they are expected to pay the brothel room and board and a percentage of their earnings—sometimes up to 50 percent. They also must pay for mandatory extras such as medical exams, assigned clothing and fines incurred for breaking house rules. And, contrary to the common claim that the brothel will protect women from the dangerous, crazy clients on the streets, rapes and assaults by customers are covered up by the management.

Local ordinances of questionable constitutionality restrict the women's activities even outside the brothel. They may be confined to certain sections of town and permitted out only on certain days, according to Barbara Hobson, author of *Uneasy Virtue*. Ordinances require that brothels must be located in uninhabited areas at least five miles from any city, town, mobile-home park or residential area. Physically isolated in remote areas, their behavior monitored by brothel managers, without ties to the community and with little money or resources of their own, the Nevada prostitutes often are virtual prisoners. Local legal codes describe the woman as "inmates."

Merely decriminalizing prostitution would not remove its stigma and liberate women in the trade. Rather, the fiction that prostitution is freely chosen would become encoded into the law's approach to prostitution. Decriminalization would render prostitution an invisible crime without a name. "The exchange of money [in prostitution] somehow makes the crime of rape invisible" to society, says Hunter.

Amy Fries, director of the National Organization for Women's International Women's Rights Task Force, speaks from experience in studying and combating the sex trade both internationally and in the Washington area. Decriminalization, she says, does not address the market forces at work in prostitution: "[Prostitution] is based on supply and demand. As the demand goes way up, [the pimps] have to meet it with a supply by bringing in more girls."

Ultimately, changing the laws will benefit the customer, not the prostitute. Legalization advocates identify the arrest as the most obvious example of the abuse of prostitutes. But, surprisingly, former prostitutes and prostitutes' advocates say the threat of jail is not a top concern. Considering the absence of any other refuge or shelter, jail provides a temporary safe haven, at the very least providing a bunk, a square meal and a brief respite from johns, pimps and drugs. This is not to make light of abuses of state and police power or the seriousness of jail—the fact that for many women jail is an improvement speaks volumes about their lives on the streets.

It is the customers who have the most to lose from arrest, who fear jail, the stigma of the arrest record and the loss of their anonymity. The argument that prostitution laws invade the privacy of consenting adults is geared toward protecting customers. Prostitutes, working on the streets or in brothels controlled by pimps, have little to no privacy. Furthermore, decriminalization of prostitution is a gateway to decriminalizing pandering, pimping and patronizing—together, decriminalizing many forms of sexual and economic exploitation of women. A 1986 proposal advocated by the New York Bar Association included repeal of such associated laws and the lowering of the age of consent for "voluntary" prostitution. Despite the assertion that prostitutes actively support decriminalization, many women who have escaped prostitution testify that their pimps coerced them into signing such petitions.

Of the many interests contributing to the power of the sex industry—the pimps, the panderers and the patrons—the acts of individual prostitutes are the least influential. Yet, unfortunately, there are incentives for law enforcement to target prostitutes for arrest, rather than aggressively enforcing laws against pimps, johns and traffickers. It is quicker and less costly to round up the women than to pursue pimps and traffickers in elaborate sting operations. The prostitutes are relatively powerless to fight arrest; it is the pimps and johns who can afford private attorneys. And, sadly, it is easier to get a public outcry and convictions against prostitutes, who are marginalized women, than against the wealthier males who are the majority of pimps and johns.

Prostitution is big business. Right now, economics provide an incentive for procuring and pimping women. In all the debates about prostitution, the factor most ignored is the demand. But it is the customers—who have jobs, money, status in the community, clean arrest records and anonymity—who have the most to lose. New legal reforms are beginning to recognize that. An increasing number of communities across the country, from Portland to Baltimore, are adopting car-seizure laws, which allow police to impound the automobiles of those who drive around soliciting prostitutes. This approach recognizes that johns degrade not only women who are prostitutes, but also others by assuming that any females in a given area are for sale. Other towns have instituted legally, or as community efforts, measures designed to publicize and shame would-be johns by publishing their names or pictures and stepping up arrests.

Globally, a pending U.N. Convention Against All Forms of Sexual Exploitation would address the modern forms of prostitution with mechanisms that target pimps and johns and that hold governments accountable for their policies.

Hunter supports the use of civil as well as criminal sanctions against johns, modeled after sexual harassment lawsuits. "People will change their behavior because of economics," she points out, using recent changes in governmental and corporate policy toward sexual harassment as an example of how the fear of lawsuits and financial loss can create social change.

At the heart of the matter, prostitution is buying the right to use a woman's body. The "profession" of prostitution means bearing the infliction of repeated, unwanted sexual acts in order to keep one's "job." It is forced sex as a condition of employment, the very definition of rape and sexual harassment. Cecilie Hoigard and Liv Finstad, who authored the 1992 book *Backstreets*, chronicling 15 years of research on prostitution survivors, stress that it is not any individual act, but the buildup of sexual and emotional violation as a daily occurrence, that determines the trauma of prostitution.

Cleaning up the surrounding conditions won't mask the ugliness of a trade in human beings.

Debate Presenter Form

Follow the guidelines for debate presenters contained in the introduction of this text and those given to you by your instructor. Use the format below to organize the material for your debate. Remember to include all relevant citation information and to present the related information in your own words. Give credit to authors when you cite a quote and be as thorough as possible when writing about your points so you will be prepared for your debate.

Reference citation #1:

Author: _____

Title: _____

Date: _____

Source: _____

_____

Content from reference citation #1: _____

_____

_____

_____

_____

_____

_____

_____

_____

_____

_____

_____

Reference citation #2:

Author: _____

Title: _____

Date: _____

Source: _____

_____

Content from reference citation #2: _____

_____

_____

_____

_____

_____

Reference citation #3:

Author: _____

Title: _____

Date: _____

Source: _____

_____

Content from reference citation #3: _____

_____

_____

_____

_____

Audience Preparation Form

Follow the guidelines for preparing to be an informed audience member on the day of the debate included in the introduction to this text. After reading both sides of the debate from this chapter, answer the following questions. Be as thorough as possible so that you will be able to make a contribution to the debate by asking informed questions or making provocative comments. This form is usually due on the day of the debate.

State the issue in your own words. Do not plagiarize the text. Demonstrate that you understand the topic and it's relevant arguments.

_____

_____

_____

_____

_____

Discuss two points on the "yes" side of the debate.

Point #1: _____

_____

Point #2: _____

_____

Discuss two points on the "no" side of the debate.

Point #1: _____

_____

Point #2: _____

_____

What is your opinion on this topic?

_____

_____

_____

_____

_____

_____

_____

What has contributed to the development of your views about this topic?

_____

_____

_____

_____

_____

_____

_____

_____

What information would be necessary to cause you to change your thinking about this topic?

_____

_____

_____

_____

_____

_____

Debate Response Form

Follow the guidelines for responding to the debates in the introductory chapter of this text. Complete this form and submit your answers at the class following the debate. Try to be thorough and convince your instructor that you were an active listener during the debate.

List a quote from a debate presenter that you think was important and explain why you think this comment was significant.

_____

_____

_____

_____

Which side of the debate do you think made the most convincing arguments, why?

_____

_____

_____

_____

After hearing the debate, in what way has your thinking been affected?

_____

_____

_____

_____

_____

ISSUE 10

Is Abstinence-Only Education Effective?

⸺∞∞⸺

YES Thomas Lickona, *Where Sex Education Went Wrong*

NO Peggy Brick and Deborah M. Roffman, *Abstinence, No Buts' Is Simplistic*

Thomas Lickona, advocate of abstinence only sex education, describes the history of models of sex education in his article. He divides these models into directive and non-directive approaches.

"Comprehensive" and the "abstinence, but" models fall short of achieving what Lickona believes should be the goal of sex education in our schools: to protect the safety, happiness and character of our teenagers.

Directive or "abstinence, no buts" sex education suggests that sexual abstinence is the only safe and moral choice for teens who are not married, condoms are not a responsible choice, and sex is only safe within monogamy. Lickona believes that these messages are the only way that sex education becomes part of the solution to teen sexual behavior, moral conduct, and pregnancy prevention.

Peggy Brick and Deborah Roffman favor comprehensive sex education and explain why directive approaches fail. These authors also cite flaws in research reporting the effectiveness of directive sex education. They suggest that comprehensive sex education has not been applied consistently or widely enough to receive proper program evaluation. Brick and Roffman conclude with a reminder that comprehensive sex education alone will not be miraculous, but it is the best tool at present.

Applications

1. What type of sex education program did you receive, directive or non-directive? Describe your reasons for placing the program at your school into one of these types.

2. What type of sex education do you think would really work to prevent spread of sexually transmitted disease, pregnancy and the psychological complications of premature sexual behavior?

3. Are there any conditions under which you think it would be acceptable for teenagers to be sexual? Explain.

Issue 10
YES

Where Sex Education Went Wrong

Thomas Lickona

Most of us are familiar with the alarming statistics about teen sexual activity in the United States. Among high school students, 54 percent (including 61 percent of boys and 48 percent of girls) say they have had sexual intercourse, according to a 1992 Centers for Disease Control study. The number of 9th graders who say they have already had sex is 40 percent.

In the past two decades, there has been an explosion in the number of sexually transmitted diseases. Twelve million people are infected each year; 63 percent of them are under 25.

Each year, 1 of every 10 teenage girls becomes pregnant, and more than 400,000 teenagers have abortions. One in 4 children is born out of wedlock, compared to 1 in 20 in 1960.

But statistics like these do not tell the whole story. The other side—one that should concern us deeply as moral educators—is the debasement of sexuality and the corruption of young people's character

A Legacy of the Sexual Revolution

A 1993 study by the American Association of University Women found that four out of five high school students say they have experienced sexual harassment ("unwanted sexual behavior that interferes with your life") in school. Commented one 14-year-old girl: "All guys want is sex. They just come up to you and grab you."

In suburban Minneapolis, a mother filed state and federal complaints because 3rd and 4th grade boys on the school bus had tormented her 1st grade daughter daily with obscene comments and repeated demands for sexual acts. A 6th grade teacher taking my graduate course in moral education said, "The boys bring in *Playboy*, the girls wear make-up and jewelry, and the kids write heavy sexual notes to each other."

At an Indiana high school, a teacher said, "Kids in the halls will call out—boy to girl, girl to boy—'I want to f--- you.'" At Lakewood High School in an affluent Los Angeles suburb, a group of boys formed the "Spur Posse," a club in which participants competed to see how many girls they could sleep with.

Growing up in a highly eroticized sexual environment—a legacy of the sexual revolution—American children are preoccupied with sex in developmentally distorted ways and increasingly likely to act out their sexual impulses. The widespread sexual harassment in schools and the rising rates of teen sexual activity are not isolated phenomena but an outgrowth of the abnormal preoccupation with sex that children are manifesting from the earliest grades.

The sexual corruption of children reflects an adult sexual culture in which the evidence continues to mount that sex is out of control. In 1990, 29 states set records for the sex-and-violence crime of rape. By age 18, more than a quarter of girls and one-sixth of boys suffer sexual abuse. One in four female students who say they have been sexually harassed at school were victimized by a teacher, coach, bus driver, teacher's aide, security guard, principal, or counselor. By various estimates, sexual infidelity now occurs in a third to one-half of U.S. marriages.

Sex is powerful. It was Freud who said that sexual self-control is essential for civilization. And, we should add, for character.

Any character education worthy of the name must help students develop sexual self-control and the ability to apply core ethical values such as respect and responsibility to the sexual domain. Against that standard, how do various contemporary models of sex education measure up?

The history of modern sex education offers three models. The first two are variations of the nondirective approach: the third, by contrast, is a directive approach.

Comprehensive Sex Education

"Comprehensive sex education," which originated in Sweden in the 1950s and quickly became the prototype for the Western world, was based on four premises:

1. Teenage sexual activity is inevitable.

2. Educators should be value-neutral regarding sex.

3. Schools should openly discuss sexual matters.

4. Sex education should teach students about contraception.

The value-neutral approach to sex soon showed up in American sex education philosophy, as in this statement by the author of the *Curriculum Guide for Sex Education in California:* "'Right' or 'wrong' in so intimate a matter as sexual behavior is as personal as one's name and address. No textbook or classroom teacher can teach it."

What was the impact of nondirective, value-neutral, comprehensive sex education on teenage sexual behavior?

- From 1971 to 1981, government funding at all levels for contraceptive education increased by 4,000 percent. During that time teen pregnancies increased by 20 percent and teen abortions nearly doubled.

- A 1986 Johns Hopkins University study concluded that comprehensive sex education did not reduce teen pregnancies, a finding replicated by other studies.

- A 1986 Lou Harris Poll, commissioned by Planned Parenthood (a leading sponsor of comprehensive sex education), found that teens who took a comprehensive sex education course (including contraceptive education) were significantly *more likely* to initiate sexual intercourse than teens whose sex education courses did not discuss contraceptives.

The "Abstinence, But" Model

Negative results like those cited did not lead comprehensive sex educators to alter their approach—but AIDS did. AIDS led to two modifications: (1) teaching students to practice "safe [or "safer"] sex" through the use of barrier contraception (condoms); and (2) grafting an abstinence message onto the old comprehensive model. These changes resulted in what can be called the "Abstinence, But" approach, which says two things to students:

- Abstinence is the only 100 percent effective way to avoid pregnancy, AIDS, and other sexually transmitted diseases.

- But if you are sexually active, you can reduce these risks through the consistent, correct use of condoms.

This hybrid model, still found in many public and private schools, seems to many like a "realistic" compromise. But closer examination revels fundamental problems in the "Abstinence, But" model.

1. It sends a mixed message.   "Don't have sex, but here's a way to do it fairly safely" amounts to a green light for sexual activity. The problem is that "Abstinence, But" is still nondirective sex education. Abstinence is presented as the safest contraceptive option, but "protected sex" is offered as a "responsible" second option. The emphases is on "making your own decision" rather than on making the right decision.

As a rule, if educators believe that a given activity is ethically wrong—harmful to self and others (as teen sexual activity clearly is)—we help students understand why that is so and guide them toward the right decision. We don't say, for example, "Drug abuse is wrong, but make your own decision, and here's how to reduce the risks if you decide to become drug active."

2. *An abstinence message is further weakened when schools provide how-to condom instructions and/or distribute condoms.* Teachers providing condom instruction will commonly demonstrate how to fit a condom to a model (or students may be asked to put a condom on a banana). In the same nonjudgmental atmosphere, discussion often includes the pros and cons of different lubricants, special precautions for oral and anal sex, and so on. Some schools also take what seems like the next logical step of actually distributing condoms to students. Both actions signal approval of "protected sex" and further undermine an abstinence message.

3. *Condoms do not make sex physically safe.* For all age groups, condoms have a 10 percent annual failure rate in preventing pregnancy; for teens (notoriously poor users), the figure can go as high as 36 percent. By one estimate, a 14-year-old girl who relies on condoms has more that a 50 percent chance of becoming pregnant before she graduates from high school.

Contraceptive sex educators often cite AIDS as the main justification for "safe sex" education, but research shows that condoms do *not* provide adequate protection against AIDS (and, especially among teens, may generate a false sense of security). In a 1993 University of Texas study, the average condom failure rate for preventing AIDS was 31 percent.

While AIDS is still relatively infrequent among teens, other sexually transmitted diseases are epidemic. Many of these diseases—and 80 percent of the time there are no visible symptoms—can be transmitted by areas of the body that are not covered by contraceptive barriers. Human Papilloma Virus, once very rare, is perhaps the most common STD among teens, infecting 38 percent of sexually active females ages 13 to 21. Victims may suffer from venereal warts, painful intercourse, or genital cancer. The virus can also cause cancer of the penis. Condoms provide no protection against this virus.

Chlamydia infects 20 to 40 percent of sexually active singles; teenage girls are most susceptible. In men, chlamydia can cause infertile sperm; in women, pelvic inflammatory disease and infection of the fallopian tubes. A single infection in a woman produces a 25 percent chance of infertility; a second infection, a 50 percent chance. Medical research has found that condoms do not significantly reduce the frequency of tubal infection and infertility stemming from this disease.

Given teenagers' vulnerability to pregnancy despite the use of condoms and the fact that condoms provide inadequate protection against AIDS and no protection against many STDs, it is irresponsible to promote the myth that condoms make sex physically safe.

4. *Condoms do not make sex emotionally safe.*   The emotional and spiritual dimensions of sex are what make it distinctively human. If we care about young people, we will help them understand the destructive emotional and spiritual effects that can come from temporary, uncommitted sexual relationships.

These psychological consequences vary among individuals but include: lowered self-esteem (sometimes linked to sexually transmitted diseases), a sense of having been "used," self-contempt for being a "user," the pain of loss of reputation, compulsive sexual behavior to try to shore up one's damaged self-image, regret and self-recrimination,.rage over rejection or betrayal, difficulty trusting in future relationships, and spiritual guilt if one has a faith tradition that prohibits sex outside marriage (as world religions typically do). Condoms provide zero protection against these emotional consequences.

5. *Nondirective sex education undermines character.*   From the standpoint of character education, the nondirective "Abstinence, But" model fails on several counts:

- It doesn't give unmarried young people compelling ethical reasons to abstain from sexual intercourse until they are ready to commit themselves to another person. Instead, students learn that they are being "responsible" if they use contraception.

- It doesn't help students develop the crucial character quality of self-control—the capacity to curb one's desires and delay gratification. To the extent that sex education is in any way permissive toward teenage sexual activity, it fosters poor character and feeds into the societal problem of sex-out-of-control.

- It doesn't develop an ethical understanding of the relationship between sex and love.

- It doesn't cultivate what young people desperately need if they are to postpone sex: a vision of the solemn, binding commitment between two people in which sex is potentially most meaningful, responsible, and safe (physically and emotionally)— namely, marriage.

Directive Sex Education

By any ethical, educational, or public health measure, nondirective sex education has been a failure. As a result, schools are turning increasingly toward directive sex education— just as the national character education movement is embracing a more directive approach to promoting core ethical values as the basis of good character.

A directive approach means helping young persons—for the sake of their safety, happiness, and character—to see the logic of an "Abstinence, No Buts" standard, often called "chastity education." This standard says three things:

1. Sexual abstinence is the *only* medically safe and morally responsible choice for unmarried teenagers.

2. Condoms do not make premarital sex responsible because they don't make it physically safe, emotionally safe, or ethically loving.

3. The only truly safe sex is having sex *only* with a marriage partner who is having sex *only* with you. If you avoid intercourse until marriage, you will have a much greater chance of remaining healthy and being able to have children.

There are now many carefully crafted curriculums, books, and videos that foster the attitudes that lead teens to choose chastity—a moral choice and a lifestyle that is truly respectful of self and others. Here are some examples:

1. Decision-making: Keys to total success. Facing a serious teen pregnancy problem (147 high school girls known to be pregnant in 1984-85), the San Marcos, California, school system implemented a multifaceted program, which included six-week courses for junior high students on developing study skills, self esteem, and positive moral values; daily 10-minute lessons on "how to be successful"; a six-week course for 8th graders using Teen Aids's curriculum on the advantages of premarital abstinence and how to regain them (for example, self-respect and protection against pregnancy and disease) after having been sexually active; *Window to the Womb*, a video providing ultrasound footage of early fetal development to show students the power of their sexuality to create human life; and summaries of all lessons for parents plus a parent workshop on teaching sexual morality to teens.

After San Marcos implemented this program, known pregnancies at the high school dropped from 20 percent in 1984 to 2.5 percent in 1986 to 1.5 percent in 1988. Meanwhile scores in tests of basic skills went up, and in 1988 San Marcos won an award for the lowest drop-out rate in California.

2. Teen S.T.A.R. (Sexuality Teaching in the context of Adult Responsibility) is currently used with more than 5,000 teens in various regions of the United States and in other countries. The program teaches that fertility is a gift and a power to be respected. Its premise is that "decisions about sexual responsibility will arise from inner conviction and knowledge of the self." More than half of the teens who enter the program sexually active stop sexual activity; very few initiate it.

3. The loving well curriculum, a literature-based program, uses selections from the classics, folktales, and contemporary adolescent literature to examine relationships from family love to infatuation and early romance to marriage. An evaluation finds that of those students who were not sexually active when they started the curriculum, 92 percent are still students who were not sexually active when they started the curriculum, 92 percent are still abstinent two years later, compared to 72 percent abstinent in a control group not exposed to the curriculum.

4. *Postponing sexual involvement* was developed by Emory University's Marion Howard specifically for low-income, inner-city 8th graders at risk for early sexual activity. Of students in the program, 70 percent said it taught them that they "can postpone sexual activity without losing their friends' respect." Participants were *five times less likely* to initiate sexual activity than students who did not take the program.

Other useful resources for directive sex education include:

• *Safe Sex: A Slide Program.* This extremely persuasive slide picture/audiotape presentation argues from medical facts alone that the only safe sex is within marriage. Available from the Medical Institute for Sexual Health, P.O. Box 4919, Austin, TX 78765-4919.

• *Let's Talk—Teens and Chastity.* In this humorous, dynamic video, Molly Kelly—an award-winning educator and mother of eight—addresses a high school assembly on safe sex and chastity. Available from the Center for Learning, Box 910, Villa Maria, PA 16155.

• *Sex, Lies, and the Truth* is a riveting, for-teens video that stresses the hard truths about sex in the '90s. Available from Focus on the Family, Colorado Springs, CO 90955. Also excellent and available from Focus on the Family is *Has Sex Education Failed Our Teenagers?* A Research Report by Dinah Richard.

• *Foundations for Family Life Education: A Guidebook for Professionals and Parents,* by Margaret Whitehead and Onalee McGraw, includes abstinence-based sex education objectives for grades K-10 and a superb annotated bibliography of age-appropriate curriculums and videos. Available from Educational Guidance Institute, 927 S. Walter Reed Dr., Suite 4, Arlington, VA 22204. Forthcoming from the same Institute: *Love and Marriage at the Movies: Educating for Character Through the Film Classics.*

• George Eager's *Love, Dating, and Sex* is one of the best-written books for teens. Available from Mailbox Club Books, 404 Eager Rd., Valdosta, GA 31602.

Answers to Common Questions

Educators committing to directive sex education must be prepared to answer some common questions. Among them:

What about all the teens who will remain sexually active despite abstinence education? Shouldn't they be counseled to use condoms? Obviously, if a person is going to have sex, using a condom will reduce the chance of pregnancy and AIDS, but not to an acceptable level. Condoms offer no protection against many other STDs and their long-term consequences, such as infertility. Schools have the mission of teaching the truth and developing right values—which means helping students understand why the various forms of contraception do not make premarital sex physically or emotionally safe and how premature sexual activity will hurt them now and in the future.

Isn't premarital sexual abstinence a religious or cultural value, as opposed to universal ethical values like love, respect, and honesty? Although religion supports premarital abstinence, it can be demonstrated, through ethical reasoning alone, that reserving sex for marriage is a logical application of ethical values. If we love and respect another, we want what is in the person's best interest. Does sex without commitment meet that criterion? Can we say that we really love someone if we gamble with that criterion? Can we say that we really love someone if we gamble with that person's physical health, emotional happiness, and future life? Given the current epidemic of sexually transmitted diseases, it's possible to argue on medical grounds alone that premarital sexual abstinence is the only ethical choice that truly respects self and other.

Isn't the recommendation to save sex for marriage prejudicial against homosexual persons, since the law does not permit them to marry? All students can be encouraged to follow the recommendation of the U.S. Department of Education's guidebook, *AIDS and the Education of Our Children*:

> Regardless of sexual orientation, the best way for young people to avoid AIDS and other STDs is to refrain from sexual activity until as adults they are ready to establish a mutually faithful monogamous relationship.

Is abstinence education feasible in places, such as the inner city, where poverty and family breakdown are harsh realities? Programs like Atlanta's Postponing Sexual Involvement have a track record of making abstinence education work amid urban poverty. Virginia Governor Douglas Wilder has argued that "the black family is teetering near the abyss of self-destruction" and that "our young, male and female alike, must embrace the self-discipline of abstinence." Sylvia Peters, who won national acclaim for her work as principal of the Alexander Dumas School (K-8) in inner-city Chicago, made the decision to tell her students (6th graders were getting pregnant before she arrived), "Do not have sex until you are married—you will wreck your life." These two black leaders know that the problem of black illegitimate births—up from 35 to 65 percent in little more than two decades—won't be solved until there is a new ethic of sexual responsibility.

Sexual behavior is determined by value, not mere knowledge. Studies show that students who have value orientations (for example, get good grades in school, have high self-regard, consider their religious faith important, have strong moral codes), are significantly less likely to be sexually active than peers who lack these values. These internally held values are more powerful than peer pressure.

Our challenge as educators is this: Will we help to develop these values and educate for character in sex, as in all other areas? If we do not move decisively—in our schools, families, churches, government, and media—to promote a higher standard of sexual morality in our society, we will surely see a continued worsening of the plague of sex-related problems—promiscuity, sexual exploitation and rape, unwed pregnancy, abortions, sexually transmitted diseases, the emotional consequences of uncommitted sex, sexual harassment in schools, children of all ages focused on sex in unwholesome ways, sexual infidelity in marriages, pornography, the sexual abuse of children, and the damage to families caused by many of these problems.

Non directive sex education obviously didn't cause all of these problems, and directive sex education won't solve all of them. But at the very least, sex education in our schools must be part of the solution, not part of the problem.

"Abstinence, No Buts" Is Simplistic

Peggy Brick
Deborah M. Roffman

There are no easy answers to the sexual health crisis afflicting our society, including those advocated by Thomas Lickona. The "Abstinence, No Buts" approach does not adequately address the development needs of children and adolescents, the reality of their lives, or the societal forces that condition their view of the world.

First, Lickona undermines rational dialogue by dividing educators into artificial, polar camps: "values-free-intercourse promoters," who push for contraception-based "comprehensive" sex education (the bad guys), and "values-based-intercourse preventers," who espouse chastity-based "character" education (the good guys). It is neither accurate nor helpful for him to imply that one particular interest group has a corner on instilling character, core values, and ethical thought; on wanting young people to grow up emotionally, socially, physically, and spiritually healthy; on working toward a day when developmental and social problems—such as premature sexual activity, teenage pregnancy, abortion, STD, HIV, sexism, and sexual harassment/abuse/exploitation—no longer threaten our children.

Second, Lickona's definition of "comprehensive" sex education bears little resemblance to the actual approach. Comprehensive sexuality education encompasses not only the complexities of sex and reproduction, but the enormously complicated subjects of human growth and development, gender roles, intimacy, and social and cultural forces that influence our development as males and females (Roffman 1992). Such an approach seeks to help young people understand sexuality as integral to their identity and enables them to make responsible lifelong decisions (SIECUS 1991).

More than 60 mainstream organizations support this approach through membership in the National Coalition to Support Sexuality Education. These include the American Medical Association, American School Health Association, American Association of School Administrators, National School Boards Association, and the Society for Adolescent Medicine. The majority of American adults support such a strategy as well. For example, recent surveys in New Jersey and North Carolina found that at least 85 percent of those surveyed approved of comprehensive sexuality education (Firestone 1993, North Carolina Coalition on Adolescent Pregnancy 1993).

A truly comprehensive approach is on-going and begins during the preschool and elementary years (Montfort, 1993). Curriculum of this type educate, rather than propagandize, children about sexuality. Youngsters learn to ask questions, predict consequences, examine values, and plan for the future. They confront real-life dilemmas: What would happen if? What would you do if? By the middle grades, students learn to take action on issues such as: What can we do to reduce teen pregnancies in this school? To educate students about HIV/AIDS? (See Reis, 1989) Kirby, et al. 1991, Center for Population Options 1992, O'Neill and Roffman 1992, SEICUS 1993). Ideally, this approach to sexuality education will be integrated throughout the entire curriculum (Brick, 1991).

Why Directive Approaches Fail

Those of us committed to comprehensive sex education and to public education in a pluralistic society are not persuaded by the arguments for "directive," ideological sex education for several reasons.

1. It is hypocritical and futile to expect efforts directed at adolescents to solve the nation's myriad sexual problems. Powerful social forces contribute to the early development of unhealthy sexual scripts—about who we are as males or females, how we should act, and issues of right and wrong.

For example, the early learning of male gender roles, often linked with violence and the need to dominate, is fundamentally related to problems of rape and harassment (Miedzian 1991). The manipulation of the sexuality of both males and females from an early age, and the stimulation of sexual desires by advertising and other media, are fundamental to the operation of our economic system (D'Emilio and Freedman, 1988). Adolescent child-bearing, sexually transmitted diseases, and the spread of HIV are highly correlated with poverty and lack of hope for the future (National Research Council, 1987). Further, many problems attributed to teens are not just teen problems: the majority of *all* pregnancies in this country are unplanned (Heller, 1993). Seventy percent of adolescent pregnancies are fathered by adult men (Males, 1993).

2.   Directive approaches require a delay of intercourse 10 or more years beyond biological maturity, which is contrary to practice in virtually all societies—unless there is a strict tradition segregating unmarried males and females and chaperoning women (Francoeur, 1991).

3.   The success of these proposals requires an immediate, fundamental change in the sexual attitudes and behaviors of a society through mere educational intervention. Such a radical change has never been accomplished. Traditionally, the majority of American males have accepted premarital intercourse, and as early as 1973, a study showed 95 percent of males and 85 percent of females approved of it (DeLamater and MacCorquodale, 1979).

4.   Advocates of the directive approach do not prepare youth to make decisions in a highly complex world. They permit no choice but *their* choice and deliberately deny potentially life-saving information to those who do not conform to their viewpoint.

5.   The curriculums espoused are fear-based, characterized by devastating descriptions of the dangers of all nonmarital intercourse and medical misinformation about abortion, sexually transmitted diseases, HIV/AIDS, and the effectiveness of condoms. For example, the major cause of condom failure is incorrect usage. Knowledge of proper condom use, of the variations in quality among brands, and of the substantial increase if effectiveness when condoms are used in combination with spermicides greatly reduces the risk for those who choose to have sexual intercourse. (Kestelman and Trussell, 1991). These sex-negative, emotionally overwhelming, and potentially guilt-producing strategies may well induce problems rather than ameliorate them by leading to unhealthy sexual attitudes, irrational decision making, denial, or rebellion (Fisher, 1989).

Moreover, these curriculums are promoted by groups such as Concerned Women for America, the Eagle Forum, Focus on the Family, and the American Life League, which are lobbying heavily to impose Fundamental Christian doctrine on public schools (Kantor, 1993, Hart, 1993).

Distorted and Misrepresented Data

Given these concerns, claims about the success of abstinence-only programs must be examined with extreme caution. Take, for example, the claim that a program in San Marcos, California, greatly reduced teen pregnancies in the mid-80s. In fact, this claim was not based on a scientific study but on the observation of the high school principal reporting the number of students who *told* the school counselor they were pregnant. After a much-publicized program condemning premarital intercourse, far fewer students reported their pregnancies to school staff; actual census figures for San Marcos indicated that from 1980–1990, the birth rate for mothers aged 14–17 more than doubled (Reynolds, 1991). Many other evaluators have challenged the integrity of research documenting these extraordinary claims in support of abstinence-only curriculums (Trudell and Whatley, 1991. Kirby, et al. 1991, Alan

Guttmacher Institute, 1993). Such programs may change attitudes temporarily (at least as reported to a teacher), but they do not change behavior in any significant way.

Similar statistical distortions have been used to discredit programs that are not abstinence-only in approach. Seriously flawed is the conclusion, based on data collected in a 1986 Lou Harris Poll, that "teens who took a comprehensive sex education course (defined as one including contraceptive education) were subsequently 53 percent more likely to initiate intercourse than teens whose sex education courses did not discuss contraceptives."

First, the survey did not ask when intercourse was initiated in relation to the timing of the program; therefore, the word "subsequently" (implying causation) is patently misleading. Second, the analysis ignored the crucial variable of chronological age. Sexual intercourse among teenagers increases with age, as does the experience of having had a "comprehensive" program. Therefore, causation was implied, when in reality, correlation was the appropriate interpretation.

Besides the use of distorted data, groups demanding an abstinence-only approach dismiss people whose values regarding sexual behaviors differ from their own, asserting that these people are "without values." In fact, comprehensive sex education is based upon core human values that form the foundation of all ethical behavior, such as personal responsibility, integrity, caring for others, and mutual respect in relationships.

Moreover, comprehensive sex education is based on values appropriate to our democratic and pluralistic society—including respect for people's diverse viewpoints about controversial issues.

A Wake-up Call for Society

Our entire society, not just sex education, has failed to provide children and youth with the educational, social, and economic conditions necessary to grow toward sexual health. In fact, truly comprehensive K-12 sexuality education, which at most exists in only 10 percent of schools nationwide, has hardly been tried (Donovan, 1989). Sexuality education—of whatever kind— is neither the cause, nor the cure, for our nations's sexual malaise.

In a society where children's consciousness is permeated by virulent images of sex—where their sexuality is manipulated by advertising and the media, where few adults provide helpful role models—we cannot expect sex education to perform a miracle. Curriculums that provide as their primary or sole strategy admonitions against nonmarital intercourse are destined to be ineffective and, in fact, insult the real-life needs of children and youths. In a society that conveys complex, confusing messages about sexuality, only comprehensive sexuality education can begin to address the diverse needs of youth and promote healthy sexual development.

Debate Presenter Form

Follow the guidelines for debate presenters contained in the introduction of this text and those given to you by your instructor. Use the format below to organize the material for your debate. Remember to include all relevant citation information and to present the related information in your own words. Give credit to authors when you cite a quote and be as thorough as possible when writing about your points so you will be prepared for your debate.

Reference citation #1:

Author: _____

Title: _____

Date: _____

Source: _____

_____

Content from reference citation #1: _____

_____

_____

_____

_____

_____

_____

_____

_____

_____

_____

_____

_____

Reference citation #2:

Author: _____

Title: _____

Date: _____

Source: _____

_____

Content from reference citation #2: _____

_____

_____

_____

_____

_____

_____

Reference citation #3:

Author: _____

Title: _____

Date: _____

Source: _____

_____

Content from reference citation #3: _____

_____

_____

_____

_____

_____

Name _____

Section _____

Audience Preparation Form

Follow the guidelines for preparing to be an informed audience member on the day of the debate included in the introduction to this text. After reading both sides of the debate from this chapter, answer the following questions. Be as thorough as possible so that you will be able to make a contribution to the debate by asking informed questions or making provocative comments. This form is usually due on the day of the debate.

State the issue in your own words. Do not plagiarize the text. Demonstrate that you understand the topic and it's relevant arguments.

_____
_____
_____
_____
_____

Discuss two points on the "yes" side of the debate.

Point #1: _____
_____

Point #2: _____
_____

Discuss two points on the "no" side of the debate.

Point #1: _____
_____

Point #2: _____
_____

What is your opinion on this topic?

_____

_____

_____

_____

_____

_____

_____

What has contributed to the development of your views about this topic?

_____

_____

_____

_____

_____

_____

_____

What information would be necessary to cause you to change your thinking about this topic?

_____

_____

_____

_____

_____

Debate Response Form

Follow the guidelines for responding to the debates in the introductory chapter of this text. Complete this form and submit your answers at the class following the debate. Try to be thorough and convince your instructor that you were an active listener during the debate.

List a quote from a debate presenter that you think was important and explain why you think this comment was significant.

_____

_____

_____

_____

Which side of the debate do you think made the most convincing arguments, why?

_____

_____

_____

_____

_____

After hearing the debate, in what way has your thinking been affected?

_____

_____

_____

_____

_____

_____

Human Sexual Behavior

ISSUE 11

Is Sexual Harassment a Pervasive Problem?

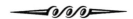

YES Catharine R. Stimpson, *Over-Reaching: Sexual Harassment and Education*

NO Gretchen Morgenson, *May I Have the Pleasure*

As the graduate dean of a large public university, Catharine Stimpson experiences first hand the pervasiveness of sexual harassment. She attributes this behavior to inequities of power; the male most often in the powerful position, the female more powerless.

Because of the prevalence of sexual harassment, four elements of a solution have been implemented on Stimpson's campus: recognition of the problem, administrative leadership in addressing the problem, workshops to raise consciousness about harassment and grievance procedures.

Gretchen Morgenson does not believe that sexual harassment pervades our work places and that the perception that it does is a product of media hype and public hysteria. She cites studies demonstrating a reduction in the number of incidences of sexual harassment. Also, of the cases filed, few result in benefits to the complainant.

Morgenson suggests that it is consulting companies who provide educational workshops to prevent sexual harassment that promote the belief in its existence for profit. In addition to this issue, Morgensen says a major complication in the estimates of the prevalence of sexual harassment is the lack of a clear definition of the term. She also suggests that as women become a greater percentage of our workforce, the incidents of sexual harassment will be even fewer in number than we experience today.

Applications

1. How has your definition of the term "sexual harassment" been influenced?

2. What do you think is the cause of sexual harassment?

3. Outline a program for sixth grade aimed at eliminating sexual harassment.

Issue 11
YES

Over-Reaching
Sexual Harassment and Education

Catherine R. Stimpson

Sexual harassment is an ancient shame that has become a modern embarrassment. Largely because of the pressure of feminism and feminists, such a shift in status took place during the 1970s. Today, the psychological and social pollution that harassment spews out is like air pollution. No one defends either of them. We have classified them as malaises that damage people and their environments. For this reason, both forms of pollution are largely illegal. In 1986, in *Meritor Savings Bank v. Vinson*, the Supreme Court held an employer liable for acts of sexual harassment that its supervisory personnel might commit.

Yet, like air pollution, the psychological and social pollution of sexual harassment persists. In the stratosphere, chlorofluorocarbons from aerosol sprays and other products break apart and help to destroy the ozone layer. Well below the stratosphere, in classrooms and laboratories sexual louts refuse to disappear, imposing themselves on a significant proportion of our students.[1] As the graduate dean at a big public university, I experience, in my everyday life, the contradiction between disapproval of sexual harassment and the raw reality of its existence. I work, with men and women of good will, to end harassment. We must work, however, because the harassers are among us.

Inevitably, then, we must ask why sexual harassment persists, why we have been unable to extirpate this careless and cruel habit of the heartless. As we know, but must continue to repeat, a major reason is the historical strength of the connections among sexuality, gender, and power. But one demonstration of the force of these connections, sexual harassment, floats at the mid-point of an ugly, long-lasting continuum. At the most glamorous end of the continuum is a particular vision of romance, love, and erotic desire. Here men pursue women for their mutual pleasure. That promise of pleasure masks the inequities of power. "Had we but world enough, and time," a poet [Andrew Marcell] sings, "The coyness, Lady, were no crime." But for the poet, there is not enough world, not enough time. The lady, then, must submit to him before"... Worms shall try/That long preserv'd Virginity." At the other end of the continuum is men's coercion of women's bodies, the brutalities of incest and of rape, in which any pleasure is perverse.

In the mid-nineteenth century, Robert Browning wrote a famous dramatic monologue, "Andrea Del Sarto." In the poem, a painter is using his wife as a model. As he paints, he speaks, muses, and broods. He is worried about his marriage, for his model/wife is apparently faithless, a less than model wife. He is worried about his art, for his talents many be inadequate. He is, finally, worried about his reputation, for other painters may be gaining on and surpassing him. In the midst of expressing his fears, he declares, "Ah, but a man's reach should exceed his grasp/Or what's a heaven for...." Traditional interpretations of his poem have praised Browning for praising the necessity of man's ambitions, of man's reaching out for grandeur. Indeed, Del Sarto, in an act of minor blasphemy, casts heaven not as God's space but as man's reminder that he has not yet achieved his personal best. Unhappily, these interpretations go on, women can hurt men in the noble quests. Fickle, feckless, the feminine often embarks on her own quest, a search-and-destroy mission against male grandeur.

A revisionary interpretation of "Andrea Del Sarto," however, can find the poem a different kind of parable about sexuality, gender, and power. In this reading, a man has at least two capacities. First, he can reach out and move about in public space and historical time. Del Sarto goes after both canvas and fame. Next, he can define a woman's identity, here through talking about her and painting her portrait. Del Sarto literally shapes the image of his wife. Ironically, he wants to believe that he is a victim. He exercises his powers in order to demonstrate that he is powerless. A man, he projects himself as a poor baby who cannot shape up his mate.

A sexual harasser in higher education reveals similar, but more sinister, capacities. The hierarchical structure of institutions sends him a supportive message: the arduous climb up the ladder is worth it. The higher a man goes, the more he deserves and ought to enjoy the sweetness and freedoms of his place.[2] First, a man reaches out for what he wants. He makes sexual "advances." His offensive weapons can be linguistic (a joke, for example) or physical (a touch). He warns the powerless that he has the ability to reach out in order to grasp and get what he wants. He also demonstrates to himself that he is able to dominate a situation. As the psychoanalyst Ethel Spector Person has pointed out, for many men, sexuality and domination are inseparable. To be sexual is to dominate and to be reassured of the possession of the power to dominate (Person, 1980).[3]

Usually, women compose the powerless group, but it may contain younger men as well, the disadvantages of age erasing the advantages of gender. One example: a 1986 survey at the University of Illinois/Champaign-Urbana found that 19 percent of the female graduate students, 10 percent of the undergraduates, and 8 percent of the professional school students had experienced harassment. So, too, had 5 percent of the male respondents. In all but one incident, the harasser was another man (Allen & Okawa, 1987).

Second, the harasser assumes the right to define the identity of the person whom he assaults. To him, she is not mind, but body; not student, not professional, but sexual being. She is who and what the harasser says she is. Ironically, like Andrea Del Sarto, many academics project their own power onto a woman and then assert that she, not he, has power.[4] He, not she, is powerless. Her sexuality seduces and betrays him. This psychological maneuver must help to explain one fear that people express about sexual harassment policies—that such policies will permit, even encourage, false complaints against blameless faculty and staff. A recent study found 78 percent of respondents worried about loss of due process and about the fate of innocent people who might be accused of misconduct. Yet, the study concluded, less than 1 percent of all sexual harassment complaints each year *are* false. The deep problem is not wrongful accusations against the innocent, but the refusal of the wronged to file any complaint at all. In part they believe they should handle sexual matters themselves. In part, they hope the problem will go away if they ignore it. In part, they fear retaliation, punishment for stepping out of line (Robertson, Dyer, & Campbell, 1988).

The unreasonable fear about false complaints is also a symptom of the blindness of the powerful to the realities of their own situation. They enjoy its benefits but are unable to see its nature and costs to other people. They are like a driver of an inherited sports car who loves to drive but refuses to learn where gas and oil come from, who services the car when it is in the garage, or why pedestrians might shout when he speeds through a red light. In a probing essay, Molly Hite (1988) tells a story about a harasser on a United States campus, a powerful professor who abused his authority over female graduate students. He damaged several women, psychologically and professionally. Yet even after that damage became public knowledge, he survived, reputation intact, although he did discreetly move to another campus. Hite inventories the responses of her colleagues to this event. Men, no matter what their academic rank, tended to underplay the seriousness of his behavior. They thought that he had acted "normally," if sometimes insensitively, that the women had acted abnormally and weakly. Women, no matter what their academic rank, tended to sympathize with the female victims. They could identify with powerlessness. Hite writes, "The more the victim is someone who could be you, the easier it is to be scared. By the same reasoning, it's possible to be cosmically un-scared, even to find the whole situation trival the point of absurdity, if you can't imagine ever being the victim" (p.9).

So far, higher education has participated in building at least four related modes of resistance to sexual harassment. First, we have named the problem *as a problem*. We have pushed it into public consciousness as an issue. The Equal Employment Opportunity Commission guidelines, in particular, have provided a citable, national language with which to describe harassment, a justifiable entry in the dictionary of our concerns. Next, we have learned how much administrative leadership has mattered in urging an institution to address this concern. Not surprisingly, faculties have not moved to reform themselves. Next, workshops that educate people about the nature of harassment do seem to reduce its virulence. Finally, we have created grievance procedures with which we can hear complaints, investigate them, and punish harassers.[5] The most carefully designed in themselves help to empower women. The process does not itself perpetuate her sense of self as victim (Hoffman, 1986).

These modes of resistance, good in themselves, have also done good. They have shown an institution's commitment to a fair, non-polluting social environment. They have warned potential harassers to stop. They have offered some redress to the harassed. Resistance will, however, be of only limited good unless a rewriting of the historical connections among sexuality, gender, and power accompanies it. Similarly, putting up traffic lights on crowded streets is good. Lights are, however, of only limited good unless drivers believe in the rights of other drivers, in safety, and in the limits of their machines.

In such a rewriting, an act of "over-reaching" will be interpreted not as aspiration and desire, but as an invasion of another person's body, dignity, and livelihood. No one will feel the approaching grasp of the harasser as a welcome clasp. Over-reaching will be a sign not of grace but of disgrace, not of strength but of callousness and, possible, anxiety, not of virility but of moral and psychological weakness. It will not be a warm joke between erotic equals, but a smutty titter from an erotic jerk. The rhetoric of neither romance nor comedy will be able to paint over the grammar of exploitation.[6]

One consequence of this rewriting will be to expand our modes of resistance to include a general education curriculum, not simply about harassment as a phenomenon, but about power itself, which harassment symptomizes. This will mean teaching many men to cut the ties among selfhood, masculinity, and domination. It will mean teaching many women to cut the ties among self, femininity, and intimacy at any price, including the price of submission. Occasionally, reading a sexual harassment complaint from a young woman, I have asked myself, in some rue and pain, why she has acted *like a woman*. By that, I have meant that her training for womanhood has taught her to value closeness, feeling, relationships. Find and dandy, but too often, she takes this lesson to heart above all others.

The first part of the curriculum, for women, will remind them of their capacity for resistance, for saying no. Telling a harasser to stop can be effective.[7] Speaking out, acting verbally, can also empower an individual woman. Less fortunately, these speech acts reconstitute the traditional sexual roles of man as hunter, woman as prey. Unlike a rabbit or doe, she is responsible for setting the limits of the hunt, for fencing in the game park. If the hunter violates these limits, it is because she did not uphold them firmly enough. Moreover, saying no to the aggressor also occurs in private space. Because of this location, both harasser and harassed can forget that these apparently private actions embody, in little, grosser structures of authority.

The second part of the curriculum will be for men and women. Fortunately, women's studies programs are not developed enough to serve as a resource for an entire institution that chooses to offer lessons about gender and power. These lessons will do more than anatomize abuses. They will also present an ethical perspective, which the practices of college and universities might well represent. This ethic will cherish a divorce between sexuality and the control of another person, an unbridgeable distance between a lover's pleasure and a bully's threat. This ethic will also ask us to cherish our capacities to care for each other, to attend to each other's needs without manipulating them.[8] We will reach out to each other without grasping, hauling, pushing, mauling.

The struggle against sexual harassment, then, is part of a larger struggle to replant the moral grounds of education. Our visionary hope is that we will, in clear air, harvest new gestures, laws, customs, and practices. We will still take poets as our prophets. When we do so, however, we might replace the dramatic monologue of a fraught, Renaissance painter with that of a strong-willed, late twentieth-century feminist. In 1977, in "Natural Resources?" Adrienne Rich spoke for those who stubbornly continue to believe in visionary hope:

> *"My heart is moved by all I cannot save: so much has been destroyed. I have to cast my lot with those who age after age, perversely, with no extraordinary power, reconstitute the world."*

Notes

1.   The authors of a survey of 311 institutions of higher education, conducted in 1984, estimate that one woman out of four experiences some form of harassment as a student (Robertson et al., 1988). A survey of a single institution, a large public research university, found that 31 percent of the more than 700 respondents had been subjected to "sex-stereotyped jokes, remarks, references, or examples" ("Survey documents," 1988, pp. 41–42).

2.   As Robertson et al. comment, "individuals in positions of authority... (are) used to viewing professional status as expanding privilege rather than increasing responsibility and obligation" (p. 808). An anecdote illustrates this generalization. Recently, I was chairing a meeting of the graduate faculty of my university. Our agenda item was a proposal to conduct a periodic review of faculty members, program by program, to help insure they were still qualified to be graduate teachers. A professor, well-known for his decency, stood up in opposition. He said, "When I got tenure, I became a member of a club, and no one is going to tell me what to do. If I don't want to publish, that's my business."

3.   Not coincidentally, most of the sexual harassers whom I have had to investigate as graduate dean have had streaks of arrogance, flare-ups of vanity. In contrast, the men who have been most sympathetic to the necessity of my investigations have had a certain ethical poise, a balance of standards and stability.

4.   An obvious parallel is a traditional response to rape, in which women are held culpable for being raped. Moreover, like versions of Jezebel, they are thought only too likely to cry rape in order to cover up their own sins.

5.   I am grateful to Robertson et. al. (1988) for their description of various modes of resistance to harassment. Their study also explores the reasons why public institutions have been more sensitive than private institutions. More specifically, Beauvais (1986) describes workshops that deal with harassment for residence hall staff at the University of Michigan.

6.   Disguising the language of harassment as humor has several advantages. First, it draws on our old, shrewd assessment of much sexual behavior as funny and comic. Next, it simultaneously inflates the harasser to the status of good fellow, able to tell a joke, and deflates the harassed to the status of prude, unable to take one.

7. Allen and Okawa (1987) say that this worked for two-thirds of the respondents in their study of harassment at the University of Illinois.

8. Tronto (1987) suggestively outlines a theory of care that educational institutions might adopt.

References

Allen, D., & Okawa, J.B. (1987). A counseling center looks at sexual harassment. *Journal of the National Association for Women Deans, Administrators, and Counselors*, 51(1), 9–16.

Beauvais, K. (1986). Workshops to combat sexual harassment: A case study of changing attitudes. *Signs*, 12(1), 130–145.

Hite, M. (1988). Sexual harassment and the university community. Unpublished manuscript.

Hoffman, F.L. (1986). Sexual harassment in academia. *Harvard Education Review*, 56(2), 105–121.

Person, E. (1980). Sexuality as the mainstay of identity. In C.R. Stimpson & E.S. Person (eds.), *Women: Sex and sexuality*. Chicago: University of Chicago Press.

Robertson, C., Dyer, C.C., & Campbell, D.A. (1988). Campus harassment: Sexual harassment policies and procedures at institutions of higher learning. *Signs*, 13(4), 792–812.

Survey documents sexual harassment at U. Mass. (1988). *Liberal Education*, 74(2), 41–2.

Tronto, J.C. (1987). Beyond gender differences to a theory of care. *Signs*, 12(4), 644–663.

May I Have the Pleasure

Gretchen Morgenson

On October 11 [1991], in the middle of the Anita Hill/Clarence Thomas contretemps, the *New York Times* somberly reported that sexual harassment pervades the American workplace. The source for this page-one story was a *Times*/CBS poll conducted two days earlier in which a handful (294) of women were interviewed by telephone. Thirty-eight percent of respondents confirmed that they had been at one time or another "the object of sexual advances, propositions, or unwanted sexual discussions from men who supervise you or can affect your position at work." How many reported the incident at the time it happened? Four percent.

Did the *Times* offer any explanation for why so few actually reported the incident? Could it be that these women did not report their "harassment" because they themselves did not regard a sexual advance as harassment? Some intelligent speculation on this matter might shed light on a key point: the vague definitions of harassment that make it easy to allege, hard to identify, and almost impossible to prosecute. Alas, the *Times* was in no mood to enlighten its readers.

It has been more than ten years since the Equal Employment Opportunity Commission (EEOC) wrote its guidelines defining sexual harassment as a form of sexual discrimination and, therefore, illegal under Title VII of the Civil Rights Act of 1964. According to the EEOC there are two different types of harassment: so-called *quid pro quo* harassment, in which career or job advancement is guaranteed in return for sexual favors, and environmental harassment, in which unwelcome sexual conduct "unreasonably interferes" with an individual's working environment or creates an "intimidating, hostile, or offensive working environment."

Following the EEOC's lead, an estimated three out of four companies nationwide have instituted strict policies against harassment; millions of dollars are spent each year educating employees in the subtleties of Title VII etiquette. Men are warned to watch their behavior, to jettison the patronizing pat and excise the sexist comment from their vocabularies.

Yet, if you believe what you read in the newspapers, we are in the Stone Age where the sexes are concerned. A theme common to the media, plaintiff's lawyers, and employee-relations consultants is that male harassment of women is costing corporations millions each year in lost productivity and low employee morale. "Sexual harassment costs a typical Fortune 500 Service or Manufacturing company $6.7 million a year" says a sexual-harassment survey conducted late in 1988 for *Working Woman* by Klein Associates. This Boston consulting firm is part of a veritable growth industry which has sprung up to dispense sexual-harassment advice to worried companies in the form of seminars, videos, and encounter groups.

But is sexual harassment such a huge problem in business? Or is it largely a product of hype and hysteria? The statistics show that sexual harassment is less prevalent today than it was five years ago. According to the EEOC, federal cases alleging harassment on the job totaled 5,694 in 1990, compared to 6,342 in 1984. Yet today there are 17 percent more women working than there were then.

At that, the EEOC's figures are almost certainly too high. In a good many of those complaints, sexual harassment may be tangential to the case; the complaint may primarily involve another form of discrimination in Title VII territory: race, national origin, or religious discrimination, for example. The EEOC doesn't separate cases involving sexual harassment alone; any case where sexual harassment is mentioned, even in passing, gets lumped into its figures.

Many of the stories depicting sexual harassment as a severe problem spring from "consultants" whose livelihoods depend upon exaggerating its extent. In one year, DuPont spent $450,000 on sexual-harassment training programs and materials. Susan Webb, president of Pacific Resources Development Group, a Seattle consultant, says she spends 95 percent of her time advising on sexual harassment. Like most consultants, Miss Webb acts as an expert witness in harassment cases, conducts investigations for companies and municipalities, and teaches seminars. She charges clients $1,500 for her 35-minute sexual-harassment video program and handbooks.

Unfelt Needs

Corporations began to express concern on the issue back in the early Eighties, just after the EEOC published its first guidelines. But it was *Meritor Savings Bank v. Vinson*, a harassment case that made it to the Supreme Court in 1985, that really acted as an employment act for sex-harassment consultants. In *Vinson*, the Court stated that employers could limit their liability to harassment claims by implementing anti-harassment policies and procedures in the workplace. And so, the anti-harassment industry was born.

Naturally, the consultants believe they are filling a need, not creating one. "Harassment is still as big a problem as it has been because the workplace is not integrated," says Susan Webb. Ergo, dwindling numbers of cases filed with the EEOC are simply not indicative of a diminution in the problem.

Then what do the figures indicate? Two things, according to the harassment industry. First, that more plaintiffs are bringing private lawsuits against their employers than are suing through the EEOC or state civil-rights commissions. Second, that the number of cases filed is a drop in the bucket compared to the number of actual, everyday harassment incidents.

It certainly stands to reason that a plaintiff in a sexual-harassment case would prefer bringing a private action against her employer to filing an EEOC claim. EEOC and state civil-rights cases allow plaintiffs only compensatory damages, such as back pay or legal fees. In order to collect big money—punitive damages—from an employer, a plaintiff must file a private action.

Yet there's simply no proof that huge or increasing numbers of private actions are being filed today. No data are collected on numbers of private harassment suits filed, largely because they're brought as tort actions—assault and battery, emotional distress, or breach of contract. During the second half of the Eighties, the San Francisco law firm of Orrick, Herrington, and Sutcliffe monitored private sexual-harassment cases filed in California. Its findings: From 1984 to 1989, the number of sexual-harassment cases in California that were litigated through a verdict totaled a whopping 15. That's in a state with almost six million working women.

Of course, cases are often settled prior to a verdict. But how many? Orrick, Herrington partner Ralph H. Baxter Jr., management co-chairman of the American Bar Association's Labor Law Committee on Employee Rights and Responsibilities, believes the number of private sexual-harassment cases launched today is greatly overstated. "Litigation is not as big a problem as it's made out to be; You're not going to see case after case," says Mr. Baxter. "A high percentage of matters go to the EEOC and a substantial number of cases get resolved."

Those sexual-harassment actions that do get to a jury are the ones that really grab headlines. A couple of massive awards have been granted in recent years—five plaintiffs were awarded $3.8 million by a North Carolina jury—but most mammoth awards are reduced on appeal. In fact, million-dollar sexual-harassment verdicts are still exceedingly rare. In California, land of the happy litigator, the median jury verdict for all sexual-harassment cases litigated between 1984 and 1989 was $183,000. The top verdict in the state was just under $500,000, the lowest was $45,000. And California, known for its sympathetic jurors, probably produces higher awards than most states.

Now to argument number two: that the number of litigated harassment cases is tiny compared to the number of actual incidents that occur. Bringing a sexual-harassment case is similar to filing a rape case, consultants and lawyers say; both are nasty proceedings which involve defamation, possible job loss, and threats to both parties' family harmony.

It may well be that cases of perceived harassment go unfiled, but is it reasonable to assume that the numbers of these unfiled cases run into the millions? Consider the numbers of cases filed that are dismissed for "no probable cause." According to the New York State human-rights commission, almost two-thirds of the complaints filed in the past five years were dismissed for lack of probable cause. Of the two hundred sexual-harassment cases the commission receives a year, 38 percent bring benefits to the complainant.

What about private actions? No one keeps figures on the percentage of cases nationwide won by the plaintiff versus the percentage that are dismissed. However, the outcomes of private sexual-harassment suits brought in California from 1984 to 1989 mirror the public figures from New York. According to Orrick, Herrington, of the 15 cases litigated to a verdict in California from 1984 to 1989, slightly less than half were dismissed and slightly more than half (53 per cent) were won by the plaintiff.

Are California and New York anomalies? Stephen Perlman, a partner in labor law at the Boston firm of Ropes & Gray, who has 15 years' experience litigating sexual-harassment cases, thinks not: "I don't suppose I've had as many as a dozen cases go to litigation. Most of the cases I've seen—the vast majority—get dismissed. They don't even have probable cause to warrant further processing."

What Is Harassment?

A major problem is the vague definition of harassment. If "environmental harassment" were clearly defined and specifiable, lawyers would undoubtedly see more winnable cases walk through their doors. Asking a subordinate to perform sexual favors in exchange for a raise is clearly illegal. But a dirty joke? A pin-up? A request for a date?

In fact, behavior which one woman may consider harassment could be seen by another as a non-threatening joke. The closest thing to harassment that I have experienced during my 15-year career occurred in the early Eighties when I was a stockbroker-in-training at Dean Witter Reynolds of New York City. I had brought in the largest personal account within Dean Witter's entire retail brokerage system, an account which held roughly $20 million in blue-chip stocks. Having this account under my management meant I had a larger capital responsibility than any of my colleagues, yet I was relatively new to the business. My fellow brokers were curious, but only one was brutish enough to walk right up to me and pop the question: "How did you get that account? Did you sleep with the guy?"

Instead of running away in tears, I dealt with him as I would any rude person. "Yeah," I answered. "Eat your heart out." He turned on his heel and never bothered me again. Was my colleague a harasser, or just practicing Wall Street's aggressive humor, which is dished out to men in other ways? Apparently, I am in the minority in thinking the latter. But the question remains. Whose standards should be used to define harassment?

Under tort law, the behavior which has resulted in a case—such as an assault or the intent to cause emotional distress—must be considered objectionable by a "reasonable person." The EEOC follows this lead and in its guidelines defines environmental harassment as that which "unreasonably interferes with an individual's job performance."

Yet, sexual-harassment consultants argue that any such behavior—even that which is perceived as harassment only by the most hypersensitive employee—ought to be considered illegal and stamped out. In fact, they say, the subtler hostile-environment cases are the most common and cause the most anguish. Says Frieda Klein, the Boston consultant: "My goal is to create a corporate climate where every employee feels free to object to behavior, where people are clear about their boundaries and can ask that objectionable behavior stop."

Sounds great. But rudeness and annoying behavior cannot be legislated out of existence; nor should corporations be forced to live under the tyranny of a hypersensitive employee. No woman should have to run a daily gauntlet of sexual innuendo, but neither is it reasonable for women to expect a pristine work environment free of coarse behavior.

Susan Hartzoge Gray, a labor lawyer at Haworth, Riggs, Kuhn, and Haworth in Raleigh, North Carolina, believes that hostile-environment harassment shouldn't be actionable under Title VII. "How can the law say one person's lewd and another's nice? she asks. "There are so many different taste levels.... We condone sexual jokes and innuendoes in the media—a movie might get a PG rating—yet an employer can be called on the carpet because the same thing bothers someone in an office."

But changing demographics may do more to eliminate genuine sexual harassment than all the apparatus of law and consultancy. As women reach a critical mass in the workforce, the problem of sexual harassment tends to go away. Frieda Klein says the problem practically vanishes once 30 percent of the workers in a department, an assembly line, or a company are women.

Reaching that critical mass won't take long. According to the Bureau of Labor Statistics, there will be 66 million women to 73 million men in the workplace by 2000. They won't all be running departments of heading companies, of course, but many will.

So sexual harassment will probably become even less of a problem in the years ahead than it is today. But you are not likely to read that story in a major newspaper anytime soon.

Debate Presenter Form

Follow the guidelines for debate presenters contained in the introduction of this text and those given to you by your instructor. Use the format below to organize the material for your debate. Remember to include all relevant citation information and to present the related information in your own words. Give credit to authors when you cite a quote and be as thorough as possible when writing about your points so you will be prepared for your debate.

Reference citation #1:

Author: _____

Title: _____

Date: _____

Source: _____

_____

Content from reference citation #1: _____

_____

_____

_____

_____

_____

_____

_____

_____

_____

_____

_____

Reference citation #2:

Author: _____

Title: _____

Date: _____

Source: _____

_____

Content from reference citation #2: _____

_____

_____

_____

_____

_____

_____

Reference citation #3:

Author: _____

Title: _____

Date: _____

Source: _____

_____

Content from reference citation #3: _____

_____

_____

_____

_____

Audience Preparation Form

Follow the guidelines for preparing to be an informed audience member on the day of the debate included in the introduction to this text. After reading both sides of the debate from this chapter, answer the following questions. Be as thorough as possible so that you will be able to make a contribution to the debate by asking informed questions or making provocative comments. This form is usually due on the day of the debate.

State the issue in your own words. Do not plagiarize the text. Demonstrate that you understand the topic and it's relevant arguments.

_____

_____

_____

_____

_____

Discuss two points on the "yes" side of the debate.

Point #1: _____

_____

Point #2: _____

_____

Discuss two points on the "no" side of the debate.

Point #1: _____

_____

Point #2: _____

_____

What is your opinion on this topic?

_____
_____
_____
_____
_____
_____
_____

What has contributed to the development of your views about this topic?

_____
_____
_____
_____
_____
_____
_____

What information would be necessary to cause you to change your thinking about this topic?

_____
_____
_____
_____
_____

Name _____

Section _____

Debate Response Form

Follow the guidelines for responding to the debates in the introductory chapter of this text. Complete this form and submit your answers at the class following the debate. Try to be thorough and convince your instructor that you were an active listener during the debate.

List a quote from a debate presenter that you think was important and explain why you think this comment was significant.

_____

_____

_____

_____

Which side of the debate do you think made the most convincing arguments, why?

_____

_____

_____

_____

_____

After hearing the debate, in what way has your thinking been affected?

_____

_____

_____

_____

_____

_____

Human Sexual Behavior

ISSUE 12

Can Sex Be an Addiction?

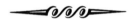

YES Patrick Carnes, *Progress in Sex Addiction: An Addiction Perspective*

NO Marty Klein, *Why There's No Such Thing as Sexual Addiction—And Why It Really Matters*

Patrick Carnes believes strongly that people can be addicted to sexual behavior. As an addictionologist, Carnes has contributed a definition of "sex addict" as: "people whose sexual behavior has become 'unstoppable' despite serious consequences."

Carnes has also described the addictive cycle as: belief system → impaired thinking → preoccupation → ritualization → sexual compulsivity → despair → unmanageability → belief system. As a treatment approach, family system theory can be successfully used according to Carnes. He concludes that additional research is needed to verify the encouraging preliminary results of family systems focused therapy for sex addicts.

Marty Klein, a sexologist, says that in order for sex to be an addiction it would have to be dangerous. Since he and his colleagues in sexology do not see danger in sex, he believes that sex cannot be an addiction. Rather than send someone with sexual problems to a 12-step program, Klein suggests psychotherapy with a trained sexologist not an addictionologist.

He sees the message of sex as an addiction for addictionologists as a threat to the patient, who may not receive appropriate and effective treatment. And to sexologists, whose professional credibility is diminished because he or she might not be "in recovery" from a sexual addiction and therefore, might be disqualified as a therapist. The sexual addiction approach is replacing sexologists as the relevant experts with addictionologists who have less professional training to work with people with sexual problems.

Applications

1. What would you say to a person who told you they feared he or she might be a sex addict?

2. Can the addiction model explain sexually compulsive behavior?

3. What are the problems with defining sexual compulsions as addictions?

Issue 12
YES

Progress in Sex Addiction
An Addiction Perspective

Patrick Carnes

Over the last fifteen years the new professional discipline of addictionology has emerged from the extensive foundations laid in both research and treatment of alcohol and drug addictions. Led by organizations like the American Academy of Addictionology and scholarly publications like the *Journal of Addictive Behaviors*, researchers have found that different addictive behaviors (e.g. compulsive eating, alcoholism, compulsive gambling, smoking) have much in common. It is not surprising that sex has only recently been added to the list, given the guilt and shame still attached to the subject. Nor should it surprise us that the professional controversy far exceeds that of other forms of addiction.

Defining Sexual Addiction

The fact remains that a significant number of people have identified themselves as sexual addicts: people whose sexual behavior has become "unstoppable" despite serious consequences. These consequences include the physical (self-mutilation, sexual violence, disease, unwanted pregnancy), occupational (large financial losses, job losses, sexual abuse and harassment, withdrawal of professional licenses), and familial (loss of relationships, impaired family functioning, sexual abuse, sexual dysfunction). In addition to those problems, one of the most frequent mental health complaints of sexual addicts is suicidal ideation.

Another frequent complaint of "recovering" sex addicts is that the mental health community does not acknowledge their problem. They become enraged when sexologists dismiss sexual addiction as a problem of sexual misinformation, or excessive guilt due to a cultural dissonance, or not a serious or widespread problem. I recently spoke at a Sexaholics Anonymous convention in which participants were rageful and moved to tears over statements made by professionals in a *New York Times* article. Stepping back from the intensity of their feelings, I had to reflect that compared to the amount of time to gain acceptance for the concept of alcoholism, the progress made in sexual addiction is remarkable.

My purpose here is to summarize this progress from an addictionologist's point of view and to specify further challenges which will require the close cooperation of specialists in addiction and professionals in human sexuality.

Case Study

Consider the case of Larry, a 45-year-old manager of a computer programming department. Larry was arrested for exhibitionism and sent to a court-mandated group for eight sessions. The group focused on the exposing behavior, but from Larry's point of view it was merely the tip of the iceberg. He had a 15-year collection of pornography, carefully cataloged and indexed. He saw prostitutes three to four times a month and masturbated daily—sometimes five times in one day. His sexual relationship with his wife, Joan, had diminished largely due to her rage at his increasing sexual demands and his sexual affairs with other women. Part of her response was to overeat so much that she gained over 125 pounds.

Larry also used marijuana and cocaine, ironic considering his intense hatred of his dad's drinking problem, another form of substance abuse. A further irony was that his wife bought the drugs for Larry because, as she later reported, it was better to have him stoned at home than out cruising around.

Larry lived in constant fear of discovery that his children, wife, or church community should find out about the range of his activities. He hated his life and was constantly trying to cope financially to support his sexual activities and drug use.

Venereal disease created a crisis in the marriage, and with the help of their physician, Larry and Joan entered a hospital outpatient program for sexual addiction. Larry found that he was not alone in his problems. Many of the patients had the same or similar issues. In an interview with Larry two-and-a-half years later, upon completion of his treatment, he recounted that there were three main changes in his life since he began treatment. First, his sexuality had shifted dramatically. No longer was he pursuing a desire that he never seemed able to satisfy. Now he and Joan were learning and enjoying sex in different ways than they had believed possible. Second, he had time for work and play. And third, he was no longer living in constant jeopardy of being discovered or running out of money.

In *Out of the Shadows: Understanding Sexual Addiction*, I describe a model (see Figure 1) in which the principle momentum for the addiction in addicts like Larry comes from a per-

Figure 1
The Addictive System

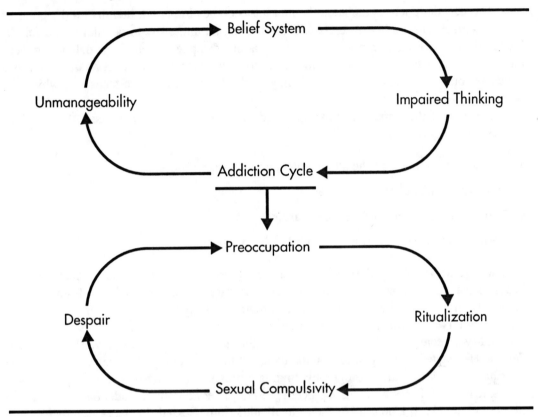

From Patrick Carnes, *Out of the Shadows: Understanding Sexual Addiction* (Minneapolis, MN: CompCare Publishers, 1983). Copyright © 1983 by Patrick Carnes, Ph.D. Reprinted by permission of CompCare Publishers.

sonal belief system. This belief system captures all the cultural and familial messages about sex and relationships. When these messages are very sex negative and are coupled with low self esteem, core beliefs about one's own innate shamefulness emerge. Shame is basically a problem of mastery (why is it other kids can do this and I can't?). When the shame is sexual (why is it other people seem to be in control of their sexual feelings and I am not?), the environment for obsessive behavior is at its optimum.

Impaired Thinking

Through these lenses the addict's thinking becomes impaired, literally, to the point of loss of contact with reality. Addicts talk of entering an altered state parallel to the Jekyll-Hyde shift where even common sense considerations disappear. Denial and delusion govern their lives. One addict, for example, told of following a woman into what he thought was a restaurant only to discover himself standing in the lobby of a police station to which the woman had fled.

Because of the impaired thinking, an addiction cycle perpetuates itself through four phases:

- preoccupation in which the addict enters a trance-like obsession

- ritualization that enhances the trance

- sexual behavior that is often not rewarding

- despair that, once again, the behavior has been repeated.

One way to stave off the despair is to start the preoccupation over again. And the cycle becomes the recursive series of events which dominates the addict's life. With this process underway, the addict's life becomes more and more unmanageable, thus confirming the basic feelings of unworthiness that are the core of the addict's belief system.

Larry's secretive life was embedded in this process of shame, powerlessness, and despair. He wanted very much to stop the pain, but the only things that seemed to help were his rituals of indexing his pornography, finding a prostitute, or, when unable to pay for sex, exposing himself. Larry's addictive process presents a very common model familiar to addiction professionals. Shame is a key factor in all addictions. Sexual shame, especially in a sex-negative culture, is particularly virulent.

Multiple Addictions

Other familiar factors in Larry's case are multiple addictions, both in the addict and his immediate family members. Golden Valley Health Center, a suburban Minneapolis hospital, has a twenty bed in-patient treatment program for sexual addiction called the Sexual Dependency Unit. I serve as a program consultant to that facility. Seventy-one percent of the patient population reports multiple addiction or compulsive behaviors. In fact, thirty-eight percent of the program's patients are chemically dependent; another thirty-eight percent have eating disorders. Compulsive gambling, spending, caffeine use, and smoking are also frequent complaints.

The Golden Valley Program represents, in a concrete manner, the emerging recognition among addictionologists that not only do addictions occur concurrently, but in mutually reinforcing ways. Clinicians often observe that the treatment of one addiction will result in the flourishing of another. Patients, for example, who have both alcoholism and sexual addiction often observe that their alcohol use was a way to anesthetize their pain around their out-of-control sexual behavior. They further comment that their alcoholism was relatively easy to deal with compared to their sexual acting out.

Such observations are at odds significantly with the traditional "disease" model of chemical dependency in which alcoholism and drug addiction are perceived as the primary "illness" and the sexual behavior as resulting from it. Unfortunately, there are still alcoholism treatment centers where patients are told that their sexual behavior will straighten out once they get sober.

Major progess is being made, however, in terms of understanding the relationships among the various addictions. One exciting example is the research of Milkman and his colleagues (*Advances in Alcohol and Substance Abuse*, 1983) on the psychobiological impact of hormone interactions on addiction pathology. For their research purposes, they use a matrix developed around three categories of addictions (e.g., gambling, sex, stimulant drugs, and high risk behaviors), the satiation addictions (e.g., overeating, depressant drugs, and alcohol), and the fantasy addictions (e.g., psychedelic drugs, marijuana, and mystical/artistic preoccupations). Beyond their research method of categorization, the conceptualization of models of poly-addiction will go far in broadening traditional models of addiction. They will also assist in answering the questions many practitioners have about cross-tolerance effects.

Family System Theory

Many addiction professionals are using systems theory as a conceptual foundation for their work not only because it is an integrative paradigm but also because it is a *growth* versus *illness* model. One of the systems identified, for example, by most addiction specialists as key to the self-defeating patterns of the addiction is the family system. Note in Larry's story how other family members had their own addiction patterns (father's drinking and wife's overeating). Observe also Joan's co-participation in the illness through the purchasing of Larry's drugs. Even her weight gain was a statement about their sexuality.

As part of the etiology of the addictive system, extreme family behavior such as extreme rigidity or chaos are common to people who have dependency problems. Further, I describe in a new book now in press a survey of 300 sexual addicts and the incidence of childhood sexual abuse. Sixty-five percent of the women and forty-five percent of the men report having been sexually abused. For a number of reasons I specify in the book, I believe that this is, in fact, underreported.

As part of treatment, the family or significant others are vital to the recovery process. When Golden Valley Health Center staff conducted six-month post-treatment evaluations, they discovered only one common denominator to all the patients who suffered relapse: no family members, partners, or significant others had participated in the family week of treatment.

System theory also allows a more organic approach to treatment. For example, comparisons between alcoholism and sexual addiction treatment can create misperceptions about the course of treatment. A better comparison can be made by looking at eating disorders. There are 34 million obese and 14 million morbidly obese persons in the United States. Yet, like sexual addiction, we have been very slow to address this problem. In compulsive overeating, patients are not asked to give up eating, but rather to learn how to eat differently. Eating patterns, environments, foods, and rituals shift so that they enhance rather than destroy the patient's life.

Similarly, sexual addiction treatment helps patients reclaim their sexuality by a primary refocusing of their sexual behavior. Some have assumed that the abstinence focus of alcohol programs has been directly translated to sex addiction programs, and they feared that treatment in these programs would be a sex-negative experience. Of the four hospital based programs I know, treatment staff work very hard to help their patients achieve the goal of sexual enhancement. Part of review criteria for all such programs should include treatment goals that encourage healthy and varied forms of sexual expression.

Treatment Outcome

In terms of treatment outcomes, the early six-month evaluation of Golden Valley Health Center patients is encouraging. This internal study of 30 patients has all the obvious limitations of a preliminary study done on the first patient cohort to reach six months. It is also not a large sample, nor is it conducted over a long period of time. Nor were the forms consistently completed. But the information obtained from this preliminary study is positive. For quality of life indicators, patients reported significant improvement in the following areas:

- Family Life 76%

- Job Performance 81%

- General Physical Health 80%

- Self-Image 71%

For program outcomes, patients reported:

- Having no or minimal problems maintaining recovery 86%

- Recommending program to others 100%

- Attending regular or frequent 12-step meetings 76%

The last program outcome requires some explanation. Addiction programs often rely on community support groups based on the 12 steps of Alcoholics Anonymous or as they are translated (e.g., Overeaters Anonymous, Gamblers Anonymous). In the case of sexual addiction, there are a number of groups, such as Sex Addicts Anonymous or Sexaholics Anonymous. The fact that 76 percent of Golden Valley's patients could find local groups is remarkable, given that the majority of them came from all over the United States and Canada. It is a testimony to the rapid expansion of resources for this problem.

Conclusion

Some professionals are mistrustful of self-help groups, especially when they have had no experience with them. The fact is they are of uneven quality. However, a good group is hard to beat in terms of helping addicts cope with their shame. The 12 steps are particularly effective with shame-based addictive disorders. Perhaps the best brief explanation of the process is Ernst Kurtz's class article "Why AA Works" (*Journal of Studies on Alcohol*, 43:38–80) for those readers with no 12-step group experience.

Definitional problems abound in sexual addiction. Eli Coleman elaborates upon them in his companion article to this piece. Questions of normalcy, cross-cultural comparisons, special populations are all familiar terrain to the addiction specialist. In fact, Jim Orford, one of the very first to articulate a theory on sexual dependency, comments in his recent book *Excessive Appetites* (1985):

> Debate over definitions in this area is intriguingly reminiscent of debates on the same subject when drugtaking, drinking, or gambling are under discussion. In none of these areas is there agreement about the precise points on the continuum at which normal behavior, heavy use, problem behaviors, excessive behavior, "mania" or "ism" are to be distinguished one from another. When reading of the supposed characteristics of the "real nymphomaniac," one is haunted by memories of attempts to define the "real alcoholic" or the "real compulsive gambler."

Current research trends are abandoning the traditional disease oriented typologies in favor of recognizing that natural systems are varied even in pathologies. To find the model "sex addict" that everyone can agree on will take us down a trail the professional addictionologist has been on before. There is not one kind of alcoholic but actually a variety of types who have excessive use of alcohol in common. So I believe that we will find similar patterns in sexual addiction.

The risk is that addiction specialists look skeptically at sex therapists and their lack of training in addictive delusional thought processes and relapse prevention while sexual scientists criticize addictionologists as having inadequate knowledge of sexuality. Meanwhile, people who are struggling with the issue are asking for help. And no progress will be made.

Therein is the opportunity. Some years ago the Italian psychiatrist Mara Palazolli (1981) appealed for professionals to work for what she termed "transdisciplinary" knowledge as contrasted with interdisciplinary efforts in which different specialists focused on a common problem. From her point of view "transdisciplinary" meant creating a new body of knowledge through the cooperation of different disciplines. Sexual addiction presents us with a great challenge and opportunity for addictionologists and sexual scientists to develop the new body of knowledge that Palazolli envisioned.

Why There's No Such Thing as Sexual Addiction — And Why It Really Matters

— Marty Klien

If convicted mass murdered Ted Bundy had said that watching Bill Cosby reruns motivated his awful crimes, he would have been dismissed as a deranged sociopath. Instead, Bundy said his pornography addiction made him do it—which many people treated as the conclusions of a thoughtful social scientist. Why?

There's a phenomenon emerging in America today that affects us and our profession whether we like it or not. Not caring about it, or having no opinion about it, is no longer an option for us.

I am not interested, by the way, in trashing 12-step programs. AA performs a great service every year in helping people handle their addiction to alcohol and other drugs. The two-part question that has been put to us—again, whether we like it or not—is, is the addiction model a good one for diagnosing sexual problems, and is the 12-step model a good one for treating sexual problems?

If it is, is it as appropriate for treating rapists as it is for people who masturbate too much?

How the Sexual Addiction Movement Affects Professionals

*People are now self-diagnosing as "sex-addicts."

They're also diagnosing their partners. Non-sexologist professionals such as ministers and doctors are diagnosing some of their clientele as sex addicts, too. As a result of these

From Annual Meeting of the Society for the Scientific Study of Sex, November 1989 by Marty Klein. Copyright © 1989 by Annual Meeting of the Society for the Scientific Study of Sex. Reprinted by permission.

trends, many people who should be seeing therapists or sexologists are not. And many who don't need "treatment" *are* getting it.

*The sexual addiction movement is aggressively training non-sexologists, such as marriage counselors, in the treatment of sexual problems.

Many professionals are now taking these programs instead of those offered by sexologists. Also, some professionals now feel incompetent to treat certain systemic problems without this sexual addiction "training."

It is important to note that the content of this sexual addiction training is sexologically inadequate: there is little or no discussion of systems, physiology, diagnoses, cultural aspects, etc.

*The concept of sexual addiction affects the sexual climate of the new society in which we work—negatively.

This negativity is reflected in anti-sex education legislation, anti-pornography ordinances, homophobic industry regulations, etc.

*Sex addicts now have cachet as sex experts.

Mass murderer Ted Bundy, widely quoted as an expert on the effects of pornography, is only one example. Right-wing crusaders now routinely quote "sex addicts" to justify repressive beliefs and public policy suggestions.

Defining Sexual Addiction

In the literature, the sex addict is typically described as:

- Someone who frequently does or fantasizes sexual things s/he doesn't like

- Someone whose sexual behavior has become unstoppable despite serious consequences (including, according to Patrick Carnes, unwanted pregnancy)

- Someone whose sexual behavior and thoughts have become vastly more important than their relationships, family, work, finances, and health

- Someone whose sexual behavior doesn't reflect her/his highest self, the grandest part of her/his humanness

- According to the National Association of Sexual Addiction Problems, "6% or 1 out of 17 Americans are sexual addicts." That's about 14 million people.

From this literature and from meetings of groups like Sexaholics Anonymous (SA), the beliefs of people committed to the sexual addiction model appear to include:

- Sex is most healthy in committed, monogamous, loving, heterosexual relationships;

- The "goal" of sex should always be intimacy and the expression of our highest self;

- There are limits to healthy sexual expression, which are obvious (e.g., masturbation more than once a day);

- Choosing to use sex to feel better about yourself or to escape from problems is unhealthy.

Clinical Implications of the Concept

*It sees powerlessness as a virtue.

Step 1 of the traditional "12 steps" of all AA-type groups is "we admitted we were powerless over X (alcohol, our sexual impulses, etc.)..."

Controlling our sexuality can be painful, not because we lack self-control or will power, but because sexual energy is powerful and demands expression. The primitive, infantile forces behind those demands often make sexuality feel like a matter of life and death—which, in the unconscious, it is.

"Sex addicts" say they are "out of control," but this is just a *metaphor*—i.e., they *feel* out of control; controlling their impulses is very painful. We've all had that experience, with sex and with other things. *Virtually everyone* has the ability to choose how to control and express their sexual impulses (we'll discuss the small group who can't later).

The concept of sexual addiction concludes with peoples' desire to shirk responsibility for their sexuality. But powerlessness is far too high a price to pay.

*It prevents helpful analysis by patients and therapists.

The concept of sexual addiction prevents any examination of the personality dynamics underlying sexual behavior. It prevents the assessment and treatment of sexual or personality problems, because identifying and dealing with the "addiction" is the goal.

By encouraging people to "admit" that they *are* powerless, the concept of sexual addiction prevents people from examining how they can come to *feel* powerless—and what they can do about that feeling. This careful examination, ultimately, is the source of personality growth and behavior change.

The expression "That's my addiction talking" is creeping into the popular vocabulary. This translates into "don't confront or puncture my defenses."

*It trivializes sexuality.

The concept of sexual addiction ignores the childhood passions at the source of sexual guilt. Aggression, lust for power, and greedy demands to be pleasured are all part of normal sexuality, which every adult needs to broker in some complex fashion.

People learn to feel guilty about their sexual impulses as infants. "Sex addicts" are told they have nothing to feel guilty about, and they can learn to feel better one day at a time. But people know all the "good" reasons they have for feeling sexual guilt. By denying the dark side of normal, healthy sexuality that most people know they have, the concept of sexual addiction *increases* guilt.

Self-identified "sex addicts" want us to remove the darkness from their sexuality, leaving only the wholesome, non-threatening part—which would, of course, also leave them as non-adults. Rather than collude with this understandable desire, competent therapists are willing to confront this darkness. Instead of snatching it away from patients, we can help them approach it, understand it, and ultimately feel less afraid of it.

Another way to describe this is that

*It lets people split—i.e., externalize their "bad" sexuality.

Once a person describes her/himself as a "sex addict," s/he can say "I don't want that sexual feeling or behavior over there; *the disease* wants it. Good therapists know how to recognize splitting, how it blocks adult functioning, and how to move patients away from it.

*It makes a disease out of what is often within reasonable limits of sexual behavior.

High levels of masturbating and *any* patronage of prostitutes, for example, are typically condemned as "abnormal" and reflecting a "disease," according to SA-type groups. Which experts get to make judgments about acceptable sexual behavior? Exactly where do their criteria come from?

*It doesn't teach sexual decision-making skills, or how to evaluate sexual situations.

Rather, the concept uses a "just say no" approach. As Planned Parenthood's Faye Wattleton says, "just say no" helps people abstain from self-destructive sex about as well as "have a nice day" helps people deal with depression.

SA-type groups say that ultimately, sexual abstinence is more like abstinence from compulsive eating—that is, moderation—than it is like abstinence from compulsive drinking—that is, zero participation. On what theoretical basis has this critical judgment been made? Simple expediency.

*Where is the healthy model of sexuality?

The sexual addiction model of human sexuality is moralistic, arbitrary, misinformed, and narrow. *Excluded* from this model are using sex to feel good; having "bad" fantasies; and enjoying sex without being in love. Where is the theoretical justification for this moralistic position?

We've seen this before: the concept of sin as sickness. It has led to sincere attempts to "cure" homosexuality, nymphomania, and masturbation—by the world's leading social scientists, within our own lifetime.

It is outrageous to treat sexual problems without a healthy model of sexuality that relates to most people's experience. The sexual addiction concept shows a dramatic ignorance of the range of typical human sexuality.

At the end of competent sex therapy or psychotherapy treatment, the patient is a grown-up, able to make conscious sexual choices. Sex addition treatment offers a patient the chance to be a recovering sex addict. Which would you rather be?

Professional Implications of the Concept

*It reduces the credibility of sexologists.

Prospective patients are now asking therapists a new kind of question: "Are you in recovery yourself?" "Have you treated sex addicts before?" What if a therapist is emotionally/sexually healthy and therefore *not* "in recovery"? Is s/he then disqualified as a professional?

The public, I'm afraid, is also getting a picture of us as being ivory tower types out of touch with the real—i.e., *destructive*—sexuality out on the street. They're feeling "You want to waste time discussing systems, regression, defenses, and meanwhile there are kids buying *Playboy* out there!"

*It replaces professional sexologists as relevant sex experts.

There are two groups of people behind this:

a) Addictionologists, often in recovery themselves (i.e., they have unresolved sexual and impulse control issues). They typically have little or no training in sexuality (e.g., I am told that Patrick Carnes' Ph.D. is in Counselor Education and Staff Development); and

b) 12-steppers themselves, lay people who love being in recovery. Their missionary zeal has nothing to do with science or clinical expertise. They freely generalize their own experience with sexual problems and "recovery" to all people and to human sexuality.

Both groups of people are now being quoted—and are actively portraying themselves—as sex experts.

By offering training from people with little or no sexological background, the concept suggests that all we offer is just another "theory" about sexual functioning. Just as creationists now want (and frequently get) "equal time" when scientists teach or discuss evolution, addictionologists now want—and are beginning to get—"equal time" regarding sexual functioning.

Graduates of such training programs believe that they have learned something about sexuality, when they haven't. They have learned something about *addiction*. And they are taught that they are competent to treat addiction in any form, whether its vehicle alcohol, food, gambling, love, or sex.

Addictionologists admit they lack skills in differential diagnosis. They and their 12-step programs let anyone define him/herself as a "sex addict." How many personality disorders, how much depression, how many adjustment reactions are being treated as "sex addiction"?

Political Implications of the Concept

*It strengthens society's anti-sex forces.

"Sexual addiction" is the Right's newest justification for eliminating sex education, adult bookstores, and birth control clinics. They are using the same arguments to eliminate books like *The Color Purple* from school libraries. Businessman Richard Enrico, whose group Citizens Against Pornography eliminated the Sale of *Playboy* magazine from all 1800 7–11 stores, did so, he says, "because smut causes sex addiction." And he was able to convince one of America's largest corporations of this complete fiction.

We should not be colluding with this destructive force.

*It emphasizes negative aspects of sex.

Sex addiction treatment is essentially creating a special interest group of people who feel victimized by their own sexuality. Not *others'* sexuality, like rape victims—their *own* sexuality. This lobby/interest group is growing as increasing numbers of people are recruited into identifying themselves as sex addicts. With the agenda of protecting people from their *own* sexuality, they are a dangerous group, easily exploited by the Right and other sex-negative points of view.

*It frightens people about the role of sexuality in social problems.

Increasingly, "sex addicts" and trainers are talking in public about how sexual impulses took over their lives and made them do things like steal money, take drugs, and see prostitutes.

This also frightens people about their ability to control their own sexuality—as if they're vulnerable to being taken over.

*It supports public ignorance about sexuality.

"Sex addicts" and trainers spread stories about how childhood masturbating to *Playboy* leads to porn addiction, and about how prostitutes become so alluring that people destroy their marriages. The public, of course, takes the additional step that this could happen to anyone—even though there is no data to support this idea.

The movement continues to spread dangerous lies about sex, even though the ultra-conservative Meese Commission was unable to find any evidence that pornography leads to child molestation, and even though no medical society in the world has ever proven that masturbation of any kind is harmful.

*It focuses on the "dignified" "purpose" of sex.

These words always seem to mean a rigid sex role system, with sex needing love to give it meaning. Sweating and moaning never seem dignified to people concerned with the dignity of sex. Ultimately, the "purpose" of sex can only be a political, rather than scientific, concept.

*It obscures the role of society in distorting our sexuality.

Sexologists understand that our moralistic American society constricts healthy sexual expression. We all know the sexual and intimacy problems this creates; in fact, we are now beginning to understand how such distortion even helps create sex offenders.

But the sexual addiction movement only sees society as encouraging promiscuity, instead of discouraging pleasure and healthy sexuality. This simplistic analysis cannot see how the media and other institutions make guilt-free sex almost impossible.

The sexual addiction concept attempts to heal society's sexual pain while keeping its economic, political, and social foundations intact. This is not only naive and ineffective, but dangerous.

Why Is the Sexual Addiction Concept So Popular?

*It distances personal responsibility for sexual choices.

As Dr. Domeena Renshaw says, "my illness makes me have affairs" is a very popular concept.

The concept seems to allow sexual expression without the punishment our infantile side fears. This is a great childhood fantasy. But the price is too high.

*It provides fellowship.

SA-type meetings provide structure and relaxed human contact for people who have trouble finding these in other ways.

The program also allows alcoholics in AA to work the steps again. This is one of the single biggest sources of self-described "sex addicts." In fact, Patrick Carnes claims that 83% of all sex addicts have some other kind of addiction.

*It provides pseudo-"scientific" support for the intuitive belief that sex is dangerous.

In doing so it legitimizes sex-negative attitudes, and supports sexual guilt.

*It lets people self-diagnose.

This is very American, very democratic. People like to feel they are taking charge of their lives, and self-diagnosing gives them the illusion that they are.

*It encourages people to split.

When people are troubled by their sexuality, it is comforting to imagine the problem "out there" rather than "in here." A striking example is Jimmy Swaggart, who railed against immorality out in the world, while behaving in the very ways he was condemning.

It also encourages a kind of splitting among *non*-"sex addicts." In answering the defensive question "how can people be sexual like *that*?," it makes people who behave in certain ways essentially *different* (they're "addicted") from us "normal" folk. Basically, people use the concept of sexual addiction as a projection of their fear about their own sexuality. Its very existence is sort of an exorcism of sexuality on a societal level.

*It helps people get distance from their sexual shame.

Most of us have deep shame about our sexuality—either our overt behavior, or the more primitive urges and images left over from childhood that we've never accepted. This profound sense of shame is what people would really like to get rid of; the behavioral symptons they're supposedly addicted to are just a symbol of that shame.

SA-type groups reframe this shame into a positive thing. It becomes a badge for membership; it lets "addicts" know they're heading toward a solution; it affirms that a sex-crazed society is victimizing them; and it suggests they're being too hard on themselves.

Good therapy does the opposite. It helps people feel their shame, relate it to an even deeper pain, and temporarily feel worse—before helping them resolve it.

Why Do So Many People Claim to Get Relief from Sexual Addiction Programs?

First, we should keep in mind that simply because people claim that something gives them emotional relief doesn't mean it works in the way they claim. Astrology apparently helped reduce Nancy Reagan's anxiety about Ron's career; but that doesn't mean it actually helped him make better decisions.

*The recovery process can be emotionally reassuring for many people.

It offers structure, goals, fellowship, and an accepting social environment. In fact, since most of the talk at SA-type groups is about sex and relationships, it's a relatively easy place to meet people for dating. And that *does* go on.

Conversation at SA-type meetings is exclusively about material that each individual is already focusing on. Thus, *all* conversation feels like it's about the individual "addict," and so participants can feel connected with others without having to abandon their own narcissistic focus. This feels intimate, and gives the illusion that an individual is making progress.

And, of course, virtually everyone gets to hear stories of people who are worse off than they are, and so they feel better.

*People enjoy feeling like they're heading somewhere.

While "addicts" learn to enjoy the *process* of recovery, they also learn they're never going to fully *get* there. So they set their sights lower—and *do* accomplish never being cured.

Because the sexual addiction movement is not interested in personality change, it can offer symptom relief without any ethical conflicts. In many cases people do get that relief— although it's at the expense of the rest of their character structure.

Finally, as "addicts" continue learning how to distance themselves from their "bad" sexuality, they feel an increasing sense of direction and relief.

*Addicts transfer some of their compulsivity to the SA-type group meeting itself.

For many "sex addicts," meetings (sometimes many times per week) are the most important part of the week. In a predictable setting and way, with comforting regularity, they get to listen to and talk about sexual feelings and behavior they dislike.

The feeling is perfectly conveyed by a "sex addict" quoted in *Contemporary Sexuality*. He notes that "Every Thursday night for the past year and a half I have repeated that statement [about his so-called "addiction"] to my 12-step support group." By itself this is a trivial point; in the context of a program supposed to heal compulsive behavior, it is troubling.

What about Sexual Compulsivity?

Most self-described sex addicts aren't out of control; they are relatively "normal" neurotics for whom being in control is *painful*. In fact, as the National Association of Sexual Addiction Problems says, "most addicts do not break the law, nor do they satisfy their need by forcing themselves upon others."

Those who are *really* sexually compulsive are typically psychotic, sociopathic, character-disordered, etc. Some of these people have impaired reality testing. Others have absolutely no concern about the consequences of their behavior. Dr. Renshaw states that "undifferentiated sexual urgency is a symptom of manic-depression."

These people don't need help laying off one day at a time. They need deep therapy, medication, structured behavioral interventions, or other intensive modalities. Dr. Eli Coleman, for example, reports treatment success with lithium, comparable to the clinical results lithium produces with other compulsives.

It is absolutely indefensible to suggest that the same mechanism is operating in the rapist and the guy who masturbates "too often." The concept of sexual addiction does nothing to diagnose serious problems, assess danger, discuss beliefs about sex, take a history, or change personality. There are no treatment statistics on *true* obsessive-compulsives via the sexual addiction model.

We must also, and this is much harder, continue to resist and interpret society's demand for simple answers and easy solutions about sex offenders.

Sexual energy scares people; distorted expressions of that energy terrify people. We need to continually educate policymakers and the public as to why the treatment of sex offenders is so complex and difficult, and why quick-fix solutions are worse than partial solutions. We must find a way to say "I don't know" or "We're still working on it" without apologizing. Cancer researchers, for example, have done a good job of making partial answers—like early detection and quitting smoking—acceptable.

Summary

The concept of "sex addiction" really rests on the assumption that sex is dangerous. There's the sense that we frail humans are vulnerable to the Devil's temptations of pornography, masturbation, and extramarital affairs, and that if we yield, we become "addicted."

Without question, being a sexual person is complex, and we *are* vulnerable—to our sex-negative heritage, shame about our bodies, and conflict about the exciting sexual feelings we can't express without risking rejection. Sexuality per se, however, is not dangerous—no matter how angry or frightened people are.

Professional sexologists should reject any model suggesting that people must spend their lives 1) in fear of sexuality's destructive power; 2) being powerless about sexuality; 3) lacking the tools to relax and let sex take over when it's appropriate.

Addictionologists have cynically misled the public into thinking that "sexual addiction" is a concept respected and used by professional therapists and educators. Even a brief look at our literature, conferences, and popular writing shows how rarely this is true. But addictionologists don't care about sexual truth or expertise—only about addiction.

The sexual addiction movement is not harmless. These people are missionaries who want to put everyone in the missionary position.

In these terrible anti-sex times, one of our most important jobs is to reaffirm that sexuality—though complicated—is precious, not dangerous. Now more than ever, our job is to help people just say yes.

Debate Presenter Form

Follow the guidelines for debate presenters contained in the introduction of this text and those given to you by your instructor. Use the format below to organize the material for your debate. Remember to include all relevant citation information and to present the related information in your own words. Give credit to authors when you cite a quote and be as thorough as possible when writing about your points so you will be prepared for your debate.

Reference citation #1:

Author: _____

Title: _____

Date: _____

Source: _____

_____

Content from reference citation #1: _____

_____

_____

_____

_____

_____

_____

_____

_____

_____

_____

_____

Reference citation #2:

Author: _____

Title: _____

Date: _____

Source: _____

_____

Content from reference citation #2: _____

_____

_____

_____

_____

_____

_____

Reference citation #3:

Author: _____

Title: _____

Date: _____

Source: _____

_____

Content from reference citation #3: _____

_____

_____

_____

_____

_____

270

Audience Preparation Form

Follow the guidelines for preparing to be an informed audience member on the day of the debate included in the introduction to this text. After reading both sides of the debate from this chapter, answer the following questions. Be as thorough as possible so that you will be able to make a contribution to the debate by asking informed questions or making provocative comments. This form is usually due on the day of the debate.

State the issue in your own words. Do not plagiarize the text. Demonstrate that you understand the topic and it's relevant arguments.

_____
_____
_____
_____
_____

Discuss two points on the "yes" side of the debate.

Point #1: _____
_____

Point #2: _____
_____

Discuss two points on the "no" side of the debate.

Point #1: _____
_____

Point #2: _____
_____

What Is your opinion on this topic?

_____

_____

_____

_____

_____

_____

_____

What has contributed to the development of your views about this topic?

_____

_____

_____

_____

_____

_____

_____

_____

What information would be necessary to cause you to change your thinking about this topic?

_____

_____

_____

_____

_____

Debate Response Form

Follow the guidelines for responding to the debates in the introductory chapter of this text. Complete this form and submit your answers at the class following the debate. Try to be thorough and convince your instructor that you were an active listener during the debate.

List a quote from a debate presenter that you think was important and explain why you think this comment was significant.

_____

_____

_____

_____

Which side of the debate do you think made the most convincing arguments, why?

_____

_____

_____

_____

_____

After hearing the debate, in what way has your thinking been affected?

_____

_____

_____

_____

_____

_____

Children

ISSUE 13

Does Divorce Place Children at Risk for Social and Psychological Problems?

YES Judith S. Wallerstein, *Children of Divorce: The Dilemma of a Decade*

NO David H. Demo and Alan C. Acock, *The Impact of Divorce on Children*

With the high rate of divorce concerns about the welfare of children are raised. Judith Wallerstein describes several research studies that conclude that children of divorce are at higher risk for mental illness. She discusses three stages that children from divorced families go through: the acute initial stage, a transitional phase, and a post-divorce stage. She also illuminates the differing responses to divorce based on the child's age.

Wallerstein concludes with a plea for more research on children as a special group at risk for psychological and emotional problems due to their parent's divorce. The goal of this research being to offer parents responsible advice on how best to help children through this challenging and very common event in their family life.

David H. Demo and Alan C. Acock begin by stating several assumptions that underlie research on the effects of divorce on children. The primary assumption suggests that a set of two parents is the minimal unit for rearing a healthy child.

After citing several flaws in the focus of existing research on the topic, Demo and Acock discuss research outcomes on personal adjustment in children of divorce. Their conclusions are that after the initial trauma of divorce, which is affected by the extent of marital discord, the child's gender and age, children indicate that they prefer the conditions of divorce to the adverse conditions of the marriage.

These authors conclude with a discussion of the positive outcomes of divorce on children. These include increased androgyny, assumption of domestic responsibility, greater maturity, feelings of efficacy and internal locus of control. Demo and Acock suggest that it is simplistic to think that divorce could have any type of uniform effect on children.

Applications

1. Is it possible that the negative outcomes related to divorce are not an issue for today's children because of the frequency of divorce today? Explain your answer.

2. From your own experience with friends who have both intact and divorced families, what do you think has been the overall effect of divorce?

3. What do you think researchers might discover as "responsible advice" for parents in divorce situations to follow?

Children of Divorce
The Dilemma of a Decade

Judith S. Wallerstien

It is now estimated that 45% of all children born in 1983 will experience their parents' divorce, 35% will experience a remarriage, and 20% will experience a second divorce (A.J. Norton, Assistant Chief, Population Bureau, United States Bureau of the Census, personal communication, 1983)....

Although the incidence of divorce has increased across all age groups, the most dramatic rise has occurred among young adults (Norton, 1980). As a result, children in divorcing families are younger than in previous years and include more preschool children....

Although many children weather the stress of martial discord and family breakup with psychopathological sequelae, a significant number falter along the way. Children of divorce are significantly overrepresented in outpatient psychiatric, family agency, and private practice populations compared with children in the general population (Gardner, 1976; Kalter, 1977; Tessman, 1977; Tooley, 1976). The best predictors of mental health referrals for school-aged children are parental divorce or parental loss as a result of death (Felner, Stolberg, & Cowen, 1975). A national survey of adolescents whose parents had separated and divorced by the time the children were seven years old found that 30% of these children had received psychiatric or psychological therapy by the time they reached adolescence compared with 10% of adolescents in intact families (Zill, 1983).

A longitudinal study in northern California followed 131 children who were age 3 to 18 at the decisive separation. At the 5-year mark, the investigators found that more than one-third were suffering with moderate to severe depression (Wallerstein & Kelly, 1980a). These findings are especially striking because the children were drawn from a nonclinical population and were accepted into the study only if they had never been identified before the divorce as needing psychological treatment and only if they were performing at age-appropriate levels in school. Therefore, the deterioration observed in these children's adjustment occurred largely following the family breakup....

Divorce is a long, drawn-out process of radically changing family relationships that has several stages, beginning with the material rupture and its immediate aftermath, continuing over several years of disequilibrium, and finally coming to rest with the stabilization of a new postdivorce or remarried family unit. A complex chain of changes, many of them unanticipated and unforeseeable, are set into motion by the marital rupture and are likely to occupy a significant portion of the child or adolescent's growing years. As the author and her colleague have reported elsewhere, women in the California Children of Divorce study required three to three-and-one-half years following the decisive separation before they achieved a sense of order and predictability in their lives (Wallerstein & Kelly, 1980a). This figure probably underestimates the actual time trajectory of the child's experience of divorce. A prospective study reported that parent-child relationships began to deteriorate many years prior to the divorce decision and that the adjustment of many children in these families began to fail long before the decisive separation (Morrison, 1982). This view of the divorcing process as long lasting accords with the perspective of a group of young people who reported at a 10-year follow-up that their entire childhood or adolescence had been dominated by the family crisis and its extended aftermath (Wallerstein, 1978).

Stages in the Process

The three broad, successive stages in the divorcing process, while they overlap, are nevertheless clinically distinguishable. *The acute phase* is precipitated by the decisive separation and the decision to divorce. This stage is often marked by steeply escalating conflict between the adults, physical violence, severe distress, depression accompanied by suicidal ideation, and a range of behaviors reflecting a spilling of aggressive and sexual impulses. The adults frequently react with severe ego regression and not unusually behave at odds with their more customary demeanor. Sharp disagreement in the wish to end the marriage is very common, and the narcissistic injury to the person who feels rejected sets the stage for rage, sexual jealousy, and depression. Children are generally not shielded from this parental conflict or distress. Confronted by a marked discrepancy in images of their parents, children do not have the assurance that the bizarre or depressed behaviors and moods will subside. As a result, they are likely to be terrified by the very figures they usually rely on for nurturance and protection.

As the acute phase comes to a close, usually within the first 2 years of the divorce decision, the marital partners gradually disengage from each other and pick up the new tasks of reestablishing their separate lives. *The transitional phase* is characterized by ventures into new, more committed relationships; new work, school, and friendship groups; and sometimes new settings, new lifestyles, and new geographical locations. This phase is marked by alternating success and failure, encouragement and discouragement, and it may also last for several years. Children observe and participate in the many changes of this period. They share the trials and errors and the fluctuations in mood. For several years life may be unstable, and home may be unsettled.

Finally, *the postdivorce phase* ensues with the establishment of a fairly stable single-parent or remarried household. Eventually three out of four divorced women and four out of five divorced men reenter wedlock (Cherlin, 1981). Unfortunately, though, remarriage does not bring immediate tranquility in the lives of the family members. The early years of the remarriage are often encumbered by ghostly presences from the earlier failed marriages and by the actual presences of children and visiting parents from the prior marriage or marriages. Several studies suggest widespread upset among children and adolescents following remarriage (Crohn, Brown, Walker, & Beir, 1981; Goldstein, 1974; Kalter, 1977). A large-scale investigation that is still in process reports long-lasting friction around visitation (Jacobson, 1983).

Changes in Parent-Child Relationships

Parents experience a diminished capacity to parent their children during the acute phase of the divorcing process and often during the transitional phase as well (Wallerstein & Kelly, 1980a). This phenomenon is widespread and can be considered an expectable, divorce-specific change in parent-child relationships. At its simplest level this diminished parenting capacity appears in the household disorder that prevails in the aftermath of divorce, in the rising tempers of custodial parent and child, in reduced competence and a greater sense of helplessness in the custodial parent, and in lower expectations of the child for appropriate social behavior (Hetherington, Cox, & Cox, 1978; 1982). Diminished parenting also entails a sharp decline in emotional sensitivity and support for the child; decreased pleasure in the parent-child relationship; decreased attentiveness to the child's needs and wishes; less talk, play, and interaction with the child; and a steep escalation in inappropriate expression of anger. One not uncommon component of the parent-child relationship coincident with the marital breakup is the adult's conscious or unconscious wish to abandon the child and thus to erase the unhappy marriage in its entirety. Child neglect can be a serious hazard.

In counterpoint to the temporary emotional withdrawal from the child, the parent may develop a dependent, sometimes passionate, attachment to the child or adolescent, beginning with the breakup and lasting throughout the lonely post-separation years (Wallerstein, 1985). Parents are likely to lean on the child and turn to the child for help, placing the child in a wide range of roles such as confidante, advisor, mentor, sibling, parent, caretaker, lover, concubine, extended conscience or ego control, ally within the marital conflict, or pivotal supportive presence in staving off depression or even suicide. This expectation that children should not only take much greater responsibility for themselves but also should provide psychological and social support for the distressed parent is sufficiently widespread to be considered a divorce-specific response along with that of diminished parenting. Such relationships frequently develop with an only child or with a very young, even a preschool, child. Not accidentally, issues of custody and visitation often arise with regard to the younger children. While such disputes, of course, reflect the generally unresolved anger of the marriage and the divorce, they may also reflect the intense emotional need of one or both parents for the young child's constant presence (Wallerstein, 1985).

Parents may also lean more appropriately on the older child or adolescent. Many young-sters become proud helpers, confidantes, and allies in facing the difficult postdivorce period (Weiss, 1979b). Other youngsters draw away from close involvement out of their fears of engulfment, and they move precipitously out of the family orbit, sometimes before they are developmentally ready....

Children's Reactions to Divorce

Initial Responses

Children and adolescents experience separation and its aftermath as the most stressful period of their lives. The family rupture evokes an acute sense of shock, intense anxiety, and profound sorrow. Many children are relatively content and even well-parented in families where one or both parents are unhappy. Few youngsters experience any relief with the divorce decision, and those who do are usually older and have witnessed physical violence or open conflict between their parents. The child's early responses are governed neither by an understanding of issues leading to the divorce nor by the fact that divorce has a high inci-dence in the community. To the child, divorce signifies the collapse of the structure that pro-vides support and protection. The child reacts as to the cutting of his or her lifeline.

The initial suffering of children and adolescents in response to a marital separation is compounded by realistic fears and fantasies about catastrophes that the divorce will bring in its wake. Children suffer with a pervasive sense of vulnerability because they feel that the protective and nurturant function of the family has given way. They grieve over the loss of the noncustodial parent, over the loss of the intact family, and often over the multiple losses of neighborhood, friends, and school. Children also worry about their distressed parents. They are concerned about who will take care of the parent who has left and whether the cus-todial parent will be able to manage alone. They experience intense anger toward one or both parents whom they hold responsible for disrupting the family. Some of their anger is reactive and defends them against their own feelings of powerlessness, their concern about being lost in the shuffle, and their fear that their needs will be disregarded as the parents give priority to their own wishes and needs. Some children, especially young children, suffer with guilt over fantasied misdeeds that they feel may have contributed to the family quarrels and led to the divorce. Others feel that it is their responsibility to mend the broken marriage (Wallerstein & Kelly, 1980a).

The responses of the child also must be considered within the social context of the divorce and in particular within the loneliness and social isolation that so many children experience. Children face the tensions and sorrows of divorce with little help from anybody else. Fewer than 10% of the children in the California Children of Divorce study had any help at the time of the crisis from adults outside the family although many people, including neighbors, pediatricians, ministers, rabbis, and family friends, knew the family and the children (Wallerstein & Kelly, 1980a). Thus, another striking feature of divorce as a childhood stress is that it occurs in the absence of or falling away of customary support.

Developmental factors are critical to the responses of children and adolescents at the time of the marital rupture. Despite significant individual differences in the child, in the family, and in parent-child relations, the child's age and developmental stage appear to be the most important factors governing the initial response. The child's dominant needs, his or her capacity to perceive and understand family events, the central psychological preoccupation and conflict, the available repertoire of defense and coping strategies, and the dominant patterning of relationships and expectations all reflect the child's age and developmental stage.

A major finding in divorce research has been the common patterns of response within different age groups (Wallerstein & Kelly, 1980a). The age groups that share significant commonalities in perceptions, responses, underlying fantasies, and behaviors are the preschool ages 3 to 5, early school age or early latency ages 5-1/2 to 8, later school age or latency ages 8 to 11, and, finally, adolescent ages 12 to 18 (Kelly & Wallerstein, 1976; Wallerstein, 1977, Wallerstein & Kelly, 1974; 1975; 1980a). These responses, falling as they do into age-related groupings, may reflect children's responses to acute stress generally, not only their responses to marital rupture.

Observations about preschool children derived from longitudinal studies in two widely different regions, namely, Virginia and northern California, are remarkably similar in their findings (Hetherington, 1979; Hetherington et al., 1978; 1982; Wallerstein & Kelly, 1975, 1980a). Preschool children are likely to show regression following one parent's departure from the household, and the regression usually occurs in the most recent developmental achievement of the child. Intensified fears are frequent and are evoked by routine separations from the custodial parent during the day and at bedtime. Sleep disturbances are also frequent, with preoccupying fantasies of many of the little children being fear of abandonment by both parents. Yearning for the departed parent is intense. Young children are likely to become irritable and demanding and to behave aggressively with parents, with younger siblings, and with peers.

Children in the 5- to 8-year old group are likely to show open grieving and are preoccupied with feelings of concern and longing for the departed parent. Many share the terrifying fantasy of replacement. "Will my daddy get a new dog, a new mommy, a new little boy?" were the comments of several boys in this age group. Little girls wove elaborate Madame Butterfly fantasies, asserting that the departed father would some day return to them, that he loved them "the best." Many of the children in this age group could not believe that the divorce would endure. About half suffered a precipitous decline in their school work (Kelly & Wallerstein, 1979).

In the 9- to 12-year-old group the central response often seems to be intense anger at one or both parents for causing the divorce. In addition, these children suffer with grief over the loss of the intact family and with anxiety, loneliness, and the humiliating sense of their own powerlessness. Youngsters in this age group often see one parent as the "good" parent and the other as "bad," and they appear especially vulnerable to the blandishments of one or the other parent to engage in marital battles. Children in later latency also have a high potential for assuming a helpful and empathic role in the care of a needy parent. School performances and peer relationships suffered a decline in approximately one-half of these children (Wallerstein & Kelly, 1974).

Adolescents are very vulnerable to their parents' divorce. The precipitation of acute depression, accompanied by suicidal preoccupation and acting out, is frequent enough to be alarming. Anger can be intense. Several instances have been reported of direct violent attacks on custodial parents by young adolescents who had not previously shown such behavior (Springer & Wallerstein, 1983). Preoccupied with issues of morality, adolescents may judge the parents' conduct during the marriage and the divorce, and they may identify with one parent and do battle against the other. Many become anxious about their own future entry into adulthood, concerned that they may experience marital failure like their parents (Wallerstein & Kelly, 1974). By way of contrast, however, researchers have also called attention to the adolescent's impressive capacity to grow in maturity and independence as they respond to the family crisis and the parents' need for help (Weiss, 1979a)....

Long-Range Outcomes

The child's initial response to divorce should be distinguished from his or her long-range development and psychological adjustment. No single theme appears among all of those children who enhance, consolidate, or continue their good development after the divorce crisis has finally ended. Nor is there a single theme that appears among all of those who deteriorate either moderately or markedly. Instead, the author and her colleague (Wallerstein & Kelly, 1980a) have found a set of complex configurations in which the relevant components appear to include (a) the extent to which the parent has been able to resolve and put aside conflict and anger and to make use of the relief from conflict provided by the divorce (Emery, 1982; Jacobson, 1978 a, b, c); (b) the course of the custodial parent's handling of the child and the resumption or improvement of parenting within the home (Hess & Camara, 1979); (c) the extent to which the child does not feel rejected by the non-custodial or visiting parent and the extend to which this relationship has continued regularly and kept pace with the child's growth; (d) the extent to which the divorce has helped to attenuate or dilute a psychopathological parent-child relationship; (e) the range of personality assets and deficits that the child brought to the divorce, including both the child's history in the predivorce family and his or her capacities in the present, particularly intelligence, the capacity for fantasy, social maturity, and the ability to turn to peers and adults; (f) the availability to the child of a supportive human network (Tessman, 1977): (g) the absence in the child of continued anger and depression; and (h) the sex and age of the child....

Future Directions

Despite the accumulating reports of the difficulties that many children in divorced families experience, society has on the whole been reluctant to regard children of divorce as a special group at risk. Notwithstanding the magnitude of the population affected and the widespread implications for public policy and law, community attention has been very limited; research has been poorly supported; and appropriate social, psychological, economic, or preventive measures have hardly begun to develop. Recently the alarm has been sounded in the national press about the tragically unprotected and foreshortened childhoods of children of divorce and their subsequent difficulties in reaching maturity (Winn, 1983). Perhaps this reflects a long-overdue awakening of community concern.

The agenda for research on marital breakdown, separation, divorce, and remarriage and the roads that families travel between each of these way stations [are] long and [have] been cited repeatedly in this [article]. The knowledge that we have acquired is considerable but the knowledge that we still lack is critical. More knowledge is essential in order to provide responsible advice to parents; to consult effectively with the wide range of other professionals whose daily work brings them in contact with these families; to design and mount education, treatment, or prevention programs; and to provide guidelines for informed social policy.

Author's Note: The Center for the Family in Transition, of which the author is the Executive Director, is supported by a grant from the San Francisco Foundation. The Zellerback Family Fund supported the author's research in the California Children of Divorce Project, one of the sources for this [article]. A slightly different version of this paper has been published in *Psychiatry Update: The American Psychiatric Association Annual Review, Vol. III.* L. Grinspoon (Ed.), pp. 144–158, 1984.

References

Cherlin, A. J. (1981). *Marriage, divorce, remarriage*. Cambridge, MA: Harvard University Press.

Crohn, H., Brown, H., Walker, L., & Beir, J. (1981). Understanding and treating the child in the remarried family. In I. R. Stuart & L. E. Abt (Eds.), *Children of separation and divorce: Management and treatment*, New York: Von Nostrand Reinhold.

Emery, R. E. (1982). Interparental conflict and children of discord and divorce. *Psychological Bulletin*, 92, 310–330.

Felner, R. D., Stolbert, A. L., & Cowen, E. L. (1975). Crisis events and school mental health referral patterns of young children. *Journal of Consulting and Clinical Psychology*, 43, 303–310.

Gardner, R. A. (1976). *Psychotherapy and children of divorce*. New York: Jason Aronson.

Goldstein, H. S. (1974) Reconstructed families: The second marriage and its children. *Psychiatric Quarterly*, 48, 433–440.

Hess, R. D., & Camara, K. A. (1979). Post-divorce relationships as mediating factors in the consequences of divorce for children. *Journal of Social Issues, 35,* 79–96.

Hetherington, E. (1979). Divorce: A child's perspective. *American Psychology, 34,* 79–96.

Hetherington, E., Cox, M., & Cox, R. (1978). The aftermath of divorce, In H. Stevens & M. Mathews (Eds.), *Mother-child relations.* Washington, DC: National Association for the Education of Young Children.

Hetherington, E. M., Cox, M., & Cox, R. (1982). Effects of divorce on parents and children. In M. E. Lamb (Ed.), *Nontraditional families: Parenting and child development.* Hillsdale, NJ: Lawrence Erlbaum Associates.

Jacobson, D. (1978a). The impact of marital separation/divorce on children: I. Parent-child separation and child adjustment. *Journal of Divorce, 1,* 341–360.

Jacobson, D. (1978b). The impact of marital separation/divorce on children: II. Interparent hostility and child adjustment. *Journal of Divorce, 2,* 3–20.

Jacobson, D. (1978c). The impact of marital separation/divorce on children: III. Parent-child communication and child adjustment, and regression analysis of findings from overall study. *Journal of Divorce, 2,* 175–194.

Jacobson, D. S. (1983). *Conflict, visiting and child adjustment in the stepfamily: A linked family system.* Paper presented at annual meeting of the American Orthopsychiatric Association, Boston.

Kalter, N. (1977). Children of divorce in an outpatient psychiatric population. *American Journal of Orthopsychiatry, 47,* 40–51.

Kelly, J. B., & Wallerstein, J. S. (1976), The effects of parental divorce: Experiences of the child in early latency. *American Journal of Orthopsychiatry, 46,* 20–32.

Kelly, J. B., & Wallerstein, J. S. (1979). The divorced child in the school. *National Principal, 59,* 51–58.

Morrison, A. L. (1982). *A prospective study of divorce: Its relation to children's development and parental functioning.* Unpublished dissertation, University of California at Berkeley.

Norton, A. J. (1980). The influence of divorce on traditional life cycle measures. *Journal of Marriage and the Family, 42,* 63–69.

Springer, C., & Wallerstein, J. S. (1983). Young adolescents' responses to their parents' divorces. In L. A. Krudek (Ed.), *Children and divorce.* San Francisco: Jossey-Bass.

Tessman, L. H. (1977). *Children of parting parents.* New York: Jason Aronson.

Tooley, J. (1976). Antisocial behavior and social alienation post divorce: The "Man of the house" and his mother. *American Journal of Orthopsychiatry, 46,* 33–42.

Wallerstein, J. S. (1977). Responses of the preschool child to divorce. Those who cope. In M. F. McMillan & S. Henao (Eds.), *Child psychiatry: Treatment and research.* New York: Brunner/Mazel.

Wallerstein, J. S. (1978). Children of divorce: Preliminary report of a ten-year follow-up. In J. Anthony & C. Chilland (Eds.), *The child in his family* (Vol 5). New York: Wiley.

Wallerstein, J. S. (1985). Parent-child relationships following divorce. In E. J. Anthony & G. Pollock (Eds.), *Parental influences in health and disease* (pp. 317–348). Boston: Little, Brown.

Wallerstein, J. S., & Kelly, J. B. (1974). The effects of parental divorce: The adolescent experience. In J. Anthony & C. Koupernik (Eds.), *The child in his family: Children at psychiatric risk* (Vol. 3). New York: Wiley.

Wallerstein, J. S. & Kelly, J. B. (1975). The effects of parental divorce: The experiences of the preschool child. *American Journal of Orthopsychiatry*, 46, 256–269.

Wallerstein, J. S., & Kelly, J. B. (1980a). *Surviving the breakup: How children and parents cope with divorce*. New York: Basic Books.

Weiss, R. S. (1979a). *Going it alone. The family life and social situation of the single parent.* New York: Basic Books.

Weiss, R. S. (1979b). Growing up a little faster. *Journal of Social Issues*, 35, 97–111.

Winn, M. (8 May 1983). The loss of childhood. *The New York Times Magazine*.

Zill, N. (22 March 1983). *Divorce, marital conflict, and children's mental health: Research findings and policy recommendations*. Testimony before Subcommittee on Family and Human Services, United States Senate Subcommittee on Labor and Human Resources.

The Impact of Divorce on Children

David H. Demo
Alan C. Acock

With the acceleration of the divorce rate from the mid-1960s to the early 1980s, the number of nontraditional families (such as single-parent families and reconstituted families) have increased relative to intact, first-time nuclear families. This article reviews empirical evidence addressing the relationship between divorce, family composition, and children's well-being. Although not entirely consistent, the pattern of empirical findings suggests that children's emotional adjustment, gender-role orientation, and antisocial behavior are affected by family structure, whereas other dimensions of well-being are unaffected. But the review indicates that these findings should be interpreted with caution because of the methodological deficiencies of many of the studies on which these findings are based. Several variables, including the level of family conflict, may be central variables mediating the effect of family structure on children.

The purpose of this article is to review and assess recent empirical evidence on the impact of divorce on children, concentrating on studies of nonclinical populations published in the last decade. We also direct attention to a number of important theoretical and methodological considerations in study of family structure and youthful well-being. We begin by briefly describing some of the theoretical propositions and assumptions that guide research in this area.

Theoretical Underpinnings

Consistent with the Freudian assumption that a two-parent group constitutes the minimal unit for appropriate sex-typed identification, anthropologists, sociologists, and social psychologists have long maintained the necessity of such a group for normal child development. Representative of structural-functional theorizing, Parsons and Bales argued that one of the basic functions of the family is to serve as a stable, organically integrated "factory" in which human personalities are formed.

Similarly, social learning theory emphasizes the importance of role models, focusing on parents as the initial and primary reinforcers of child behavior (Bandura and Walters, 1963). Much of the research adopting this perspective centers on parent-child similarities, analyzing the transmission of response patterns and the inhibitory or disinhibitory effect of parental models. The presence of the same-sex parent is assumed to be crucial in order for the child to learn appropriate sex-typed behavior. This assumption is shared by developmental and symbolic interactionist theories, various cognitive approaches to socialization, and confluence theory, as well as anthropological theories.

It logically follows that departures from the nuclear family norm are problematic for the child's development, especially for adolescents, inasmuch as this represents a crucial stage in the developmental process. Accordingly, a large body of research literature deals with father absence, the effects of institutionalization, and a host of "deficiencies" in maturation, such as those having to do with cognitive development, achievement, moral learning, and conformity. This focus has pointed to the crucial importance of both parents' presence but also has suggested that certain causes for parental absence may accentuate any negative effects....

Divorce and Family Structure

In examining [the] research,... it is important to distinguish between studies investigating the effects of family structure and those investigating the effects of divorce. Most studies compare intact units and single-parent families, guided by the assumption that the latter family structure is precipitated by divorce. Of course, this is not always the case. Single-parent families consist of those with parents who have never married, those formed by the permanent separation of parents, and those precipitated by the death of a parent. Simple comparisons between one-and *two*-parent families are also suspect in that two-parent families are not monolithic. First-time or nondivorced units differ from divorced, remarried units in which stepparents are involved. In addition, little recognition has been given to the fact that families of different types may exhibit varying levels of instability or conflict, a potentially confounding variable in establishing the effects of family structure. In short, most investigations of the linkage between family structure and youthful well-being have failed to recognize the complexity of present-day families....

Bearing in mind these conceptual distinctions, we now move to a systematic review of recent evidence on the impact of divorce on children and adolescents.

Existing Research

A substantial amount of research has examined the effects of family structure on children's social and psychological well-being. Many studies document negative consequences for children whose parents divorce and for those living in single-parent families. But most studies have been concerned with limited dimensions of a quite complex problem. Specifically, the research to date has typically *(a)* examined the effects of divorce or father absence on children, ignoring the effects on adolescents; *(b)* examined only selected dimensions of children's well-being; *(c)* compared intact units and single-parent families but not recognized important variations (e.g., levels of marital instability and conflict) within these structures; and *(d)* relied on cross-sectional designs to assess developmental processes.

Social and psychological well-being includes aspects of personal adjustment, self-concept, interpersonal relationships, antisocial behavior, and cognitive functioning....

Personal Adjustment

Personal adjustment is operationalized in various ways by different investigators but includes such variables as self-control, leadership, responsibility, independence, achievement orientation, aggressiveness, and gender-role orientation....

On the basis of her review of research conducted between 1970 and 1980, Cashion (1984: 483) concludes: "The evidence is overwhelming that after the initial trauma of divorce, the children are as emotionally well-adjusted in these [female-headed] families as in two-parent families." Investigations of long-term effects (Acock and Kiecolt, 1988; Kulka and Weingarten, 1979) suggest that, when socioeconomic status is controlled, adolescents who have experienced a parental divorce or separation have only slightly lower levels of adult adjustment.

While their findings are not definitive, Kinard and Reinherz speculate that either "the effects of parental divorce on children diminish over time; or that the impact of marital disruption is less severe for preschool-age children and for school-age children" (1986: 291). Children's age at the time of disruption may also mediate the impact of these events on other dimensions of their well-being (e.g., self-esteem or gender-role orientation) and thus will be discussed in greater detail below.... But two variables that critically affect children's adjustment to divorce are marital discord and children's gender.

Marital discord.   ...[E]xtensive data on children who had experienced their parents' divorce indicated that, although learning of the divorce and adjusting to the loss of the non-custodial parent were painful, children indicated that these adjustments were preferable to living in conflict. Many studies report that children's adjustment to divorce is facilitated under conditions of low parental conflict—both prior to *and* subsequent to the divorce (Guidubaldi, Cleminshaw, Perry, Nastasi, and Lightel, 1986; Jacobson, 1978; Lowenstein and Koopman, 1978; Porter and O'Leary, 1980; Raschke and Raschke, 1979; Rosen, 1979).

Children's gender. Children's gender may be especially important in mediating the effects of family disruption, as most of the evidence suggests that adjustment problems are more severe and last for longer periods of time among boys (Hess and Camara, 1979; Hetherington, 1979; Hetherington, Cox, and Cox, 1978, 1979, 1982; Wallerstein, 1984; Wallerstein and Kelly, 1980b). Guidubaldi and Perry (1985) found, controlling for social class, that boys in divorced families manifested significantly more maladaptive symptoms and behavior problems than boys in intact families. Girls differed only on the dimension of locus of control; girls in divorced households scored significantly higher than their counterparts in intact households....

While custodial mothers provide girls with same-sex role models, most boys have to adjust to living without same-sex parents. In examining boys and girls living in intact families and in different custodial arrangements, Santrock and Warshak (1979) found that few effects could be attributed to family structure per se, but that children living with opposite-sex parents (mother-custody boys and father-custody girls) were not as well adjusted on measures of competent social behavior....

Along related lines, a number of researchers have examined gender-role orientation and, specifically, the relation of father absence to boys' personality development. Most of the evidence indicates that boys without adult male role models demonstrate more feminine behavior (Biller, 1976; Herzog and Sudia, 1973; Lamb, 1977a), except in lower-class families (Biller, 1981b). A variety of studies have shown that fathers influence children's gender role development to be more traditional because, compared to mothers, they more routinely differentiate between masculine and feminine behaviors and encourage greater conformity to conventional gender roles (Biller, 1981a; Biller and Davids, 1973; Bronfenbrenner, 1961; Heilbrun, 1965; Lamb, 1977b; Noller, 1978).... But it should be reiterated that these effects have been attributed to father absence and thus would be expected to occur among boys in all female-headed families, not simply those that have experienced divorce....

[M]ost of the research on boys' adjustment fails to consider the quality or quantity of father-child contact or the availability of alternative male role models (e.g., foster father, grandfather, big brother, other male relatives, coach, friend, etc.), which makes it difficult to assess the impact of changing family structure on boys' behavior. There are also limitations imposed by conceptualizing and measuring masculinity-femininity as a bipolar construct (Bem, 1974; Constantinople, 1973; Worell, 1978), and there is evidence that boys and girls in father-absent families are better described as androgynous (Kurdek and Siesky, 1980a).

Positive outcomes of divorce. ...[T]he tendency of children in single-parent families to display more androgynous behavior may be interpreted as a beneficial effect. Because of father absence, children in female-headed families are not pressured as strongly as their counterparts in two-parent families to conform to traditional gender roles. These children frequently assume a variety of domestic responsibilities to compensate for the absent parent (Weiss, 1979), thereby broadening their skills and competencies and their definitions of gender-appropriate behavior. Divorced parents also must broaden their behavioral patterns to meet increased parenting responsibilities, thereby providing more androgynous role models.

Kurdek and Siesky (1980a: 250) give the illustration that custodial mothers often "find themselves needing to acquire and demonstrate a greater degree of dominance, assertiveness, and independence while custodial fathers may find themselves in situations eliciting high degrees of warmth, nurturance, and tenderness."

Aside from becoming more androgynous, adolescents living in single-parent families are characterized by greater maturity, feelings of efficacy, and an internal locus of control (Guidubaldi and Perry, 1985; Kalter, Alpern, Spence, and Plunkett, 1984; Wallerstein and Kelly, 1974; Weiss, 1979). For adolescent girls this maturity stems partly from the status and responsibilities they acquire in peer and confidant relationships with custodial mothers....

There is evidence (Kurdek et al., 1981) that children and adolescents with an internal locus of control and a high level of interpersonal reasoning adjust more easily to their parents' divorce and that children's divorce adjustment is related to their more global personal adjustment.

Self-Concept. . .

Marital discord. ...[F]amily structure is unrelated to children's self-esteem (Feldman and Feldman, 1975; Kinard and Reinherz, 1984; Parish, 1981; Parish, Dostal, and Parish, 1981), but parental discord is negatively related (Amato, 1986; Berg and Kelly, 1979; Cooper, Holman, and Braithwaite, 1983; Long, 1986; Raschke and Raschke, 1979; Slater and Haber, 1984). Because this conclusion is based on diverse samples of boys and girls of different ages in different living arrangements, the failure to obtain effects of family structure suggests either that family composition really does not matter for children's self-concept or that family structure alone is an insufficient index of familial relations. Further, these studies suggest that divorce per se does not adversely affect children's self-concept. Cashion's (1984) review of the literature indicates that children living in single-parent families suffer no losses to self-esteem, except in situations where the child's family situation is stigmatized (Rosenberg, 1979)....

Cognitive Functioning

... Many ... studies find that family conflict and disruption are associated with inhibited cognitive functioning (Blanchard and Biller, 1971; Feldman and Feldman, 1975; Hess and Camara, 1979; Kinard and Reinherz, 1986; Kurdek, 1981; Radin, 1981).... In this section we summarize the differential effects of family disruption on academic performance by gender and social class and offer some insights as to the mechanisms by which these effects occur.

Children's gender. Some studies suggest that negative effects of family disruption on academic performance are stronger for boys than for girls (Chapman, 1977; Werner and Smith, 1982), but most of the evidence suggests similar effects by gender (Hess and Camara, 1979; Kinard and Reinherz, 1986; Shinn, 1978). While females traditionally outscore males on standardized tests of verbal skills and males outperform females on mathematical skills, males who have experienced family disruption generally score higher on verbal aptitude

(Radin, 1981). Thus, the absence of a father may result in a "feminine" orientation toward education (Fowler and Richards, 1978, Herzog and Sudia, 1973). But an important and unresolved question is whether this pattern results from boys acquiring greater verbal skills in mother-headed families or from deficiencies in mathematical skills attributable to father absence. The latter explanation is supported by evidence showing that father-absent girls are disadvantaged in mathematics (Radin, 1981),

Children's race. ...[M]ost studies show academic achievement among black children to be unaffected by family structure (Hunt and Hunt, 1975, 1977; Shinn, 1978; Solomon, Hirsch, Scheinfeld, and Jackson, 1972), Svanum, Bringle, and McLaughlin (1982) found, controlling for social class, that there are no significant effects of father absence on cognitive performance for white or black children. Again, these investigations focus on family composition and demonstrate that the effects of family structure on academic performance do not vary as much by race as by social class, but race differences in the impact of divorce remain largely unexplored....

Family socioeconomic status. ...When social class is controlled, children in female-headed families fare no worse than children from two-parent families on measures of intelligence (Bachman, 1970; Kopf, 1970), academic achievement (Shinn, 1978; Svanum et al., 1982), and educational attainment (Bachman, O'Malley, and Johnston, 1978).... In order to disentangle the intricate effects of family structure and SES [socioeconomic status] on children's cognitive performance, family researchers need to examine the socioeconomic history of intact families and those in which disruption occurs, to examine the economic resources available to children at various stages of cognitive development, and to assess changes in economic resources and family relationships that accompany marital disruption.

Family processes. ...First, family disruption alters daily routines and work schedules and imposes additional demands on adults and children living in single-parent families (Amato, 1987; Furstenberg and Nord, 1985; Hetherington et al., 1983; Weiss, 1979). Most adolescents must assume extra domestic and child care responsibilities, and financial conditions require some to work part-time. These burdens result in greater absenteeism, tardiness, and truancy among children in single-parent households (Hetherington et al., 1983). Second, children in recently disrupted families are prone to experience emotional and behavioral problems such as aggression, distractibility, dependency, anxiety, and withdrawal (Hess and Camara, 1979; Kinard and Reinherz, 1984), factors that may help to explain problems in school conduct and the propensity of teachers to label and stereotype children from broken families (Hess and Camara, 1979; Hetherington et al., 1979, 1983). Third, emotional problems may interfere with study patterns, while demanding schedules reduce the time available for single parents to help with homework....

Interpersonal Relationships...

Peer relations. Studies of preschool children (Hetherington et al., 1979) and preadolescents (Santrock, 1975; Wyman, Cowen, Hightower, and Pedro-Carroll, 1985) suggest that children in disrupted families are less sociable: they have fewer close friends, spend less time with friends, and participate in fewer shared activities. Stolberg and Anker (1983) observe that children in families disrupted by divorce exhibit psychopathology in interpersonal relations, often behaving in unusual and inappropriate ways. Other studies suggest that the effects are temporary. Kinard and Reinherz (1984) found no differences in peer relations among children in intact and disrupted families, but those in recently disrupted families displayed greater hostility. Kurdek et al. (1981) conducted a two-year follow-up of children whose parents had divorced and showed that relationships with peers improved after the divorce and that personal adjustments was facilitated by opportunities to discuss experiences with peers, some of whom had similar experiences....

Dating patterns. Hetherington (1972) reported that adolescent girls whose fathers were absent prior to age 5 had difficulties in heterosexual relations, but Hainline and Feig's (1978) analyses of female college students indicated that early and later father-absent women could not be distinguished on measures of romanticism and heterosexual attitudes.

An examination of dating and sexual behavior among female college students found that women with divorced parents began dating slightly later than those in intact families, but women in both groups were socially active (Kalter, Riemer, Brickman, and Chen, 1985). Booth, Brinkerhoff, and White (1984) reported that, compared to college students with intact families, those whose parents were divorced or permanently separated exhibited higher levels of dating activity, and this activity increased further if parental or parent-child conflict persisted during and after the divorce... Regarding adolescent sexual behavior, the findings consistently demonstrate that males and females not living with both biological parents initiate coitus earlier than their counterparts in intact families (Hogan and Kitagawa, 1985; Newcomer and Udry, 1987). But Newcomer and Udry propose that, because parental marital status is also associated with a broad range of deviant behaviors, these effects may stem from general loss of parental control rather than simply loss of control over sexual behavior. Studies of antisocial behavior support this interpretation.

Antisocial Behavior

Many studies over the years have linked juvenile delinquency, deviancy, and anti-social behavior to children living in broken homes (Bandura and Walters, 1959, Glueck and Glueck, 1962; Hoffman, 1971; McCord, McCord, and Thurber, 1962; Santrock, 175; Stolberg and Anker, 1983; Tooley, 1976; Tuckman and Regan, 1966). Unfortunately, these studies either relied on clinical samples or failed to control for social class and other factors related to delinquency. However, ...a number of studies involving large representative samples and controlling for social class provide similar findings (Dormbusch, Carlsmith, Bushwall, Ritter, Leiderman, Hastorf, and Gross, 1985; Kalter et al., 1985; Peterson and Zill, 1986; Rickel and Langer, 1985). Kalter et at. (1985) studied 522 teenage girls and found that girls in divorced families committed more delinquent acts (e.g., drug use, larceny, skipping school) than their counterparts in intact families. Dornbusch et al. (1985) examined a representative national sample of male and female youth aged 12–17 and found that adolescents in mother-only households were more likely than their counterparts in intact families to engage in deviant acts, partly because of their tendency to make decisions independent of parental input. The presence of an additional adult (a grandparent, an uncle, a lover, a friend) in mother-only households increased control over adolescent behavior and lowered rates of deviant behavior, which suggests that "there are functional equivalents of two-parent families—nontraditional groupings that can do the job of parenting" (1985: 340)....

A tentative conclusion based on the evidence reviewed here is that antisocial behavior is less likely to occur in families where two adults are present, whether as biological parents, stepparents, or some combination of biological parents and other adults. Short-term increases in anti-social behavior may occur during periods of disruption, however, as children adjust to restructured relationships and parents struggle to maintain consistency in disciplining (Rickel and Langner, 1985).... Peterson and Zill (1986) demonstrated that, when social class was controlled, behavior problems were as likely to occur among adolescents living in intact families characterized by persistent conflict as among those living in disrupted families.... Peterson and Zill found that "poor parent-child relationships lead to more negative child behavior, yet maintaining good relationships with parents can go some way in reducing the effects of conflict and disruption" (1986: 306). Hess and Camara's (1979) analyses of a much smaller sample yielded a similar conclusion: aggressive behavior in children was unrelated to family type but was more common in situations characterized by infrequent or low-quality parent-child interaction and parental discord....

Conclusions

There is reason to question the validity of the family composition hypothesis. Theoretically, it has been assumed that the nuclear family is the norm and, by implication, that any departure from it is deviant and therefore deleterious to those involved. Even if this were the case, no theoretical perspective recognizes that these effects may be short-lived or otherwise mitigated by compensatory mechanisms and alternative role models. In the absence of a parent, it is possible that developmental needs are met by other factors.

It is simplistic and inaccurate to think of divorce as having uniform consequences for children. The consequences of divorce vary along different dimensions of well-being, characteristics of children (e.g., predivorce adjustment, age at the time of disruption) and characteristics of families (e.g., socioeconomic history, pre- and postdivorce level of conflict, parent-child relationships, and maternal employment). Most of the evidence reviewed here suggests that some sociodemographic characteristics of children, such as race and gender, are not as important as characteristics of families in mediating the effects of divorce. Many studies report boys to be at a greater disadvantage, but these differences usually disappear when other relevant variables are controlled. At present, there are too few methodologically adequate studies comparing white and black children to conclude that one group is more damaged by family disruption than the other.

Characteristics of families, on the other hand, are critical to youthful well-being. Family conflict contributes to many problems in social development, emotional stability, and cognitive skills (Edwards, 1987; Kurdek, 1981), and these effects continue long after the divorce is finalized. Slater and Haber (1984) report that ongoing high levels of conflict, whether in intact or divorced homes, produce lower self-esteem, increased anxiety, and loss of self-control. Conflict also reduces the child's attraction to the parents (White, Brinkerhoff, and Booth, 1985), Rosen (1979) concludes that parental separation is more beneficial for children than continued conflict.... Such conflict and hostility may account for adolescent adjustment problems whether the family in question goes through divorce or remains intact (Hoffman, 1971). The level of conflict is thus an important dimension of family interaction that can precipitate changes in family structure and affect children's well-being.

Maternal employment is another variable mediating the consequences of divorce for children. Divorced women often find the dual responsibilities of provider and parent to be stressful (Bronfenbrenner, 1976). But studies indicate that women who work prior to the divorce do not find continued employment problematic (Kinard and Reinherz, 1984); the problem occurs for women who enter the labor force after the divorce and who view the loss of time with their children as another detriment to the children that is caused by the divorce (Kinard and Reinherz, 1984). As a practical matter, the alternative to employment for single-parent mothers is likely to be poverty or, at best, economic dependency. The effects of maternal employment on children's well-being need to be compared to the effects of nonemployment and consequent poverty.

Other bases of social support for single-parent mothers and their children must also be examined. The presence of strong social networks may ease the parents' and, presumably, the child's adjustment after a divorce (Milardo, 1987; Savage et al., 1978). However, women who are poor, have many children, and must work long hours are likely to have limited social networks and few friends. Typically, the single mother and her children are also isolated from her ex-husband's family (Anspach, 1976). By reuniting with her family of origin, the mother may be isolated from her community and new social experiences for herself and her children (McLanahan, Wedemeyer, and Adelberg, 1981). Kinship ties are usually strained, as both biological parents and parents-in-law are more critical of the divorce than friends are (Spanier and Thompson, 1984). Little has been done to relate these considerations about kinship relations and social networks of divorced women to the well-being of children and adolescents. We believe that these social relations are important, but empirical verification is needed.

Debate Presenter Form

Follow the guidelines for debate presenters contained in the introduction of this text and those given to you by your instructor. Use the format below to organize the material for your debate. Remember to include all relevant citation information and to present the related information in your own words. Give credit to authors when you cite a quote and be as thorough as possible when writing about your points so you will be prepared for your debate.

Reference citation #1:

Author: _____

Title: _____

Date: _____

Source: _____

_____

Content from reference citation #1: _____

_____

_____

_____

_____

_____

_____

_____

_____

_____

_____

_____

Reference citation #2:

Author: _____

Title: _____

Date: _____

Source: _____

_____

Content from reference citation #2: _____

_____

_____

_____

_____

_____

_____

Reference citation #3:

Author: _____

Title: _____

Date: _____

Source: _____

_____

Content from reference citation #3: _____

_____

_____

_____

_____

Audience Preparation Form

Follow the guidelines for preparing to be an informed audience member on the day of the debate included in the introduction to this text. After reading both sides of the debate from this chapter, answer the following questions. Be as thorough as possible so that you will be able to make a contribution to the debate by asking informed questions or making provocative comments. This form is usually due on the day of the debate.

State the issue in your own words. Do not plagiarize the text. Demonstrate that you understand the topic and it's relevant arguments.

_____

_____

_____

_____

_____

Discuss two points on the "yes" side of the debate.

Point #1: _____

_____

Point #2: _____

_____

Discuss two points on the "no" side of the debate.

Point #1: _____

_____

Point #2: _____

_____

What is your opinion on this topic?

_____

_____

_____

_____

_____

_____

_____

What has contributed to the development of your views about this topic?

_____

_____

_____

_____

_____

_____

_____

_____

What information would be necessary to cause you to change your thinking about this topic?

_____

_____

_____

_____

_____

Debate Response Form

Follow the guidelines for responding to the debates in the introductory chapter of this text. Complete this form and submit your answers at the class following the debate. Try to be thorough and convince your instructor that you were an active listener during the debate.

List a quote from a debate presenter that you think was important and explain why you think this comment was significant.

_____

_____

_____

_____

Which side of the debate do you think made the most convincing arguments, why?

_____

_____

_____

_____

_____

After hearing the debate, in what way has your thinking been affected?

_____

_____

_____

_____

_____

_____

Children

ISSUE 14

Should Drug Use by Pregnant Women Be Considered Child Abuse?

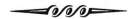

 Paul A. Logli, *Drugs in the Womb: The Newest Battlefield in the War on Drugs*

 Maureen A. Norton-Hawk, *How Social Policies Make Matters Worse: The Case of Maternal Substance Abuse*

A large number of fetuses are exposed to illicit drug use through the drug habits of their mothers. Many of these babies are actually born addicted to illegal substances. Paul A. Logli has suggested that maternal drug abuse be considered child abuse, a prosecutable charge. Logli cites pain, suffering, death and enormous economic costs as the rationale for prosecution of mothers in drug-related births.

Several cases, and common sense, indicate that children have the right to come into our world with a sound mind and body. Anyone who knowingly interferes with this right should be civilly liable according to Logli. The specific wording of the statute would be, "Conduct Injurious To A Newborn." Violation of this statute would be a class four felony resulting in a one to three year prison sentence.

Marueen A. Norton-Hawk suggests that this type of social policy, prosecution of mothers of drug-affected babies, will make the situation worse, not better. She believes that consequating prenatal drug use with criminal prosecution will exacerbate drug use by these mothers.

The concern is that not only will drug abusing pregnant women avoid drug treatment during pregnancy for fear of prosecution, they may also avoid pre-natal care for this same reason. Furthermore, jailed pregnant women are exposed to conditions that are counter to their health and that of their unborn child.

Norton-Hawk suggests that the better solution would be to increase the availability of drug treatment for these mothers. The focus of the social policies should be on reduction of the addictive behavior and prosecution is not going to bring this result.

Applications

1. Discuss whether or not you think that prosecution of pregnant women for child abuse because they have used illegal drugs would ultimately benefit the children of these women.

2. From your experience with people who use illegal drugs, what do you think would be the best approach for a pregnant drug user?

3. What rights do unborn children have? Would you support a raise in taxes if it were supposed to pay for the development of drug treatment programs for pregnant women?

4. Do you think some women might get pregnant just to get into the drug treatment programs designed for them? Why or why not?

Issue 14

YES

Drugs in the Womb
The Newest Battlefield in the War on Drugs

Paul A. Logli

Introduction

The reported incidence of drug-related births has risen dramatically over the last several years. The legal system and, in particular, local prosecutors have attempted to properly respond to the suffering, death, and economic costs which result from a pregnant woman's use of drugs. The ensuing debate has raised serious constitutional and practical issues which are far from resolution.

Prosecutors have achieved mixed results in using current criminal and juvenile statutes as a basis for legal action intended to prosecute mothers and protect children. As a result, state and federal legislators have begun the difficult task of drafting appropriate laws to deal with the problem, while at the same time acknowledging the concerns of medical authorities, child protection groups, and advocates for individual rights.

The Problem

The plight of "cocaine babies," children addicted at birth to narcotic substances or otherwise affected by maternal drug use during pregnancy, has prompted prosecutors in some jurisdictions to bring criminal charges against drug-abusing mothers. Not only have these prosecutions generated heated debates both inside and outside of the nation's courtrooms, but they have also expanded the war on drugs to a controversial new battlefield—the mother's womb.

A 1988 survey of hospitals conducted by Dr. Ira Chasnoff, Associate Professor of Northwestern University Medical School and President of the National Association for Prenatal Addiction Research and Education (NAPARE) indicated that as many as 375,000 infants may be affected by maternal cocaine use during pregnancy each year. Chasnoff's survey included 36 hospitals across the country and showed incidence rates ranging from 1 percent to 27 percent. It also indicated that the problem was not restricted to urban populations or particular racial or socio-economic groups.[1] More recently a study at Hutzel Hospital in Detroit's inner city found that 42.7 percent of its newborn babies were exposed to drugs while in their mother's wombs.[2]

The effects of maternal use of cocaine and other drugs during pregnancy on the mother and her newborn child have by now been well-documented and will not be repeated here. The effects are severe and can cause numerous threats to the short-term health of the child. In a few cases it can even result in death.[3]

Medical authorities have just begun to evaluate the long-term effects of cocaine exposure on children as they grow older. Early findings show that many of these infants show serious difficulties in relating and reacting to adults and environments, as well as in organizing creative play, and they appear similar to mildly autistic or personality-disordered children.[4]

The human costs related to the pain, suffering, and deaths resulting from maternal cocaine use during pregnancy are simply incalculable. In economic terms, the typical intensive-care costs for treating babies exposed to drugs range from $7,500 to $31,000. In some cases medical bills go as high as $150,000.[5]

The costs grow enormously as more and more hospitals encounter the problem of "boarder babies"—those children literally abandoned at the hospital by an addicted mother, and left to be cared for by the nursing staff.[6] Future costs to society for simply educating a generation of drug-affected children can only be the object of speculation. It is clear, however, that besides pain, suffering, and death the economic costs to society of drug use by pregnant women is presently enormous and is certainly growing larger.

The Prosecutor's Response

It is against this backdrop and fueled by the ever-growing emphasis on an aggressively waged war on drugs that prosecutors have begun a number of actions against women who have given birth to drug-affected children. A review of at least two cases will illustrate the potential success or failure of attempts to use existing statutes.

People vs. Melanie Green[7]   On February 4, 1989, at a Rockford, Illinois hospital, two-day old Bianca Green lost her brief struggle for life. At the time of Bianca's birth both she and her mother, twenty-four-year-old Melanie Green, tested positive for the presence of cocaine in their systems.

Pathologists in Rockford and Madison, Wisconsin, indicated that the death of the baby was the result of a prenatal injury related to cocaine used by the mother during the pregnancy. They asserted that maternal cocaine use had caused the placenta to prematurely rupture, which deprived the fetus of oxygen, the child's brain began to swell and she eventually died.

After an investigation by the Rockford Police Department and the State of Illinois Department of Children and Family Services, prosecutors allowed a criminal complaint to be filed on May 9, 1989, charging Melanie Green with the offenses of Involuntary Manslaughter[8] and Delivery of a Controlled Substance.[9]

On May 25, 1989, testimony was presented to the Winnebago County Grand Jury by prosecutors seeking a formal indictment. The Grand Jury, however, declined to indict Green on either charge. Since Grand Jury proceedings in the State of Illinois are secret, as are the jurors' deliberations and votes, the reason for the decision of the Grand Jury in this case is determined more by conjecture than any direct knowledge. Prosecutors involved in the presentation observed that the jurors exhibited a certain amount of sympathy for the young woman who had been brought before the Grand Jury at the jurors' request. It is also likely that the jurors were uncomfortable with the use of statutes that were not intended to be used in these circumstances.

It would also be difficult to disregard the fact that, after the criminal complaints were announced on May 9th and prior to the Grand Jury deliberations of May 25th, a national debate had ensued revolving around the charges brought in Rockford, Illinois, and their implications for the ever-increasing problem of women who use drugs during pregnancy.

People vs. Jennifer Clarise Johnson.[10] On July 13, 1989, a Seminole County, Florida judge found Jennifer Johnson guilty of delivery of a controlled substance to a child. The judge found that delivery, for purposes of the statute, occurred through the umbilical cord after the birth of the child and before the cord was severed. Jeff Deen, the Assistant State's Attorney who prosecuted the case, has since pointed out that Johnson, age 23, had previously given birth to three other cocaine-affected babies, and in this case was arrested at a crack house. "We needed to make sure this woman does not give birth to another cocaine baby."[11]

Johnson was sentenced to fifteen years of probation including strict supervision, drug treatment, random drug testing, educational and vocational training, and an intensive prenatal care program if she ever became pregnant again.[12].

Support for the Prosecution of Maternal Drug Abuse

Both cases reported above relied on a single important fact as a basis for the prosecution of the drug-abusing mother: that the child was born alive and exhibited the consequences of prenatal injury.

In the Melanie Green case, Illinois prosecutors relied on the "born alive" rule set out earlier in *People vs Bolar.*[13] In Bolar the defendant was convicted of the offense of reckless homicide.[14] The case involved an accident between a car driven by the defendant, who was found to be drunk, and another automobile containing a pregnant woman. As a result, the woman delivered her baby by emergency caesarean section within hours of the collision. Although the newborn child exhibited only a few heart beats and lived for approximately two minutes, the court found that the child was born alive and was therefore a person for purposes of the criminal statutes of the State of Illinois.

The Florida prosecution relied on a live birth in an entirely different fashion. The prosecutor argued in that case that the delivery of the controlled substance occurred after the live birth via the umbilical cord and prior to the cutting of the cord. Thus, it was argued, that the delivery of the controlled substance occurred not to a fetus but to a person who enjoyed the protection of the criminal code of the State of Florida.

Further support for the State's role in protecting the health of newborns even against prenatal injury is found in the statutes which provide protection for the fetus. These statutes proscribe actions by a person, usually other than the mother, which either intentionally or recklessly harm or kill a fetus.[15] In other words, even in the absence of a live birth, most states afford protection to the unborn fetus against the harmful actions of another person. Arguably, the same protection should be afforded the infant against intentional harmful actions by a drug-abusing mother.

The state also receives support for a position in favor of the protection of the health of a newborn from a number of non-criminal cases. A line of civil cases in several states would appear to stand for the principle that a child has a right to begin life with a sound mind and body, and a person who interferes with that right may be subject to civil liability. In two cases decided within months of each other, the Supreme Court of Michigan upheld two actions for recovery of damages that were caused by the infliction of prenatal injury. In *Womack vs. Buckhorn*[16] the court upheld an action on behalf of an eight-year-old surviving child for prenatal brain injuries apparently suffered during the fourth month of the pregnancy in an automobile accident. The court adopted with approval the reasoning of a New Jersey Supreme Court decision and "recognized that a child has a legal right to begin life with a sound mind and body."[17] Similarly, in *O'Neill vs. Morse*[18] the court found that a cause of action was allowed for prenatal injuries that caused the death of an eight-month-old viable fetus.

Illinois courts have allowed civil recovery on behalf of an infant for a negligently administered blood transfusion given to the mother prior to conception which resulted in damage to the child at birth.[19] However, the same Illinois court would not extend a similar cause of action for prebirth injuries as between a child and its own mother.[20] The court, however, went on to say that a right to such a cause of action could be statutorily enacted by the Legislature.

Additional support for the state's role in protecting the health of newborns is found in the principles ennunciated in recent decisions of the United States Supreme Court. The often cited case of *Roe vs. Wade*[21] set out that although a woman's right of privacy is broad enough to cover the abortion decision, the right is not absolute and is subject to limitations, "and that at some point the state's interest as to protection of health, medical standards and prenatal life, becomes dominant."[22]

More recently, in the case of *Webster vs. Reproductive Health Services*,[23] the court expanded the state's interest in protection of potential human life by setting aside viability as a rigid line that had previously allowed state regulation only after viability had been shown but prohibited it before viability.[24] The court goes on to say that the "fundamental right" to abortion, as described in *Roe,* is now accorded the lesser status of a "liberty interest."[25] Such language surely supports a prosecutor's argument that the state's compelling interest in potential human life would allow the criminalization of acts which if committed by a pregnant woman can damage not just a viable fetus but eventually a born-alive infant. It follows that, once a pregnant woman has abandoned her right to abort and has decided to carry the fetus to term, society can well impose a duty on the mother to insure that the fetus is born as healthy as possible.[26]

A further argument in support of the state's interest in prosecuting women who engage in conduct which is damaging to the health of a newborn child is especially compelling in regard to maternal drug use during pregnancy. Simply put, there is no fundamental right or even a liberty interest in the use of psycho-active drugs.[27] A perceived right of privacy has never formed an absolute barrier against state prosecutions of those who use or possess narcotics. Certainly no exception can be made simply because the person using drugs happens to be pregnant.

Critics of the prosecutor's role argue that any statute that would punish mothers who create a substantial risk of harm to their fetus will run afoul of constitutional requirements, including prohibitions on vagueness, guarantees of liberty and privacy, and rights of due process and equal protection.

> A criminal statute designed to punish reckless or negligent behavior creating a substantial risk of harm to the fetus (an objective standard of care) effectively would result in a strict liability crime that would disregard a woman's economic situation, personal values, and individual health needs. Although a narrower statute targeting intentional or knowing imposition of harm (a subjective standard of care) might avoid the problems inherent in an objective standard, it nonetheless would deter women from seeking prenatal care of substance abuse treatment. Ironically, such a statute would be so narrow that it would not reach women who are the subject of public concern: those who use drugs during pregnancy because of addiction, rather than out of a desire to harm their fetus.
>
> Even a narrow statute that only punishes women who have been informed of the risks of drug use and who were offered a voluntary treatment option nonetheless raises serious constitutional questions about fair notice, liberty and equal protection. Acts potentially harmful to a fetus cannot be defined with sufficient precision to give notice to mothers of the legal behavioral standard. The statute probably would be enforced only against poor mothers, because they often are in closer contact with government's monitors and generally are in poorer health. Further, such a vague statute would deputize the medical profession by imposing report requirements, undermining the patient-doctor privilege and deterring care, eviscerating the informed consent model of treatment, and giving fallible medical judgments the force of law. Finally, such a statute would punish women who lack notice of their own pregnancy since the most serious prenatal harms often occur very early in pregnancy before women realize that they are pregnant.[29]

In spite of such criticism, the state's role in protecting those citizens who are least able to protect themselves, namely the newborn, mandates an aggressive posture. Much of the criticism of prosecutorial efforts is based on speculation as to the consequences of prosecution and ignores the basic tenet of criminal law that prosecutions deter the prosecuted and others from committing additional crimes. To assume that will only drive persons further underground is to somehow argue that certain prosecutions of crime will only force perpetrators to make even more aggressive efforts to escape apprehension, thus making arrest and prosecution unadvisable. Neither could this be accepted as an argument justifying even the weakening of criminal sanctions. "The speculative danger of abuse is no reason to exempt children from legal protection against pregnant women who are not able to meet responsible community standards about safe conduct during pregnancy."[30]

The concern that pregnant addicts will avoid obtaining health care for themselves or their infants because of the fear of prosecution cannot justify the absence of state action to protect the newborn. If the state were to accept such reasoning, then existing child abuse laws would have to be reconsidered since they might deter parents from obtaining medical care for physically or sexually abused children. That argument has not been accepted as a valid reason for abolishing child abuse laws or for not prosecuting child abusers.[31]

> To view children as mere chattels of their parents is anachronistic. The belief that parents can best fulfill their responsibilities to their children if free from the intervention is naive in the fetal abuse context. Children have separate and distinct legal rights, and are entitled to the protection of the law, even from their parents. In extreme cases of fetal abuse, those resulting in abortion and stillbirths, parental autonomy cannot possible justify unbridled discretion... To legitimate this moral and spiritual existence of the unborn child, society must prevent fetal substance abuse by any possible means.[32]

The far better policy is for the state to acknowledge its responsibility not only to provide a deterrent to criminal and destructive behavior by pregnant addicts but also to provide adequate opportunities for those who might seek help to discontinue their addiction. Prosecution has a role in its ability to deter future criminal behavior and to protect the best interests of the child. The medical and social welfare establishment must assume an even greater responsibility to encourage legislators to provide adequate funding and facilities so that no pregnant woman who is addicted to drugs will be denied the opportunity to seek appropriate prenatal care and treatment for her addiction.

One State's Response

The Legislature of the State of Illinois, at the urging of local prosecutors, moved quickly to amend its juvenile court act in order to provide protection to those children born drug-affected. Previously, Illinois law provided that a court could assume jurisdiction over addicted minors[32] or a minor who is generally declared neglected or abused.[33]

Effective January 1, 1990, the juvenile court act was amended to expand the definition of a neglected or abused minor. That statute now provides that

> those who are neglected include...any newborn infant whose blood or urine contains any amount of a controlled substance as defined in...the Illinois Controlled Substances Act, or a metabolite of a controlled substance, with the exception of controlled substances or metabolites of such substances, the presence of which in the newborn infant is a result of medical treatment administered to the mother or the newborn infant.[34]

The purpose of the new statute is to make it easier for the court to assert jurisdiction over a newborn infant born drug-affected. The state is not required to show either the addiction of the child or harmful effects on the child in order to remove the child from a drug-abusing mother. Used in this context, prosecutors can work with the mother in a rather coercive atmosphere to encourage her to enter into drug rehabilitation and, upon the successful completion of the program, be reunited with her child.

Additional legislation before the Illinois Legislature is House Bill 2835 sponsored by Representatives John Hallock (R-Rockford) and Edolo "Zeke" Giorgi (D-Rockford). This bill represents the first attempt to specifically address the prosecution of drug-abusing pregnant women. The act would establish a new criminal statute entitled "Conduct Injurious To A Newborn," and sets out the following:

> Any woman who is pregnant and without a prescription knowingly or intentionally uses a dangerous drug or a narcotic drug and at the conclusion of her pregnancy delivers a newborn child, and such child shows signs of narcotic or dangerous drug exposure or addiction, or the presence of a narcotic or dangerous drug in the child's blood or urine, commits the offense of conduct injurious to a newborn.[35]

The statute provides for a class 4 felony disposition upon conviction. A class 4 felony is a probationable felony which can also result in a term of imprisonment from one to three years.

Subsequent paragraphs set out certain defenses available to the accused.

> It shall not be a violation of this section if a woman knowingly or intentionally uses a narcotic or dangerous drug in the first twelve weeks of pregnancy and:
> 1. She has no knowledge that she is pregnant; or
> 2. Subsequently, within the first twelve weeks of pregnancy, undergoes medical treatment for substance abuse or treatment or rehabilitation in a program or facility approved by the Illinois Department of Alcoholism and Substance Abuse, and thereafter discontinues any further use of drugs or narcotics as previously set forth.[36]

The statute clearly requires live birth consistent with the case law under *Bolar*.[37] It also requires that narcotic substances be found in the baby's system, which would presuppose that drugs were used within a short period of time prior to birth. A woman, under this statute, could not be prosecuted for self-reporting her addiction in the early stages of the pregnancy. Nor could she be prosecuted under this statute if, even during the subsequent stages of the pregnancy, she discontinued her drug use to the extent that no drugs were present in her system or the baby's system at the time of birth. The statute, as drafted, is clearly intended to allow prosecutors to invoke the criminal statutes in the most serious cases.

Conclusion

Local prosecutors have a legitimate role in responding to the increasing problem of drug-abusing pregnant women and their drug-affected children. Eliminating the pain, suffering and death resulting from drug exposure in newborns must be a prosecutor's priority. However, the use of existing statutes to address the problem may meet with limited success since they are burdened with numerous constitutional problems dealing with original intent, notice, vagueness, and due process.

The juvenile courts may offer perhaps the best initial response in working to protect the interests of a surviving child. However, in order to address more serious cases, legislative efforts may be required to provide new statutes that will specifically address the problem and hopefully deter future criminal conduct which deprives children of their important right to a healthy and normal birth.

The long-term solution does not rest with the prosecutor alone. Society, including the medical and social welfare establishment, must be more responsive in providing readily accessible prenatal care and treatment alternatives for pregnant addicts. In the short term however, prosecutors must be prepared to play a vital role in protecting children and deterring women from engaging in conduct which will harm the newborn child. If prosecutors fail to respond, then they are simply closing the doors of the criminal justice system to those persons, the newborn, who are least able to open the doors for themselves.

Notes

1 NAPARE, Update, 3/89 enclosure, and *A First: National Hospital Incidence Survey, and Substances Most Commonly Abused During Pregnancy and Their Risks to Mother and Baby* (May 1989).

2 Hundley, *Infants: A Growing Casualty of the Drug Epidemic*, Chicago Tribune, Oct. 16, 1989, at 1.

3 *See* Little, Snell, Klein & Gilstrap, *Cocaine Abuse during Pregnancy; Maternal and Fetal Implications* 73 OBST. & GYN. 2 (1989).

4 Chasnoff, Griffith, MacGregor, Dirkes & Burns, *Temporal Patterns of Cocaine Use in Pregnancy*. 261 J AM. MED. A. 12 (1989).

5   Smith, *The Dangers of Prenatal Cocaine Use*, 13 MATERNAL CHILD NURSING J. (May/June 1988).

6   Fink, *Effects of Crack and Cocaine Upon Infants: A Brief Review of the Literature*, 10 JOURNAL 4 (Fall 1989).

7   Hundley, *supra* note 2, at 2.

8   Greene, *Boarder Babies Linger in Hospitals*, Washington Post, Sept. 11, 1989, at A1 and A7.

9   ILL. REV. STAT. ch. 38, ¶ 9–3 (1987). Count I of the complaint read in part:

That between the dates of January 26, 1989, and February 2, 1989, in the County of Winnebago, State of Illinois, Melanie Green, committed the offense of involuntary manslaughter in that she unintentionally and without lawful justification killed her child, Bianca Greene, by recklessly performing the act of ingesting a controlled substance containing cocaine while pregnant with Bianca and nearly at full term of that pregnancy, that act being likely to cause death or great bodily harm to Bianca, and that act in fact caused Bianca's death.

10   ILL. REV. STAT. ch. 56 1/2, ¶ 1407 (1987). Count II of the complaint read in part:

That between the dates of January 26, 1989 and February 2, 1989 in the County of Winnebago, State of Illinois, Melanie Green committed the offense of violation of the controlled substances act in that she, a person over eighteen years of age, delivered to a person under eighteen years of age a controlled substance containing cocaine, to wit: while pregnant and nearly at full term with a child, Bianca Green, she knowingly ingested a controlled substance containing cocaine which was thereby delivered to the bloodstream and body of her fetus, Bianca.

11   Curriden, *Holding Mom Accountable*, 76 A.B.A. J., March 1990, at 51–53.

12   *Id.* at 51.

13   People vs. Bolar, 109 Ill. App.3d 384, 440 N.E. 2d639 (1982).

14   ILL. REV. STAT. ch.38, ¶ 9–3 (1979).

15.   ILL. REV. STAT. ch. 38,¶¶ 9–1.2, 9–2.1, 9–3.2, 12–3.1, 12–4.4 (1987); CAL. PENAL CODE ¶ 187 (West Supp. 1988); IOWA CODE ANN. ¶ 707.7 (West 1979); Michigan Comp.Laws Ann. ¶ 750–322 (1968); MISS. CODE ANN. ¶ 97–3–37 (1973); and several other states.

16   Womak vs Buchhorn 384 Mich. 718, 187 N.W. 2d 218 (1971).

17   *Id.* at 222.

18   O'Neill vs. Morse 385 Mich.. 130, 188 N.W. 2d 785 (1971).

19   Renslow vs. Mennonite Hospital 67 Ill. 2d 348, 367 N.E. 2d 1250 (1977).

20   Stallman vs. Youngquist 125 Ill. 2d 267, 531 N.E. 2d 355 (1988).

21   Roe vs. Wade 410 U.S. 113 (1973).

22   *Id.* at 156

23   Webster vs. Reproductive Health Services 109 S.Ct. 3040 (1989).

24   *Id.* at 3057.

25   *Id.* at 3058

26   *See* discussion in Robertson, *Procreative Liberty*, 69 VA.L. REV. 405 (1983).

27   *See* California v. LaRue, 409 U.S. 109 (1972); and City of Newport v. Iacobucci, 479 U.S. 1047 (1986) regarding local regulation of alcohol. State of Minnesota ex rel. Whipple v. Martenson, 256 U.S. 41 (1921) and Whalen v. Roe, 429 U.S. 589 (1977) regarding state regulation of the dispensing of drugs.

28   McNulty, *Pregnancy Police; The Health Policy and Legal Implications of Punishing Pregnant Women for Harm to their Fetuses*, 16 REV. OF LAW & SOC. CHANGE 277 (1987)

29   *Id.* at 318, 319.

30   Robertson, *Fetal Abuse: Should We Recognize It as a Crime?* A.B.A. J. Aug. 1989, at 38.

31   Fost, *Maternal-Fetal Conflicts: Ethical and Legal Considerations*, 562 ANNALS N.S. ACAD. SCI. 248 (1989).

32   ILL. REV. STAT., ch. 37, 804–1 (1987).

33   ILL. REV. STAT. ch. 37, 802–3 (1987).

34   ILL REV. STAT. ch. 37, 802–3 (c) (1989).

35   HB 2835, 86th General Assembly, State of Illinois (1989 and 1990), amending ch. 38, new ¶ 12-4.7 (LRB8607533RCm6).

36   *Id.*

37   *Supra* note 13.

How Social Policies Make Matters Worse
The Case of Maternal Substance Abuse

Maureen A. Norton-Hawk

This article addresses the issue of maternal substance abuse and the consequences of our current punitive approach. This article initially presents information that defines the scope of the problem and then offers case illustrations of the court's attempt to deal with women who use drugs and alcohol when pregnant. The article then focuses on characteristics of interventions that have the potential for bringing about a deterioration of the problem of maternal substance abuse.

In an attempt to address maternal substance abuse evolving social policy is relying on the criminal justice system. In fact since 1987 there have been more than 160 criminal prosecutions against women for their drug or alcohol use during pregnancy (Paltrow 1992). However, the prosecution of these women fails to rectify the problem of substance-abusing pregnant women and, in fact, this policy exacerbates the problem of drug and alcohol use during pregnancy.

Each year approximately 739,200 women use one or more illegal drugs during pregnancy (Gomby and Shiono, 1991). Calculations by the National Association for Perinatal Addiction Research and Education (NAPARE) indicate that maternal drug use annually affects 375,000 newborns (Chasnoff, 1989). Studies have indicated that a relationship exists between the use of various illicit drugs and lower birth weight and smaller head circumference, irritability, neurobehavioral dysfunction, sudden infant death syndrome (Zuckerman, 1991), negative responses to multiple stimuli (Howard and Beckwith, 1989), and a potential for malformation of developing systems (Zuckerman, 1991). It is important to note that while there exists a correlation between illicit drug use and physiological/psychological problems in newborns, neither causality nor a complete understanding of the potential harm of specific substances has been established. This difficulty in confirming a direct link between drug use and drug effect in pregnant addicts is due in part to the involvement of other extraneous variables such as the lack of prenatal care (Kronstadt, 1991) poor maternal health, inadequate maternal nutrition, and polydrug use (Zuckerman, 1991).

These physiological/psychological effects on newborns, if accurate, can result in dramatic social and medical costs. The General Accounting Office (1990) found that in one hospital the median cost for the medical care of a newborn was $4,100 higher for drug-exposed infants with the cost rising as high as $135,000 for a drug-exposed, premature infant needing intensive care for several months (Halfon, 1989). The cost climbs as we confront the problem of boarder babies—those children abandoned in the hospital at birth. Foster care for one of these children is estimated to be $6,000 annually (General Accounting Office 1990). For a group of nine thousand identified as crack-exposed infants, the Office of the Inspector General (1990) estimated that the total cost of hospital and foster care for this group until the age of five will approximate $500 million.

Prenatal exposure to illicit substances is hardly the only concern. Five to ten percent of pregnant women continue to drink heavily (Balisy, 1987) resulting in Fetal Alcohol Syndrome (FAS). Estimates of the incidence of FAS is 1 to 3 cases per 1,000 live births (Abel and Sokol 1987) or nearly 5,000 newborns annually (Office of the Inspector General, 1990). Fetal Alcohol Syndrome is marked by dysfunction of the central nervous system, prenatal and postnatal growth deficiency, and facial malformations (Warren, 1987; Abel, 1984) and is the third leading cause of birth defects associated with mental retardation (Office of the Inspector General, 1990). In 1980, the estimated cost for medical, educational and custodial services for children born with Fetal Alcohol Syndrome for Fetal Alcohol Effect in the United States was $2.7 billion (Balisy, 1987).

In an attempt to grapple with the physiological, social and economic costs of drug and alcohol use during pregnancy, twenty-six states have prosecuted these women on charges of child abuse/neglect, contributing to the delinquency of a minor, causing dependency, child endangerment, drug possession, assault with a deadly weapon, manslaughter, homicide, vehicular homicide and delivering a controlled substance to a minor (Paltrow, 1992). Though the rhetoric implies that the goal of these prosecutions is to protect the child and increase infant health, prosecution of pregnant addicts will not protect the child, nor will this policy increase the likelihood of infant health. Rather than the creation of a social policy that effectively remedies a social problem, what has emerged is a regressive intervention—an intervention that makes the original aim of the policy less attainable or cause a deterioration of the social problem one wanted to ameliorate (Sieber, 1981:10).

An example of such a failed intervention is the effect of the decision of the U.S. Supreme Court in *Brown v. Board of Education*, which held that separate schools are inherently unequal. Courts mandated that segregated schools be integrated. To comply with the Court's order, Boston, as in other areas of the country, imposed a system of busing students (Lukas, 1986).

Social Problem
Unequal Education

Goal
Integration

Intervention
Busing

The result of this social intervention was the flight of whites to the suburbs or the placement of their children in private schools as a means of avoiding, at all costs, the court-mandated busing. This "white flight" caused an even more segregated school system as the number of white students in the system dropped from 67,028 in 1967 to 11,555 in 1992 (Canellos 1993), thus making the goal of integration less attainable and making the problem of inequitable education more pronounced.

We can apply this framework of regressive interventions to maternal substance abuse.

Social Problem
Substance Abuse
by Pregnant Women

Goal
Decrease Drug
Use/Insure
Infant Health

Intervention
Prosecution

Most Americans would agree that ingestion of illicit substances by pregnant women is a social concern and many would argue that punitive sanctions need to be applied. According to a popular magazine poll, 46% favored criminal penalties for prenatal substance abuse (*Glamour,* 1988). Problematic as such popular surveys are, this poll may indicate that, at least for a portion of the population, the pervasive ideology is that prosecution and indictment of maternal substance abusers will decrease their drug use thus increase the likelihood of infant health.

But does the prosecution of pregnant substance abusers insure the health of their newborns? Brenda Vaughan, a Washington, D.C. resident who was originally arrested for writing bad checks, tested positive for cocaine and was sent to jail until the date her baby was due to protect her fetus. The judge stated:

> I'm going to keep her locked up until the baby is born because she's tested positive for cocaine. She's apparently an addictive personality, and I'll be darned if I'm going to have a baby born that way (Cassen Moss, 1988:20).

While incarcerated, Ms. Vaughn received no drug treatment, was allowed to detoxify with no medical supervision, received only spotty prenatal care (Smith, 1990), and lost weight because of improper nutrition (Cassen, Moss 1988)—hardly an environment that would insure the health of the newborn.

Does the prosecution of pregnant addicts increase the likelihood that pregnant substance abusers will avail themselves of available drug treatment thus preventing potential harm to the fetus? In May 1989, Melanie Green was indicted on charges of manslaughter and delivery of a controlled substance to a minor after the purported drug induced death of her newborn. The publicity surrounding this arrest impeded efforts to get women to seek and remain in prenatal care and drug treatment. The Prenatal Center for Chemical Dependence at Northwestern University received numerous calls from women who were frightened that they would also be arrested. These women, who up until that time had been receiving prenatal care at the facility, wanted to stop seeing the doctors rather than risk possible prosecution (Chasnoff, 1990). Thus, we can see the regressive nature of such interventions.

The question now becomes, what are the dynamics of regressive interventions? How can a social policy actually make the goal of the intervention less attainable or cause a deterioration in the original social problem? To deal with these questions one needs to understand the notion of a conversion mechanism. A conversion mechanism is a feature or characteristic of an intervention or social policy that interacts with the environment and results in a regressive intervention. At least six types of conversion mechanisms have been suggested: functional imbalance (an overemphasis on a specific goal), exploitation (the exploitation of the intervention by the target population), goal displacement (the goal of efficiency overshadows the goal of effectiveness), provocation (the stirring up of emotions), derogatory classification (consequences of labeling), and placation (interventions that are primarily a means of placating certain groups in the society (Sieber, 1981). We will now examine each of these conversion mechanisms and illustrate how a punitive approach to pregnant drug users fails to deal with the two key goals of eliminating substance abuse during pregnancy and protecting the fetus and newborn.

Conversion Mechanisms

Functional Imbalance

Social policies can have regressive effects when there is such an emphasis on a specific goal rather than other facets of the social problem. For example, the Nixon administration's War on Drugs concentrated on drug supply from Mexico. While the United States' policy was successful in diminishing the flow of marijuana across our southern borders, not only did other countries replace Mexico as our prime supplier, but domestic production increased. Thus, the intervention undertaken, to eliminate drugs at their source, while successful in one area, may have actually made the overall problem more pronounced by failing to address the "demand" side of the drug problem (Goode, 1989).

The emphasis in addressing the problem of maternal substance abuse through prosecution of these women focuses on punishment and incarceration. By concentrating almost exclusively on retribution, needs and issues that are created by this position are overlooked. There exists little consideration for the fact that there are few treatment facilities that deal with pregnant drug abusers and fewer jails and prisons that can adequately deal with an expectant mother.

In one case brought by Prisoners with Children, the plaintiff delivered her baby on the floor of the Kern County Jail in Bakersfield, California (Cassen Moss, 1988).

> Pregnant women in jail are routinely subject to conditions that are hazardous to fetal health such as gross overcrowding, 24-hour lock-up with no access to exercise or fresh air, exposure to tuberculosis, measles, and hepatitis, and a generally filthy and unsanitary environment (Cole, 1990:2667).

In the prison system health care officials warn that prisons are extremely deficient in the resources needed to accommodate pregnant women (Barry, 1989). Thus, the fetus may be as much danger, if not more, from the intervention.

Exploitation

Another aspect of social policies that may bring about regressive effects is the potential for exploitation by the target group. In other words, the group that is the target of the social policy uses an intervention, not for its intended purposes, but for personal benefit. Pregnant women who are prosecuted and incarcerated for their drug use may have little desire to stop using drugs and drugs are probably as, if not more, available in jails. Brenda Vaughn, during her incarceration, reported that on a couple of occasions she had the opportunity to use drugs (Cassen Mass, 1988). So by incarcerating these women they are being placed in an environment where their drug use can continue and potentially accelerate. Not only may the women have as great or even greater accessibility to drugs but, because of contact with a diverse inmate subculture, they may also have the opportunity to experiment with different drugs and may make drug connections in jail that can endure long after release. Thus, the potential for greater abuse of drugs by women who are reluctant to stop using is inherent in the design of this punitive approach making resolution of the problem less likely.

Goal Displacement

A regressive intervention can result when the benefits of providing an efficient and inexpensive method in dealing with a problem takes precedent over the policy's efficacy. For example, in addressing marijuana use, spraying the plant with paraquat—a toxic herbicide—may seem like an efficient strategy to deter use of the drug. However, this strategy, because it does not change patterns of use, may be less than effective in improving the health of marijuana users, decreasing social and medical costs of drug use, or decreasing the demand for the drug from other sources.

Likewise, the policy that deals with maternal substance abusers through indictments and prosecution may appear to be, at first glance, the most efficient strategy to decrease use if one assumes that fear of legal consequences can deter one from use. "What people like about doing it in this way (incarceration) is it doesn't cost any money. You don't have to raise taxes. You just have to bring down a couple of indictments" (Kennedy, 1989:1).

The question still remains is the incarceration of maternal substance abusers effective in reducing their drug use? Or is our punitive social policy simply a response that gives the picture that something is being done about the problem but a policy that never really addresses the underlying issues that are the basis of continued maternal substance abuse? The women who are prosecuted are overwhelmingly low-income, single women, primarily women of color who are dependent on public facilities for their care. Incarceration leaves unaddressed the possible roots of the problem: poverty, unemployment, and lack of educational and vocational opportunities (Smith, 1990).

Additionally, pregnant women are seldom welcome in treatment programs. Pregnant and addicted women were refused admission to 54% of seventy-eight treatment programs surveyed in New York City. Sixty-seven percent of the programs denied treatment to pregnant addicts on Medicaid and addicted specifically to crack (Chavkin, 1989). Treatment facilities justify exclusion of pregnant women arguing that their program may be unable to adequately care for the women during detoxification, may be ill equipped to provide prenatal care, and may lack the appropriate facilities and expertise to provide newborn and child care services (Kumpfer, 1991). Rather than allocate moneys for social programs and treatment or instead of demanding legislation mandating treatment facilities accept pregnant addicts, the method that appears the most efficient is prosecution and incarceration.

> The focus on maternal behavior allows the government to appear to be concerned about babies without having to spend the money, change any priorities or challenge any vested interest (Pollitt, 1990:410).

Provocation

Social policies have the potential to provoke a counterproductive emotional response in the group targeted by this intervention. If the practice of indictments and prosecution of maternal substance abusers continues, pregnant mothers who use drugs may refrain from any form of prenatal care thus increasing the risk to the child (Pollitt, 1990).

Further, when the social policy is perceived as illegitimate, this intervention can engender anger and defiance, not just on an individual level, but also on a collective scale (Sieber, 1981:119). Numerous groups have come forth to protest the prosecution of pregnant women. Paltrow, of the American Civil Liberties Union, contends that government intrusion in pregnant women's lives is unconstitutional and violates the fundamental right to privacy (Kennedy, 1989). The indictment of a Waltham woman for motor vehicle homicide after an accident where the woman was driving under the influence of alcohol and where her unborn child was killed, resulted in an outcry among advocates of women's rights. Eight groups filed an *amicus* brief. Though the goal of these groups may in fact be to protect the woman's legal rights, the focus on constitutional and legal issues detracts from some resolution of the original problem—to reduce substance abuse among pregnant women. People may become so embroiled in the controversy over women's rights that the social/medical problems confronting pregnant substance abusers and their infants becomes a secondary consideration. That is one protects rights but still offers no solution.

Additionally, subcultures may engage in certain illicit behavior primarily to symbolize their rejection of dominant group motives. Drug use among minorities may symbolize a rejection of the dominant middle-class values of health and abstinence. If this is the case, focusing on addicted babies may simply be a way of perpetrating the symbolic function of drug-using behavior.

Derogatory Classification

Derogatory classification is the regressive effect of some interventions where the societal label imposed on an individual "may reduce a change in the expectations of others, as well as a change in self-perception" (Sieber, 1981:141). This process can be examined within the context of deviance amplification.

Once a behavior is defined and accepted as deviant, the tendency of the society's non-deviant members is to isolate the individuals who fit the deviant definition. With the separation from the larger population those defined as meeting the criteria for inclusion into the deviant group, not only cease to have information regarding normal behavior and acceptable norms, but will in fact develop a value system that supports and enhances continued deviant behavior (Wilkins, 1965).

This may well be the case with the pregnant substance abuser. The pregnant addict fails to conform exclusively to any one existing deviant category for she is not simply a substance abuser nor solely a negligent parent. Placement in the special classification of pregnant drug abuser relegates the woman to the periphery of society where she will have less contact with mainstream society and its norms, where she will have access to deviant group norms that explain, rationalize, and justify her substance abuse thus decreasing the likelihood of substantive change in her drug-abusing behavior.

Placation

Placation is a characteristic of a social policy where the goal of the intervention is one of "placating certain parties whose support is considered necessary" (Sieber, 1981:65). An example of this process is the eventual support by the Reagan administration for the proposed legislation introduced by Mothers Against Drunk Driving (MADD). MADD is a group of individuals who had been negatively affected by a drunk driver and who, as a group, demanded legislative action—not against the liquor companies, but against those individuals who chose to drink and drive. In particular this group supported, and had overwhelming congressional approval for, federal legislation that would force states to increase the drinking age to twenty-one. President Reagan, who favored federal noninterference in state matters, was reluctant to sign any such legislation. Under pressure from his advisors who informed the president that he could not afford to oppose such legislation, Reagan signed the bill. Though it appears that Reagan conceded an issue to popular and political pressure, however, he effectively placated a large and vocal segment of the population (Reinarman, 1988). Thus, while MADD was successful and certainly placated, larger issues with potentially greater ramifications, such as the role of alcohol as a potentially harmful drug, were not addressed. Further, this legislative action, while potentially ineffective, gave the appearance to the general public that steps were being taken to resolve drunk driving thus allaying public concern.

This same process of placating certain groups, and at the same time scarcely addressing and possibly exacerbating the problem of maternal substance abuse, may be best examined on a macro or societal level and can be understood within the framework of our current drug policy. Since the 1960s, the U.S. government has been waging a war on drugs (Czajkoski, 1990) with questionable and variable results. Even if we are not winning the war, a war on drugs, as in any war, may serve a number of useful control purposes. For example, during a war the general population is often willing to accept an abridgment of civil liberties and a subordination of the individual. This type of abridgment would never be accepted by the general public in more stable times. Today in the name of the War on Drugs and zero tolerance the general population appears willing to accept random drug screens—what seems to many a clear violation of self-incrimination and privacy rights.

In such a war mentality the pregnant substance abuser is branded as the enemy, and is exposed and sanctioned. Through this punishment the illusion that the battle is being won is perpetuated and as a result the public is placated by war victories. Furthermore, by punishing these drug-abusing expectant mothers, usually members of poor and disenfranchised groups (National Association for Perinatal Addiction Research and Education, 1992), we are focusing on a group whose political power is minimal. The likelihood of protest of the current punitive policy or consideration of violations of civil rights are minimized. In terms of placation the punishment of pregnant substance abusers shows something is being done about the drug problem, even if nothing is being accomplished; satisfies the public; and avoids addressing central problems in the social system such as poverty, unemployment, and lack of education that may in fact exacerbate the drug problem.

Conclusion

Certainly we are dealing, in the case of pregnant substance abusers, with a very special population. Exactly what we should do seems at times problematic. What is clear, as we have shown, is what we should not do. Evidence indicates that time and time again, whether we are dealing with desegregation of schools, fighting the war on drugs, or confronting the issue of poverty, certain features of our social policies bring about a deterioration of the problem that we desire to ameliorate. This use of counterproductive social policies is certainly the case in the prosecution of alcohol- and drug-abusing pregnant women.

What we need to do now is to reexamine the policy of arresting, indicting and incarcerating pregnant substance abusers and offer some alternatives that would be more productive in dealing with the pregnant addict. If we really want to try to insure the health of infants born to alcohol- and drug-abusing mothers, rather than arrest these women, and approach that may place a woman in an environment counterproductive to infant and maternal health, we should insist instead on screening and channeling high-risk expectant mothers into appropriate social services. These services could include AFDC, WIC, Medicaid, prenatal and health care agencies, family planning services, and drug and alcohol treatment. The earlier assistance is offered the more likely this intervention can be of value to both mother and child.

Rather than arresting, indicting and incarcerating pregnant substance abusers—a practice that increases the likelihood a woman will not access prenatal care and decreases the likelihood of infant health—we need to increase appropriations for drug and alcohol treatment facilities that are geared toward substance-abusing expectant mothers. These long-term facilities, in addition to confronting the woman's drug-using behavior, would offer detoxification, prenatal care, and infant and child care services. These neonatal and pediatric services could include treatment for drug-affected babies. Experts contend that cocaine-affected babies can be greatly improved with therapy and other special attention. Dr. Chasnoff of NAPARE estimates that 300,000 children have suffered some damage due to the expectant mother's cocaine use, but that less than 10% receive treatment (Treaster, 1993).

Rather than arrest, indict and incarcerate the woman who uses drugs or alcohol when pregnant—a policy that labels then marginalizes these women and decreases the likelihood of their wholesale participation in society—we should focus on policies that may change addictive behavior. Clearly the war on drugs, while increasing the prison population, has done little to affect addiction. Certainly fear has not stopped women who are pregnant from drug use. The $7.4 billion allocated by the previous administration to enforce compliance with existing drug laws (Corn, 1990) might better be used for education and treatment. A policy that offers hope may well draw more women than our current regressive policy.

References

Abel, E. 1984. *FAS and FAE*. New York: Plenum Press

Abel E. and R. J. Sokol. 1987. Incidence of Fetal Alcohol Syndrome and economic impact of FAS-related anomalies. *Drug and Alcohol Dependence* 19:51–70.

Balisy, S. S. 1987. Maternal substance abuse: The need to provide legal protection for the fetus. *Southern California Law Review* 60:1209–38.

Barry, E. 1989. Pregnant prisoners. *Harvard Women's Law Journal* 12:199–200.

Cannellos, P. 1993. Walk to schools sought anew. *Boston Globe* 29 January.

Cassen Moss, D. 1988. Pregnant? Go directly to jail. *American Bar Association Journal* November 1:20.

Chasnoff, I. J. 1989. Drug use and women: Establishing a standard of care. *Annals of New York Academy of Sciences* 562.2008–10.

Chasnoff, I. J.1990. Testimony. The President's National Drug Abuse Strategy before the Subcommittee On Health and Environment of the U.S. House of Representatives Committee on Energy and Commerce. 30 April.

Chavkin, W.1990. Drug addiction and pregnancy: Policy crossroads. *American Journal of Public Health* 80:483–7.

Cole, H. M. 1990. Legal interventions during pregnancy. *Journal American Medical Association* 264:2667.

Corn, D. 1990. Justice's war on drug treatment. *The Nation* 14 May 250:659-62.

Czajkoski, E. H. 1990. Drugs and the warlike administration of justice. *Journal of Drug Issues* 20(1): 125–130.

General Accounting Office. 1990. Drug exposed infants: A generation at risk. (GAO/HRS–90–138) June.

Glamour. 1988. This is what you thought: 46% say prenatal abuse should be a criminal offense. 86:109.

Gomby, D. S. and P. H. Shiono. 1991. Estimating the number of drug exposed infants. *Future of Children* 1(1): 17–25.

Goode, E. 1989. *Drugs in American Society*. New York: A. A. Knopf.

Halfon, M. 1989. Testimony Born Hooked: Confronting the impact of perinatal substance abuse. The Select Committee of Children, Youth, and Families. U.S. House of Representatives. 27 April.

Howard, J. and L. Beckwith. 1989. The development of young children of substance-abusing parents: Insights from seven years of intervention and research. *Zero to Three*. 1(5):8–12.

Kennedy, J. 1989. Uncertainties surround infant cocaine case. *Boston Globe*. 23 August.

Kronstadt, D. 1991. Complex developmental issues of prenatal drug exposure. *Future of Children* 1(1):36–49.

Kumpfer, K. L. 1991. Treatment programs for drug abusing women. *Future of Children* 1(1):51–60.

Lukas, J. A. 1986. *Common ground*. New York: Vintage Books.

National Association for Perinatal Addiction Research and Education 1992. Epidemiological study of the prevalence of alcohol and other drug use among pregnant and parturient women in Illinois.

Office of the Inspector General.1990. Getting straight: Overcoming treatment barriers for addicted women and their children. Fact sheet. U.S. House of Representatives. 23 April. Hearing Select Committee on Children, Youth, and Families.

Paltrow, L. 1992. Criminal prosecutions against pregnant women. National update and overview.

Reproductive Freedom Project, American Civil Liberties Union Foundation. April.

Pollitt, K. 1990. Fetal rights—A new assault on feminism. *The Nation* 26 March: 409–18.

Reinarman, C. 1988. The social construction of an alcohol problem. *Theory and Society* 17:91–120.

Seiber, S. 1981. *Fatal remedies*. New York: Plenum Press.

Smith, B.V. 1990. Testimony. Law and policy affecting addicted women and their children. Hearing Select Committee on Children, Youth and Families. U.S. House of Representatives. 17 May.

Treaster, J. B. 1993. For children of cocaine fresh reasons for hope. *New York Times*, 16 February.

Warren, K. 1987. Alcohol and birth defects: FAS and related disorders. *National Institute on Alcohol Abuse and Alcoholism* vii.

Wilkins, L. 1965. The deviance amplifying system. In *Social deviance*, ed. Farrell and Swigert, 182–4.

Zuckerman, B. 1991. Drug exposed infants: Understanding the medical risk. *Future of Children* 1(1):26–35.

Debate Presenter Form

Follow the guidelines for debate presenters contained in the introduction of this text and those given to you by your instructor. Use the format below to organize the material for your debate. Remember to include all relevant citation information and to present the related information in your own words. Give credit to authors when you cite a quote and be as thorough as possible when writing about your points so you will be prepared for your debate.

Reference citation #1:

Author: _____

Title: _____

Date: _____

Source: _____

_____

Content from reference citation #1: _____

_____

_____

_____

_____

_____

_____

_____

_____

_____

_____

_____

_____

Reference citation #2:

Author: _____

Title: _____

Date: _____

Source: _____

_____

Content from reference citation #2: _____

_____

_____

_____

_____

_____

_____

Reference citation #3:

Author: _____

Title: _____

Date: _____

Source: _____

_____

Content from reference citation #3: _____

_____

_____

_____

_____

_____

Audience Preparation Form

Follow the guidelines for preparing to be an informed audience member on the day of the debate included in the introduction to this text. After reading both sides of the debate from this chapter, answer the following questions. Be as thorough as possible so that you will be able to make a contribution to the debate by asking informed questions or making provocative comments. This form is usually due on the day of the debate.

State the issue in your own words. Do not plagiarize the text. Demonstrate that you understand the topic and it's relevant arguments.

_____

_____

_____

_____

_____

Discuss two points on the "yes" side of the debate.

Point #1: _____

_____

Point #2: _____

_____

Discuss two points on the "no" side of the debate.

Point #1: _____

_____

Point #2: _____

_____

What is your opinion on this topic?

_____

_____

_____

_____

_____

_____

_____

What has contributed to the development of your views about this topic?

_____

_____

_____

_____

_____

_____

_____

What information would be necessary to cause you to change your thinking about this topic?

_____

_____

_____

_____

_____

Debate Response Form

Follow the guidelines for responding to the debates in the introductory chapter of this text. Complete this form and submit your answers at the class following the debate. Try to be thorough and convince your instructor that you were an active listener during the debate.

List a quote from a debate presenter that you think was important and explain why you think this comment was significant.

_____

_____

_____

_____

Which side of the debate do you think made the most convincing arguments, why?

_____

_____

_____

_____

_____

After hearing the debate, in what way has your thinking been affected?

_____

_____

_____

_____

_____

_____

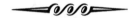

Children

ISSUE 15

Do Physically Punished Children Become Violent Adults?

 YES Murray Straus, *Discipline and Deviance: Physical Punishment of Children and Violence and Other Crime in Adulthood*

 NO Joan McCord, *Questioning the Value of Punishment*

Discipline has been a controversial issue since humans have been parents. Murray Straus reports on the irony that physical punishment, designed to induce conformity in the child, can actually produce a deviant and less conforming child and adult. After providing excellent definitions of terms relevant to this discussion, Straus presents conclusions on the effects of childhood physical corporal punishment on later adult violent behavior.

One often-overlooked outcome of being physically punished is that the child may become abusive with his or her siblings. These children are three times more likely to assault a sibling. Also, children who are physically punished are at much higher risk of abusing their spouses in later life. Physically punished children are also much more likely to engage in street crime and acts of violence. Straus' conclusion is that both corporal punishment and crime are symptoms of the undercurrent of violence in our society.

Joan McCord provides an explanation of the relationship between corporal punishment and adult violence called "Construct Theory." She proposes that it is not simply the violent punishment that leads to violent behavior, but that negative experiences for the child in general can lead to adult criminal violence. McCord emphasizes that neglected and rejected children also have high rates of violent behavior as adults. Parental affection emerges as a factor in later violence. Children who experienced corporal punishment were less likely to become violent adults when their parents were affectionate. Criminal behavior of the father was also related to commission of crimes by sons, regardless of whether or not they had been abused.

Construct Theory suggests that children learn to look for personal benefits of their behavior. Punishment, neglect, and rejection teach egocentrism. Children who experience these abuses tend not to learn to think about others welfare. Therefore, the use of punishment is short-sighted. It not only risks making the forbidden act more appealing, but it risks desensitizing children to their own pain and the pain of others.

Applications

1. Where did you get your ideas about the use of corporal punishment?

2. What do you think about the ways in which your parents disciplined you? Did these methods serve you well?

3. How have you, or do you plan to, discipline your own children if you have them? Why?

Discipline and Deviance
Physical Punishment of Children and Violence and Other Crime in Adulthood

Murray S. Straus

In this paper I present a theoretical model intended to aid research on physical punishment of children and its consequences. The model focuses primarily on the hypothesis that while physical punishment by parents or teachers may produce conformity in the immediate situation, in the long run it tends to *increase* the probability of deviance, including delinquency in adolescence, wife-beating, child abuse, and crime outside the family (such as robbery, assault, and homicide) as an adult. This hypothesis involves considerable irony since the intent of physical punishment is to increase socially *conforming* rather than deviant behavior. As shown below, almost all parents and a majority of teachers believe that physical punishment is an appropriate and effective form of discipline....

Definitions

Physical Punishment

Exploring such issues as the legitimacy of physical punishment requires some definition of terms. Physical punishment is a legally permissible physical attack on children. The most common forms are spanking, slapping, grabbing, and shoving a child "roughly"—with more force than is needed to move the child. Hitting a child with an object is also legally permissible and widespread (Wauchope and Straus, 1990). Parents in the United States and most countries have a legal right to carry out these acts, as do teachers in most U.S. states and most nations; whereas, the same act is a criminal assault if carried out by someone not in a custodial relationship to the child.

The section on "General Justification" of violence in the Texas Penal Code, for example (9.61, West Publishing Company, 1983), declares that the use of force, but not deadly force, against a child younger than 18 years is justified (1) when the actor is the child's parent or step-parent or is acting in *loco parentis* to the child, and (2) when and to the degree that the actor reasonably believes that force is necessary to discipline the child or to safeguard or promote welfare.

The New Hampshire Criminal Code (627.6:I, Equity Publishing, 1985) similarly declares that "A parent, guardian, or other person responsible for the general care and welfare of a minor is justified in using force against such a minor when and to the extent that he reasonably believes it necessary to prevent or punish such a minor's misconduct." Both these statutes cover parents and teachers, and neither sets any limit except "not deadly."

Is Physical Punishment Violence?

Since the concept of violence is used in this paper as often as physical punishment, it also needs to be defined. Though the lack of a standard definition or consensus on its meaning results in considerable confusion, the following definition makes clear the conceptual framework of this paper, even though it will not be accepted by all readers: *Violence* is an act carried out with the intention, or perceived intention, of causing physical pain or injury to another person.

This definition and alternative definitions are examined in detail in Gelles and Straus, (1979). As defined, violence is synonymous with the term "physical aggression" as used in social psychology (Bandura, 1973; Berkowitz, 1962). This definition overlaps with but is not the same as the legal concept of "assault." The overlap occurs because the definition of assault, like the definition of violence, refers to an *act*, regardless of whether injury occurred as a result of that act. However, the concept of assault is more narrow than that of violence because not all acts of violence are crimes, including acts of self-defense and physical punishment of children. Some violent acts are required by law—for example, capital punishment.[1]

The fact that physical punishment is legal is not inconsistent with the definition of violence just given, since, as noted, there are many types of legal violence. An examination of the definition shows that physical punishment of children fits every element of the definition of violence given. Thus, from a theoretical perspective, physical punishment and capital punishment are similar, despite the vast difference in level of severity.

Physical Punishment of Children as the Primordial Violence

Incidence of Physical Punishment by Parents

Ninety-nine percent of the mothers in the classic study of *Patterns of Child Rearing* (Sears, Maccoby, and Levin, 1957) used physical punishment as defined above on at least some occasions, and 95 percent of students in a community college sample reported having experienced physical punishment at some point (Bryan and Freed, 1982)....[T]he National Family Violence Surveys (Straus, 1983; Wauchope and Straus, 1990), studies of large and nationally representative samples of American children conducted in 1975 and 1985...found that almost all parents in the United States use physical punishment with young children—over 90 percent of parents of children age 3 and 4. A remarkable correspondence exists between the results of these four surveys in the near universality with which punishment was used on children age 2 to 6; and also between the two national surveys in showing that physical punishment was still being used on one out of three children at age 15.

Despite the widespread use of physical punishment, there is nonetheless considerable variation—more than enough to enable empirical study of the correlates of physical punishment. First, we see that the percentage of people experiencing physical punishment drops off rapidly with age so that by age 13 there are nearly equal numbers of children who are and who are not punished. Second, at each age, there is enormous variation in how often a specific child experiences physical punishment (Wauchope and Straus, 1990).

Incidence of Physical Punishment in Schools

In 1989 all but eleven states permitted physical punishment of children by school employees. A 1978–79 national survey of schools found an annual incidence of 2.5 instances of physical punishment per 100 children. Only five states reported no instances of physical punishment (calculated from Hyman, 1990: Appendix B). These figures are probably best interpreted as "lower bound" estimates, and the reported absence of physical punishment in five states must also be regarded with some caution.

A Theoretical Model

In the light of the above incidence rates and the previously listed reasons for the importance of research on physical punishment, a framework is needed to help stimulate and guide research. This section presents such a framework in the form of a causal model. The model was created on the basis of previous theoretical an empirical research.

Cultural Spillover Theory

An important component of the theoretical model to be presented is what I have called "Cultural Spillover Theory" (Baron and Straus, 1987; Baron, Straus, and Jaffee, 1988; Straus, 1985), which holds that violence in one sphere of life tends to engender violence in other spheres, and that *this carry-over process transcends the bounds between legitimate and criminal use of force*. Thus, the more a society uses force to secure socially desirable ends (for example, to maintain order in schools, to deter criminals, or to defend itself from foreign enemies) the greater the tendency for those engaged in illegitimate behavior to also use force to attain their own ends.

Cultural Spillover Theory was formulated as a macro-sociological theory to explain society-to-society differences in violence rates, such as the huge differences between societies in the incidence of murder and rape. My colleagues and I tested this theory using a 12 indicator index to measure the extent to which violence was used for socially legitimate purposes ranging from physical punishment of children to capital punishment of criminals. We found that the higher the score of a state on the Legitimate Violence Index, the higher the rate of criminal violence such as rape (Baron and Straus, 1987, 1989; Baron, Straus, and Jaffee, 1988) and murder (Baron and Straus, 1988).

We must also understand the individual-level processes which underlie the macro-level relationship. These can be illustrated by considering the hypothesis that use of physical punishment by teachers tends to increase the rate of violence by children in schools. The individual level aspect of this hypothesis is based on two assumptions: (1) that children often mistreat other children, (2) that teachers are important role models. Therefore, if children frequently misbehave toward other children, and if teachers who serve as role models use violence to correct misbehavior, a larger proportion of children will use violence to deal with other children whom they perceive as having mistreated them than would be the case if teachers did not provide a model of hitting wrongdoers.

The Cultural Spillover Theory overlaps with the "Brutalization" Theory of capital punishment (Bowers, 1984; Hawkins, 1989), and the "Cultural Legitimation" Theory of homicide (Archer and Gartner, 1984). All three of these theories can be considered a variant of what Farrell and Swigert (1988:295) identify as "social and cultural support" theories of crime, including the Differential Association Theory, the Delinquent Subculture Theory, and the Social Learning Theory. Each of these theories seeks to show that crime is not just a reflection of individual deviance (as in psycho-pathology theories of crime) or the absence of social control (as in Social-Disorganization Theory). Rather, crime is also engendered by social integration into groups which share norms and values that support behavior which the rest of society considers to be criminal. Thus, the processes which produce criminal behavior are structurally parallel to the processes which produce conforming behavior, but the cultural content differs.[2]

The Model

The theoretical model diagramed in Figure 1 depicts the causes and consequences of physical punishment and suggests salient issues for empirical investigation. It is a "system model" because it assumes that the use of physical punishment is a function of other characteristics of the society and its members and that physical punishment in turn influences the society and its members....

Each of the blocks in Figure 1 should also have arrows between the elements within each block; except for Block II at the center of the model, they were omitted to provide a clear picture. The arrows within Box II posit a mutually reinforcing relationship between physical punishment in the schools and by parents. It seems highly plausible that a society which approves of parents hitting children will also tend to approve of teachers doing the same, and that when physical punishment is used in the schools, it encourages parents to also hit children....

Antecedents of Physical Punishment by Parents

Block I at the left of the model identifies characteristics of the society, of the schools, of families, and of individual parents which are hypothesized to influence the extent to which physical punishment is used. This list is far from exhaustive, as are the hypotheses to be tested. Both are intended only to illustrate some of the many factors which might influence use of physical punishment.[3]

Societal Norms

Physical punishment is deeply rooted in Euro-American religious and legal traditions (Foucault, 1979; Greven, 1990). It would be difficult to find someone who could not recite the biblical phrase "spare the rod and spoil the child." The common law of every American state permits parents to use physical punishment. These are not mere vestiges of ancient but no longer honored principles. In addition to defining and criminalizing "child abuse," the child abuse legislation which swept through all 50 states in the late 1960s often reaffirmed cultural support for physical punishment by declaring that nothing in the statute should be construed as interfering with the rights of parents to use physical punishment. There is a certain irony to this legislation because, as will be suggested below, use of physical punishment is associated with an increased risk of "child abuse."[4]

Approval of physical punishment.

Attitude surveys have repeatedly demonstrated high approval of physical punishment. Ninety percent of the parents in the 1975 National Family Violence Survey expressed at least some degree of approval of physical punishment (Straus, Gelles, and Steinmetz, 1980:55). Other studies report similar percentages. For example, a 1986 NORC national survey found

Figure 1
System Model of Causes and Consequences of Physical Punishment

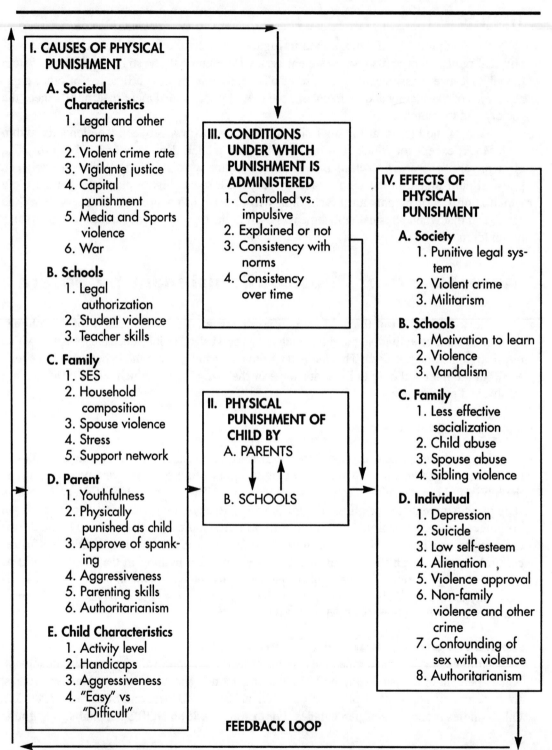

that 84 percent agreed or strongly agreed that "It is sometimes necessary to discipline a child with a *good, hard spanking* (italics added). Moreover, this approval does not apply only to small children. The New Hampshire Child Abuse Survey (described in the Methodological Appendix and in Moore and Straus, 1987) found that less than half of the parents interviewed (47 percent) strongly disagree with the statement "Parents have a right to slap their teenage children who talk back to them." When asked whether "Spanking children helps them to be better people when they grow up," only one out of six disagreed (16.7 percent).

Approval of hitting and actual hitting.

There is evidence that, as hypothesized by the path going from Block I.D2 of the theoretical model to Block II.A, parents who approve of physical punishment do it more often. Parents who approve of slapping a teenager who talks back reported hitting their teenager an average of 1.38 times during the year, about four times more often that the average of .33 for the parents who did not approve. For younger children, the frequency of physical punishment was much greater (an average of 4.9 times for preschool children and 2.9 times for 6–12 year old children), but the relationship between approval and actual hitting was almost identical.

Role Modeling

The path in Figure 1 from I.D2 to II.A, and from II.A to IV.C2 is based on the assumption that children learn by example, and we have seen that over 90 percent of parents provide examples of physical punishment. However, as noted above, there is a great deal of variation in how long physical punishment continues to be used and in the frequency with which it is used. This variation made it possible to test the hypothesis that the more a person experienced physical punishment, the more likely such persons are to use physical punishment on their own children....

Effects of Physical Punishment by Parents

Block IV on the right side of Figure 1 illustrates the hypothesized effects of physical punishment on individuals, schools, families and the society. The empirical analyses to be reported are all derived from the proposition that the "legitimate violence" of physical punishment tends to spill over to illegitimate violence and other crime. If subsequent research supports these effects, the next step will be research to identify the processes which produce them.

Physical Punishment and Physical Abuse

The basic tenant of Cultural Spillover Theory—that legitimate violence tends to increase the probability of criminal violence—is represented by the path going from II.A (physical punishment by parents) to IV.C2 (physical abuse by parents).

Analysis of the New Hampshire Child Abuse Survey (Moore and Straus, 1987) shows that parents who believe in physical punishment not only hit more often, but they more often go beyond ordinary physical punishment and assault the child in ways which carry a greater risk of injury to the child such as punching and kicking. Specifically, parents who approved of physical punishment had a child abuse rate of 99 per 1,000, which is four times the rate for parents who did not approve of physical punishment (28 per 1,000).

Assaults on Siblings and Spouses

From the 1975 National Family Violence Survey (Straus, 1983), we know that children who were physically punished during the year of that survey have also three times the rate of severely and repeatedly assaulting a sibling three or more times during the year. Though it is likely that many of these children were physically punished precisely because of hitting a sibling, it is also clear that the physical punishment did not serve to reduce the level of assaults to the rate for children who were not physically punished.

Similarly, findings from the 1975 National Family Violence Survey (Straus, 1983) clearly show that for both men and women the more physical punishment a respondent experienced as a child, the higher the probability of assaulting a *spouse* during the year of the survey. These findings are consistent with the hypothesized path from Box II.A to IV.C3.

Physical Punishment and Street Crime

The theoretical model predicts that ordinary physical punishment increases the probability of "street crime" (path from Box II.A to IV.D.4). Evidence consistent with that hypothesis is presented in Figure 2 for juveniles and Figures 3 and 4 for adults.

The juvenile crime data are from a 1972 survey of 385 college students (Straus, 1973, 1974, 1985) who completed a questionnaire referring to events when they were high school seniors. The questionnaire included an early version of the Conflict Tactics Scales and also a self-report delinquency scale. Figure 2 shows that significantly more children who were physically punished engaged in both violent crime and property crime.

The findings on crime by adults were obtained by an analysis of covariance of the 1985 National Family Violence Survey sample, controlling for socioeconomic status. Figure 3 shows that the more physical punishment experienced by the respondent as a child, the higher the proportion who as adults reported acts of physical aggression *outside the family* in the year covered by this survey. This relationship is highly significant after controlling for SES. The results are parallel when physical punishment by the father is the independent variable.

Although the arrest rate of respondents in the 1985 National Family Violence Survey was very low (1.1 percent or 1.100 per 100,000 population), this is very close to the 1,148 per 100,000 rate for the entire U.S. population (Federal Bureau of Investigation, 1985). Consequently, despite the low rate, we examined the relationship of arrests to physical punishment experienced during the teenage years. Although the differences overall are statistically significant ($F = 3.75$, $p < .001$), the graph does not show the expected difference between those who were and were not hit as a teen. Instead, only respondents who were hit

Figure 2
Juvenile Assault and Theft Rate by Physical Punishment

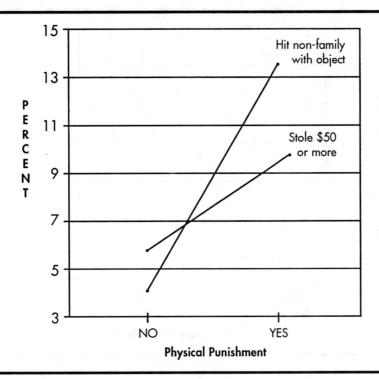

extremely often (eleven or more times during the year) had the predicted higher arrest rates. It is possible that these erratic results occur because the base rate for arrests is so low. A statistical analysis based on a characteristic which occurs in such a small percentage of the population is subject to random fluctuations unless the sample is much larger than even the 6,002 in the 1985 survey....

Summary and Conclusions

This paper formulated a theoretical model of the links between physical punishment of children and crime and also presented preliminary empirical tests of some of the paths in the model. Although the empirical findings are almost entirely consistent with the theory, they use data which cannot prove the theory because they do not establish the causal direction. Nevertheless, the fact that so many analyses which could have falsified the theory did not strengthens the case for the basic proposition of the theory: that although physical punishment may produce short term conformity, over the longer run it probably also creates or exacerbates deviance.

Figure 3
Non-Family Assaults of Adults by Physical Punishment as a Teen

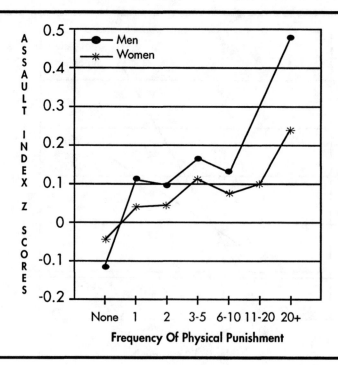

Frequency Of Physical Punishment

The Causal Direction Problem

The causal direction problem can be illustrated at the macro level by the correlation between laws authorizing physical punishment in schools and the homicide rate. It is likely that at least part of this relationship occurs because both physical punishment and crime are reflections of an underlying violent social climate. When crime and violence flourish, even ordinarily law-abiding citizens get caught up in that milieu. When crime rates are high, citizens tend to demand "getting tough" with criminals, including capital punishment and laws such as those recently enacted in Colorado and other states. These laws added protection of property to self-defense as a circumstance under which a citizen could use "deadly force." The question from the perspective of Cultural Spillover Theory is whether such laws, once in effect, tend to legitimize violence and, therefore, further increase rather than reduce violent crime.

The causal direction problem in the individual-level findings is even more obvious because it is virtually certain that part of the linkage between physical punishment and crime occurs because "bad" children are hit, and these same bad children go on to have a higher rate of criminal activity than other children.[5] However, the question is not whether misbe-

Figure 4
Arrests Per 1,000 by Physical Punishment as a Teen

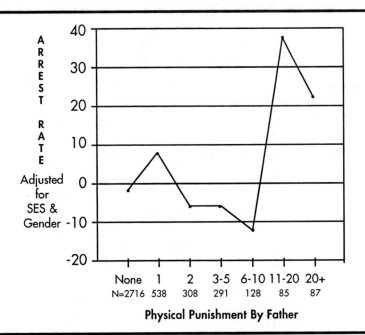

having children are spanked but whether spanking for misbehavior, despite immediate compliance, tends to have longer term negative effects. Research by Nagaraja (1984), Patterson (1982), and Patterson and Bank (1987) suggests that this is the case. This research found an escalating feedback loop which is triggered by attempts to use physical punishment or verbal aggression to control deviant behavior of the child. These processes together with the hypothesized legitimation of violence are modeled in Figure 5.

It should be noted that physical punishment usually does not set in motion the deviation amplifying process just discussed, at least not to the extent that it produced seriously deviant behavior. We must understand the circumstances or branching processes which produce these different outcomes. The variables identified in Box III of Figure 1 ("Conditions Under Which Punishment is Administered") and by the diagonal path in Figure 5, are likely to be crucial for understanding this process. Three examples can illustrate this process. (1) If physical punishment is administered "spontaneously" and as a means of relieving tension, as advocated by a number of child care "experts" (e.g., Ralph 1989), it may increase the risk of producing a person who as an adult will be explosively violent, as compared to physical punishment is administered under more controlled circumstances. The latter is assumed to provide a model of controlled use of force. (2) If physical punishment is accompanied by verbal assaults, it may increase the risk of damage to the child's self-esteem compared to phys-

Figure 5
Process Model of Effects of Corporal Punishment

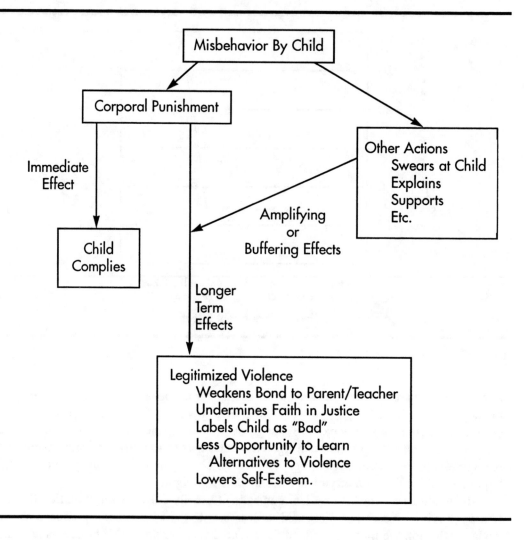

ical punishment administered in the context of a supportive relationship. (3) If physical punishment is administered along with reasoned explanations, the correlation between physical punishment and child's aggressiveness may be reduced. A study by Larzelere (1986) found such a reduction, but also found that despite the lowered relationship, a statistically significant relationship remains.

Research Implications

Both the overall theoretical model (Figure 1) and the micro-process model (Figure 5) can only be adequately investigated with longitudinal and experimental data. There are already examples of studies at the macro-level which meet these criteria, including the research of Archer and Gartner (1984) on the effects of war on the homicide rate and research on the "brutalization" effect of executions (Bowers, 1984; Hawkins, 1989). At the individual level, McCord's follow up of the Cambridge-Somerville Youth Study (1988) sample illustrates what can be done with a longitudinal design. As for experiments, it would be unethical to randomly assign groups of parents to "spanking" and "no spanking" conditions. However, the fact that almost all parents do spank makes a number of experiments possible because the treatment can be in the form of helping parents use alternatives to spanking. One example would be an interrupted time series using volunteer parents. Another example would be randomized field trial of a "no-spanking" parent education program.

There are hundreds of research questions that spring from the theoretical model presented in this paper. The process of transforming that model into meaningful research can be aided if criminologists and family violence researchers collaborate more than in the past to seek a full accounting of the links between physical punishment and crime outside the family. There are no serious structural or theoretical barriers to discourage such mutually informed work, but there is a set of beliefs that continues to define "family violence" in ways which inhibit research on physical punishment. Among family violence researchers, but especially those concerned with wife-beating, there has been a reluctance, and sometimes even condemnation, of considering ordinary physical punishment as part of the same continuum as wife-beating and child abuse (Breines and Gordon, 1983: 505, 511). Spanking children is not seen as "real family violence." Similarly, among criminologists, physical punishment of children is not seen as important for understanding "real crime."

The theory developed in this paper and the research evidence so far available on that theory support the opposite formulation. However, there is no contradiction between the idea that all violence has something in common and the idea that there are important differences between various types of violence. Both propositions can be correct, and both approaches are needed for research on this complex phenomenon. Whether one focuses on the common elements in all violence or on the unique aspects of a certain type of violence depends on the purpose of the study. Research intended to inform interventions designed to aid "battered women" or "abused children," or to deter "wife-beating" or "street crime" must focus on the specific situation of those specific types of victims and offenders (Straus, 1990c). However, for research intended to inform programs of "primary prevention" (Caplan, 1974; Cowen, 1984) of violent crime such as wife beating and homicide, it is essential to understand the social psychological process by which violence becomes an integral part of both legitimate and criminal behavior. The theoretical model presented in this paper suggests that the almost universal use of physical punishment in child rearing is part of the process.

Notes

1. This brief discussion shows that the fact of a physical assault having taken place is not sufficient for understanding violence. Several other dimensions also need to be considered. It is also important that each of these other dimensions be measured separately so that their causes and consequences and joint effects can be investigated. Other dimensions include the seriousness of the assault (ranging from a slap to shooting), whether a physical injury was produced (from none to death), the motivation (from a concern for a person's safety, as when a child is spanked for going into the street, to hostility so intense that the death of the person is desired), and whether the act of violence is normatively legitimate (as in the case of slapping a child) or illegitimate (as in the case of slapping a spouse), and which set of norms are applicable (legal, ethnic or class norms, couple norms, etc.). See Gelles and Straus (1979) for further analyses of these issues.

2. There are a number of other theories relevant to the issues discussed in this paper. The larger theoretical task will be to integrate Cultural Spillover Theory and the theories just listed with theories such as Control Theory (Hirshi, 1969), Labeling Theory (Scheff, 1966; Straus, 1973), Social Learning Theory (Bandura, 1973; Berkowitz, 1962; Eron, Walder, and Lefkowitz ,1971; Gelles and Straus, 1979; McCord, 1988), and a variety of personality mediated theories. Although space limitations required deletion of my initial attempts to specify some of the interrelationships, the concluding theoretical discussion is a small step in that direction. I argue that physical punishment might bring about changes in personality, such as lowered self-esteem or increased powerlessness and alienation. These personality variables can, by themselves, serve as "risk factors" for violence. At the empirical level, it will require a "competing theories" research design and triangulation via several different types of research to adequately investigate these issues.

3. Moreover, due to space limitations, I will only discuss the paths for which I carried out empirical tests. However, since a reader of an earlier draft of the paper questioned the hypothesized paths and feedback loop running from use of corporal punishment back to low teacher and parental skill (I.C3 and I.D5), the reasoning needs to be summarized: It is simply that to the extend parents and teachers use corporal punishment as a means of inducing appropriate behavior, they get less practice in using other means of inducing appropriate behavior and, therefore, do no enhance their skills in those techniques, thus further increasing the probability of using corporal punishment.

4. A study of the reasons for including reaffirmation of corporal punishment in the child abuse legislation might provide important insights on American attitudes about children and violence. Such a study could be undertaken by analysis of the proceedings of state legislatures. For the moment, I would like to suggest two scenarios, both of which may have been operating. The first reason is that both spring from a concern about the welfare of children, and specifically the idea that children need to be protected from abuse but also need "strong discipline" (including physical punishment "when necessary") if they are to become responsible law-abiding citizens. The second reason is that the combination reflects a political compromise which the advocates of "child protection" needed to make in order to have the legislation pass. However, these two reasons overlap to a certain extent because conservative members of the legislation who needed to be placated favor physical punishment because they deeply believe it is in the best interest of children.

5.   I emphasize "a higher *rate*" because most "bad" children, regardless of whether they have been physically punished, do not become criminals. The theory put forth in this paper does not assert that corporal punishment is a necessary and sufficient cause of violence and other crime. On the contrary, crime is a multiply determined phenomenon, and corporal punishment is assumed to be only one of these many causes. Consequently, many individuals who have not been assaulted as children engage in crime, just as many who have been assaulted by teachers or parents avoid criminal acts.

Questioning the Value of Punishment

— Joan McCord —

The author critically examines and rejects the claim that physical punishment leads to aggression through the acceptance of norms of violence. She proposes an alternate theory to account for how children acquire norms and why they become violent. The proposed Construct Theory explains why abused, neglected, and rejected children—as well as those who are punished—tend to become anti-social.

"Spare the rod and spoil the child," many have argued. "No," says others, as they refer to evidence that physical punishment leads to, rather than prevents, violent behavior. Yet only a few, it seems, have whispered that we should question the value of every type of punishment, including psychological punishments and deprivation of privileges as well as physical punishments.

When attention has been focused only on physical punishment, critics typically note that such discipline provides a model for the use of force, thereby teaching people to use force. Murray Straus, for example, argues that corporal punishment contributes to a cycle of violence that includes violent crime, child abuse, spouse abuse, non-violent crimes, ineffective family socialization, and ineffective schooling. Straus accounts for correlations between the use of physical punishment, on the one hand, and antisocial or dysfunctional behaviors on the other by means of Cultural Spillover Theory. This theory is an amalgam of explanations that consider behavior to be learned through imitation of models and adoption of norms supported by groups with whom an individual associates. In this view, individuals come to accept the use of violence—and to be violent—because they see violence as legitimated through its use by role models, and they generalize the behavioral norm to include illegitimate uses of violence.

While Straus is correct that physical punishments tend to increase aggression and criminal behavior, I believe he takes too narrow a view about the mechanisms that account for the relationships. My conclusion is grounded in evidence from longitudinal studies about the transmission of violence from one generation to the next. I offer a competing theory, one that merges evidence from experimental studies designed by psychologists to understand the conditions under which children learn and that considers critical issues related to the learning of language. The competing theory, which I call the Construct Theory, suggests how the same mechanism that links physical punishment to aggression can be triggered by nonphysical punishments and neglect. Before turning to the competing theory, I present empirical evidence that physical punishment leads to aggression and criminal behavior and then show that the Cultural Spillover Theory inadequately explains the relationship.

Problems with the Cultural Spillover Explanation

Much of the research to which Straus refers in his analysis of the relationship between physical punishment and misbehavior is cross-sectional. With such data, as Straus acknowledges, one cannot determine whether punishments were a cause or an effect of the behavior. Three longitudinal studies that measured discipline prior to the age serious antisocial behavior began, however, suggest temporal priority for punitive discipline. Comparing children whose parents depended on physical punishments with those whose parents did not in Finland (Pulkkinen, 1983), Great Britain (Farrington, 1978), and in the United States (McCord, 1988), researchers found that those parents used harsh physical punishments had greater probabilities for subsequently committing serious crimes. Longitudinal studies of victims of child abuse, too, suggest that violence tends to increase the probability that victims will commit serious crimes (McCord, 1983; Widom, 1989).

The theory of Cultural Spillover, like similar theories that attempt to explain pockets of violence, postulates acceptance of norms exhibited by the subculture using violence. Although longitudinal studies suggest that violence in the family precedes violence in society, they contain data incongruent with a theory that explains the causal mechanism as socialization into norms that legitimize violence.

One incongruence is revealed in my study of long-term effects of child abuse in which I compared abused sons with neglected and rejected and loved sons (McCord, 1983). The classifications were based on biweekly observations in the homes when the boys were between the ages of 8 and 16 years and living in high-crime areas. Records of major (FBI Index) crime convictions were collected thirty years after the study ended. Twenty-three percent of those reared in loving families and 39 percent of those reared in abusing families had been convicted; but the conviction rate was 35 percent for the neglected and 53 percent for the rejected boys. That is, the data show almost as much violence produced from neglect as from abuse, and greater violence from rejection without abuse than from abuse. Because neglect and rejection typically lead to socialization failure, these results raise doubts that acceptance of norms of violence account for transmission of violence. It would be an anomaly if the very conditions that undermine acceptance of other types of norms promoted norms of violence.

One might argue that Cultural Spillover Theory accounts for violence among the abused and some other theory accounts for violence among neglected and rejected children. Yet neglect and rejection have enough in common with abuse to suggest that a more parsimonious account would be desirable. Furthermore, as will be shown, when neglect is combined with abuse, the result is not increased violence as one would expect were there different causes involved.

My data from the Cambridge-Somerville Youth Study records permitted further checks on the Cultural Spillover Theory. The data include parental criminal records as well as coded descriptions of family life between 1939 and 1945. Sons' criminal records had, as noted, been collected in 1978, when the sons were middle-aged. Among the 130 families containing two natural parents, 22 included a father who had been convicted for an Index crime. Fifty-five percent (12) of their sons were convicted for an Index crime. In comparison, twenty-five percent (27) of the 108 sons of noncriminal men had been convicted ($X^2_{(1)} = 7.60$, P = .006). The criminal fathers were more likely to use physical punishment: 73 percent compared with 48 percent ($X^2_{(1)} = 4.43$, P = .035). Further, the combined impact of a criminal father using physical punishment appeared to be particularly criminogenic.

These data support the view that use of physical punishment increases the likelihood that sons of criminals will be criminals. Cultural Spillover Theory suggests that the increase comes about because sons adopt the norms displayed through physical punishments. If the theory were correct, then the transmission of norms of violence should be particularly effective under conditions that promote acceptance of other types of norms as well. The evidence, however, gives another picture.

Many studies have shown that warmth or affection facilitates acceptance of social norms (e.g., Austin, 1978; Bandura and Huston, 1961; Bandura and Walters, 1963; Baumrind, 1978; Bender, 1947; Bowlby, 1940; Glueck and Glueck, 1950; Goldfarb, 1945; Hirschi, 1969; Liska and Reed, 1985; Maccoby, 1980; McCord, 1979; Olsosn, Bates, and Bayles, 1990; Patterson, 1976). Parental affection for the child should increase concordance if a similar mechanism for acceptance of norms accounts for a connection between parents' and children's aggression. To test this hypothesis, the 130 families were divided into three groups: those not using physical punishment, those using physical punishment and also expressing affection for the child, and those using physical punishment and not expressing affection for the child.

The data show that parental affection did not increase acceptance of norms of violence, but the opposite. For individuals reared with physical punishment, those whose parents were affectionate were *less* likely to become criminals. This result does not easily fit an assumption that normative acquisition accounts for the violence.

Another inconsistency is apparent in a longitudinal study that at first glance might appear to support the Cultural Spillover Theory. Widom (1989) retraced children reported to have been victims of abuse or neglect prior to the age of 11. Using records from elementary schools and hospitals at birth, Widom was able to match 667 of 908 children on sex, race, and age with children not known to have been either abused or neglected. Widom's analyses, based either on aggregate data combining abuse with neglect or matched and unmatched cases, have led her to conclude that violence breeds violence. I reanalyzed her data (Widom 1990) to differentiate effects of neglect from effects of violence.

The matched pairs were divided into those in which the child had experienced sexual abuse (85 females, 15 males), neglect but not physical abuse (205 females, 254 males), physical abuse but not neglect (14 females, 35 males), and both physical abuse and neglect (29 females, 30 males). Assuming that acceptance of a norm of violence accounts for the high rates of crime that Widom found to follow abuse, crime would be considerably more prevalent among those who had been physically abused than among those who had been neglected but not abused.

Using Widom's codes of the individuals' criminal records, I compared each case with the matched control to see which had the worse criminal record. If both had been convicted of at least one crime, the one convicted for more crimes was counted as being worse.

The data shows that neglect is about as criminogenic as sexual abuse and physical abuse. Moreover, the combined effects of neglect and abuse are not worse than those of either alone as would be expected if each had separate causal impact. Comparisons of cases and controls for crimes of violence (e.g., assault, murder, attempted murder) produced similar results.

These comparisons again suggest that continuity in violence among abusing families has been mistakenly attributed to transmission of norms of violence. Among males, neglect and sexual abuse were in fact more likely than physical abuse to lead to violence. Yet if transmission of social norms accounts for violence, physical abuse should create more. The reanalysis of these data suggest that one ought to search for a common cause, for something shared by neglect and abuse that might lead to violence.

In sum, violence seems to beget violence, but studies of child abuse and of family socialization undermine the argument that violence begets violence *through acceptance of family (subcultural) norms of violence*. Because neglect, rejection, and physical abuse result in similarly high rates of crime, it seems appropriate to search for a cause in terms of what they have in common.

A sound understanding of the way children learn can explain why physical abuse, neglect, and rejection lead to antisocial behavior. Below I develop such an understanding to show that a norm of self-interest, rather than a norm of violence, underlies the education shared by those who are rejected, neglected, and abused. It is the norm of self-interest that leads to violence in some circumstances.

Undermining Some Assumptions

Side stepping the issue of how infants learn, many psychologists have simply assumed that babies are completely self-centered. In contrast, the evidence shows that how much children care about their own pleasures and pains and what they will consider pleasurable and painful is largely a function of the way they are taught.

It may, for instance, be tempting to believe that an infant "instinctively" cries for food, to be held, or to have dirty diapers removed, but evidence points to large contributions from experience. In a study of neonates, Thoman, Korner and Benson-Williams (1977) randomly assigned primiparous healthy newborns to conditions in which one third were held when they awakened. As anticipated by the authors, the babies who were held spent more time with their eyes open and cried less vigorously while being held; unexpectedly, however, they spent more time crying during non-stimulus periods. The babies had been equated for pretrial behaviors, so the authors suggest that the infants had come to associate their crying with being picked up during the 48 hour training period.

In another study also showing that neonates learn from their environments, Riese (1990) compared 47 pairs of monozygotic twins, 39 pairs of dizygotic twins of the same sex, and 72 pairs of dizygotic twins of the opposite sex. Using standardized tests for irritability, resistance to soothing, activity level when awake, activity level when asleep, reactivity to a cold disk on the thigh and to a pin prick, and response to cuddling, she found significant correlations for the dizygothic twins (both same and opposite sex), indicating shared environmental influences, but no significantly larger correlations among the monozygothic pairs. Riese concluded that "environment appears to account for most of the known variance for the neonatal temperament variables" (1236).

Just as neonates can learn to cry in order to be picked up, children learn what to consider painful. Variability in recognizing sensations as painful has been dramatically evidenced through studies of institutionalized infants, who received serious injuries without seeming to notice (Goldfarb, 1958). During the period of observation, one child caught her hand in the door, injuring a finger so severely that it turned blue; yet the child did not cry or otherwise indicate pain. Another child sat on a radiator too hot for the teacher to touch. Observed injuries also included a child who was cutting the palm of his own hand with sharp scissors and another who had removed from her cornea a steel splinter that had been embedded for two days without any report of pain. All the children, however, gave pain responses to a pin prick, dispelling the hypotheses that they had a higher than normal threshold for pain. Goldfarb reasonably concluded: "The perception of pain and the reaction to pain-arousing stimuli are episodes far more complex than is implied in the concept of pure, unencumbered sensation" (1945:780–781).

Often, children show no signs of pain after a fall until adults show that they expect a "pained" response. Studies with college students show that feeling pain is influenced by pain exhibited by models (Craig and Theiss, 1971), role playing as calm or upset (Kopel and Arkowitz, 1974), and feedback from one's own responsive behavior (Bandler, Madaras, and

Bem 1968). My personal experience and reports from students suggest that children whose mothers do not respond to their cuts with anxious concern do not exhibit such pain-behavior as crying when they fall.

Not only do children learn what is painful, but they attach pleasure to circumstances intended to result in pain. Solomon (1980) demonstrated that over a range of behaviors, pain-giving consequences acquire positive value through repetition (see Shipley, 1987; Aronson, Carlsmith, and Darley, 1963; Walster, Aronson, and Brown, 1966). Studies showing that children learn to repeat behaviors that result in "reinforcement" through negative attention demonstrate that expectations are only one basis for the attraction of "pain-giving" stimuli (Gallimore, Tharp, and Kemp, 1969; White and Grossman, 1971).

Children also learn without extrinsic reinforcement. Curious about why so many young children appeared to increase their aggressiveness in experimental situations, Siegel and Kohn (1959) measured aggression both with and without an adult in the room. Only when adults were present did escalation occur. The authors drew the sensible conclusion that young children assume that what is not forbidden is permitted.

The egocentric motivational assumption that underlies classic theories of socialization has been subjected to a series of criticism, most notably by Butler (1726) and Hume (1960 [1777]). These authors pointed out that the plausibility of the egocentric assumption rests on circular reasoning. The fact that a voluntary action must be motivated is confused with an assumption that voluntary actions must be motivated by desire to benefit from them. Often the only evidence for self-interest is the occurrence of the act for which a motive is being sought.

Raising further questions about the assumption of egocentrism in children, some studies indicate that altruistic behavior is not always egoistic behavior in disguise (Batson et. al., 1988; Grusec and Skubiski, 1970). In fact, altruistic behavior turns up at very young ages (Rheingold and Emery, 1986; Zahn-Waxler and Radke-Yarrow, 1982; Zahn-Waxler et al., 1988) suggesting that even babies are not exclusively interested in themselves.

The prevalent view that children require punishment in order to learn socialized behavior rests on three erroneous assumptions. The first two—that children are motivated by self-interest and that what gives them pain is "fixed"—have been shown to lack support in empirical research. The third—that unless there are punishments rules have no power—is addressed in my proposal of Construct Theory.

An Alternative: Construct Theory

Construct Theory states that children learn to do and what to believe in the process of learning how to use language. In simplest form, Construct Theory claims that children learn by constructing categories organized by the structure of the language in their culture. These categories can be identified by descriptions, much as one might identify a file, for example, "accounting," "things to do," "birthdays," "Parsons, T.," "true." Some categories are collections of objects, but others are actions that can be identified by such descriptions as "to be done" or "to be believed" or "to be doubted."

Learning a language requires learning more than concepts. Children learn not only what to count as tables and chairs, cars and trucks, but also what to count as painful or pleasant, undesirable or desirable, and worth avoiding or pursuing. In learning labels, in learning how to name and to re-identify objects, children are constructing classifications. The classification systems they develop will permeate what they notice and how they act as well as what they say.

Construct Theory explains the fact that different people consider similar events to have different affective characteristics—for example, as undesirable and desirable—because individuals construct different classifications of the events. This theory can account for relations between knowledge and action that have led many theorists to conjure "pro-attitudes" as the means by which some knowledge sometimes changes behavior (e.g., Kenny, 1963; Milligan, 1980; Müller, 1979; Nowell-Smith, 1954). According to Construct Theory, those reasons that move one to action are classified as "reasons worth acting upon"; no special entity need also be attached to them.[1] Construct Theory also explains how language can be learned and how people can communicate, for it shows the way in which meanings can be made public through the categories that are constructed.[2]

Learning a language involves learning to formulate sentences as well as learning how to use words. At its most fundamental level, sentences involve stringing together what logicians call "predicates" (which can be thought of as classes) and functional relations among them. Perhaps no component of a sentence is so critical to understanding how punishment works as the connective "if... then," for on this connective punishments rely. The connective also gives linguistic expression to what the neonates described above learned when they cried and were picked up (if I cry, then I will be picked up), what an infant learns by pushing a ball (if I push, then it will roll), and what the child learns when discovering natural consequences in the physical world.

Both natural and artificial contingencies provide information to the child who is learning about consequences. When a child is credibly threatened with punishment, the information conveyed extends beyond the intended message that the child ought not do something. A punishment is designed to give pain. Unless the chosen event is thought by the punisher to be painful, it would not be selected as a means for controlling the child's behavior. What is selected as a punishment, then, shows what the punisher thinks to be painful.[3]

A child also perceives the intention of the punisher to give pain (and may attempt to thwart the intention by saying such things as "I didn't like the dessert anyway" or "There's nothing good on TV anyhow"). So the use of punishment shows the child that the punisher is willing to hurt the threatened or punished child. This knowledge may decrease the child's desire to be with the punisher or to care how the punisher feels, thereby reducing the socializing agent's influence.

An interesting study illustrated another feature of punishment: it conveys information about what (according to the punisher) is valuable, thus potentially enhancing the value of the forbidden. Aronson and Carlsmith (1963) asked preschool children, individually, to compare five toys until they established stable transitive preferences. The experimenter then said he had to leave the room for a few minutes and placed on a table the toy ranked second-favorite by the child. The child was told not to play with that toy but that playing with the others was permissible. Half of the 44 children were randomly assigned to each of two conditions. In the "mild threat" condition, the experimenter said he would be annoyed if the child played with the forbidden toy. In the "severe threat" condition, the experimenter said that if the child played with the forbidden toy, the experimenter would be very angry and would take all the toys and never come back. The experimenter left the child for 10 minutes. Approximately 45 days later, the children were again asked to rank the five toys. For this ranking, 4 of the children from the mild threat condition ranked the forbidden toy as a favorite whereas 14 of those in the severe threat condition regarded the forbidden toy as the favorite. Conversely, 8 of those were merely told that the experimenter would be annoyed had decreased their preference for the forbidden toy whereas none of the children who were threatened with punishment had they played with the toy decreased their preference for it.

In a near replication, Lepper (1973) found that, two weeks later, children from his stronger threat condition were more likely to cheat in a game. There are two explanations for this. Lepper explained the findings by suggesting that the children who resisted with severe threat reasoned: "I am the sort of person who would break the rules except for the fact that I would be punished." In contrast, according to this self-referential theory, the children under mild threat defined themselves as the sorts of people who generally conform to rules and requests.

I suggest an alternative explanation: The different exposures in the experiment taught the children something about the world and about other people—not primarily something about themselves. The more severe threats taught the children that they ought to orient their behavior around estimates of consequences *to themselves*. In the process of assessing their self-interests, the children looked for attractive features of that which had been forbidden. The "mild threat" condition in both experiments, however, implied only that the child should be concerned about how the experimenter might feel.

Punishments are invoked only when rules are disobeyed, so that telling a child about rules in conjunction with information about punishments for infractions informs a child that he or she has a choice: obey, or disobey-and-accept-the-consequences named as punishment.

Negative correlations between a parent's use of punishments and insistence that rules be followed were so strong in their study of misbehavior that Patterson, Dishion, and Bank (1984) could not use both measures in their model. Believing that punishments were more important, they dropped the follow-through measure. The data, however, show equally that a parent who insists that rules be followed need not use punishments to socialize children.

It might be tempting to argue that rewards circumvent the unwanted effects of punishment as a means for teaching norms. That would be a mistake. Although using rewards does not hazard rejection of the purveyor, rewarding shares many of the characteristics of punishing. Rewards as well as punishments employ the "if... then" relationship. Laboratory studies have demonstrated, as predicted from the Construct Theory, that contingent reinforcements sometimes interfere with the discovery of general rules (Schwartz, 1982). Studies have demonstrated, also as predicted from Construct Theory, that incentives larger than necessary to produce an activity sometimes result in devaluation of the activity being rewarded (Greene and Lepper, 1974; Lepper, Greene, and Nisbett, 1973; Lepper et. al., 1982; Ross, 1975; Ross, Karniol, and Rothstein, 1976).

Like those involved in punishments, contingencies that use rewards convey more information than intended when a socializing agent uses them to convince a child to do something. A reward is designed to be attractive, so rewards contain information about what the rewarder believes to be valuable. When a reward is clearly a benefit to the person being promised the reward, rewarding teaches the child to value his or her own benefit.[4]

In addition to learning that whatever requires reward is probably considered unpleasant, children learn that the reward is something considered valuable by the reward-giver. That children *learn* to perceive rewards as valuable has been demonstrated in the laboratory (Lepper et al. 1982). Children were told a story about a mother giving her child two supposed foods; children in the study were asked which the child in the story would prefer: "hupe" or "hule". Children in the experiment group were told that the mother explained to her child that (s)he could have one ("hupe" or "hule" for different children) if (s)he ate the other. In this condition, the contingent relation led the children to suppose that the second food was a reward for eating the first. The children overwhelmingly thought the second food would be preferred—and gave grounds for the choice in terms of its tasting better. The experiment showed that the contingent relation, rather than the order of presentation, influenced preference because children in the control condition who were told only that the child's mother gave the child first one and then the other food either refused to make a choice or gave no reason for a selection (which they equally distributed between the two). In other experiments with preschool children, play objects have been manipulated similarly, showing that an activity that is arbitrarily selects as the one to be rewarded will be "discounted" whereas the arbitrarily selected inducement gains value (e.g., Lepper et al., 1982; Boggiano and Main, 1986). These studies show that children learn what to value as well as how to act from perceiving the ways in which rewards are used.[5]

The Construct Theory explains why punishments tend to increase the attraction of activities punished—and why extrinsic rewards tend to reduce the value of activities rewarded. The categorizing that children learn as they learn sentences in a language can be schematically represented by formal logic. When children become aware of the logical equivalence between the conditional (if x then y), they learn that *rewards and punishments weaken the force of a rule by introducing choices*. If rewards are designed to give pleasure to the child an punishments are designed to give the child pain, then their use teaches children that they ought to value their own pleasure and to attempt to reduce their own pain.

Conclusion

Rewards and punishments are used to manipulate others. They often result in short-term gains, but their use teaches children to look for personal benefits. Like rewards and punishments, neglect and rejection teach egocentrism. Children brought up among adults who do not attend to their well-being are given no grounds for learning to consider the welfare of others.

Using punishment seems particularly short-sighted. Punishments may increase the attraction of forbidden acts. They also risk desensitizing children both to their own pains and the pains of others (Cline, Croft, and Courrier, 1973; Pearl, 1987; Thomas et al., 1977). Although severe penalties may force compliance in specific instances, the behavior being punished is actually more likely to occur at a time or place when opportunities for detection are reduced (Bandura and Walters, 1959).

No increase in punishment or in reward can guarantee that children will make the choices adults wish them to make. Several studies show, however, that children are more likely to want to do what an adult wishes if the adult generally does as the child desires. In one study, randomly selected mothers of preschoolers were trained to respond to their children's requests and to avoid directing them during a specified period of time each day for one week. Their children complied with more of the mother's standardized requests in the laboratory than the comparison group of children whose mothers used contingency training (Papal and Maccoby, 1985). The results are mirrored in a natural setting with the discovery that children reared at pre-school age in a consensual environment were among the most likely to value autonomy, intellectual activity, and independence as well as to have high educational aspirations ten years later (Harrington, Block, and Block, 1987).

In another study, mothers and children were observed at home for three months when the children were between 9 and 12 months in age. Mothers were rated for their sensitivity to their babies, a rating based on their perceived ability to see things from the baby's perspective, positive feelings expressed toward the baby, and adaptations favoring the baby's arrangements of his or her own behavior. Discipline was rated for verbal commands as well as for frequency of any physical interventions. The baby's compliance was a simple measure of the proportion of verbal commands the baby obeyed without further action by the mother. Compliance turned out to be practically unrelated to discipline, although it was strongly related to the mother's responsiveness. The authors note: "The findings suggest that a disposition toward obedience emerges in a responsive, accommodating social environment without extensive training, discipline or other massive attempts to shape the infant's course of development" (Stayton, Hogan, and Ainsworth, 1971:1065).

Punishments—non-physical as well as physical—teach children to focus on their own pains and pleasures in deciding how to act. If parents and teachers were to substitute non-physical punishments for physical ones, they might avoid teaching children to hit, punch, and kick; yet, they would nevertheless perpetuate the idea that giving pain is a legitimate way to exercise power. If the substitute for physical punishment were to be non-physical punishments, the consequences could be no less undermining of compassion and social interests.

Children do not require punishments if their teachers will guide them consistently, and they do not require rewards if intrinsic values of what they ought to do are made apparent to them. I am not suggesting that a child will be constantly with the values of those who do not punish. No techniques will guarantee a clone. Rather, I do suggest that children can be taught to follow reasonable rules and to be considerate—and that the probabilities for their learning these things are directly related to the use of reason in teaching them and to the consideration they see in their surroundings.

Straus turns a spotlight on physical punishment, suggesting that by using violence to educate, adults legitimize the use of violence. I paint a broader canvas, suggesting that by using rewards and punishments to educate, adults establish self-interest as the legitimate grounds for choice.

Notes

1. The interpretation of language provides a modification of the Aristotelian notion that action is the conclusion of a practical syllogism; it adds a proviso that the syllogism must correctly represent the classification system of the actor, and then "straightway action follows." The interpretation also reflects the Humean claim that reason alone cannot account for action. It does so by including motivational classifications as separate from purely descriptive classifications.

2. Wittgrenstein (1958) demonstrated the implausibility of accounting for language through private identification of meanings.

3. Thus, there is the irony that when teachers use school work, parents use performing chores, and both use being by oneself as punishments, they are likely to create distaste for learning, doing chores, and being alone.

4. One could, of course, reward a child by permitting some action beneficial to others or by permitting the child a new challenge.

5. The phenomenon is well enough known to have produced several theories, ranging from balance theory (Heider, 1946) and Theory of Cognitive Dissonance (Festinger, 1957) to Psychological Reactance (Brehm, 1966; Brehm and Brehm, 1981). None to my knowledge has tied the phenomenon with language.

References

Aronson, Elliot, and J. Merrill Carlsmith 1963 "Effect of the severity of threat on the devaluation of forbidden behavior." Journal of Abnormal and Social Psychology 66:584–588.

Aronson, Elliot, J. Merrill Carlsmith, and John M. Darley, 1963. " The effects of expectancy on volunteering for an unpleasant experience." Journal of Abnormal and Social Psychology 6:220–224.

Austin, Roy L. 1978 "Race, father-absence, and female delinquency." Criminology 15:487–504.

Bandler, Richard J., George R. Madaras, and Daryl J. Bem, 1968 "Self-observation as a source of pain perception." Journal of Personality and Social Psychology 9:205–209.

Bandura, Albert and Aletha C. Huston, 1961 "Identification as a process of incidental learning." Journal of Abnormal and Social Psychology 63:311–318.

Bandura, Albert and Richard H. Walters, 1959, Adolescent Aggression. New York: Ronald. 1963 Social Learning and Personality Development. New York: Holt, Rinehart, and Winston.

Batson, C. Daniel, Janine L. Dyck, J. Randall Brandt, Judy G. Batson, Anne L. Powell, M. Rosalie McMaster, and Cari Griffitt, 1988, "Five studies testing two new egoistic alternatives to the empathy-altruism hypothesis." Journal of Personality and Social Psychology 55:52–77.

Baumrind, Diana, 1978, "Parental disciplinary patterns and social competence in children." Youth and Society 9:239–276.

Bender, Loretta, 1947, "Psychopathic behavior disorders in children." In Handbook of Correctional Psychology, ed. R. Lindner and R. Seliger, 360–377. New York: Philosophical Library.

Boggiano, Ann K., and Deborah S. Main, 1986, "Enhancing children's interest in activities used as rewards: The bonus effect." Journal of Personality and Social Psychology 31:1116–1126.

Bowlby, John, 1940, "The influence of early environment on neurosis and neurotic character." International Journal of Psychoanalysis 21:154–178.

Brehm, Jack W. 1940, A theory of Psychological Reactance. New York: Academic Press.

Debate Presenter Form

Follow the guidelines for debate presenters contained in the introduction of this text and those given to you by your instructor. Use the format below to organize the material for your debate. Remember to include all relevant citation information and to present the related information in your own words. Give credit to authors when you cite a quote and be as thorough as possible when writing about your points so you will be prepared for your debate.

Reference citation #1:

Author: _____

Title: _____

Date: _____

Source: _____

_____

Content from reference citation #1: _____

_____

_____

_____

_____

_____

_____

_____

_____

_____

_____

_____

Reference citation #2:

Author: _____

Title: _____

Date: _____

Source: _____

_____

Content from reference citation #2: _____

_____

_____

_____

_____

_____

Reference citation #3:

Author: _____

Title: _____

Date: _____

Source: _____

_____

Content from reference citation #3: _____

_____

_____

_____

_____

Audience Preparation Form

Follow the guidelines for preparing to be an informed audience member on the day of the debate included in the introduction to this text. After reading both sides of the debate from this chapter, answer the following questions. Be as thorough as possible so that you will be able to make a contribution to the debate by asking informed questions or making provocative comments. This form is usually due on the day of the debate.

State the issue in your own words. Do not plagiarize the text. Demonstrate that you understand the topic and it's relevant arguments.

_____

_____

_____

_____

_____

Discuss two points on the "yes" side of the debate.

Point #1: _____

_____

Point #2: _____

_____

Discuss two points on the "no" side of the debate.

Point #1: _____

_____

Point #2: _____

_____

What is your opinion on this topic?

_____

_____

_____

_____

_____

_____

_____

What has contributed to the development of your views about this topic?

_____

_____

_____

_____

_____

_____

_____

What information would be necessary to cause you to change your thinking about this topic?

_____

_____

_____

_____

_____

_____

Debate Response Form

Follow the guidelines for responding to the debates in the introductory chapter of this text. Complete this form and submit your answers at the class following the debate. Try to be thorough and convince your instructor that you were an active listener during the debate.

List a quote from a debate presenter that you think was important and explain why you think this comment was significant.

_____

_____

_____

_____

Which side of the debate do you think made the most convincing arguments, why?

_____

_____

_____

_____

_____

After hearing the debate, in what way has your thinking been affected?

_____

_____

_____

_____

_____

_____

_____

Drug Use

ISSUE 16

Would Our Society Benefit from a Policy Allowing Employers to Drug Test All Emloyees?

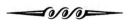

YES William J. Judge, *Drug Testing: The Legal Framework*

NO Judith Wagner DeCew, *Drug Testing: Balancing Privacy and Public Safety*

Many employees have faced drug testing to keep their jobs, many must pass a drug screening to obtain a job. William J. Judge supports employer drug testing of current and potential employees as not only a legal right, but a necessary safety practice. Judge says, "To ignore the problem is to invite disaster."

Reduced injury, increased productivity, and higher profit all result from decreased drug use on the job according to Judge. The threat of random drug screening and implementation of actual drug testing works to insure these positive outcomes in the workplace.

Judith Wagner DeCew argues against drug testing and suggests restrictions and precautions when drug testing does occur. She believes that toxic screening should be limited to cases where there is substantial evidence that drug abuse is taking place and job performance is clearly affected. Drug testing under any other circumstances constitutes ethical and constitutional violations according to DeCew. She raises numerous concerns about types of testing, including blood and urine, test accuracy, and whether tests will be truly random or possibly be targeted at particular groups of people.

The threats to individual privacy are serious violations of personal boundaries. In some cases, a urine sample is obtained while a guard observes procurement of the specimen to ensure it is untainted. When blood is drawn, the person risks the invasion to the body made by the needle. Additionally, blood and urine testing can reveal many other conditions and practices not related to substance abuse that individuals may not wish to become public.

Naturally, substance abusers have developed techniques for avoiding detection. There is even an internet site where customers can purchase "clean" urine samples for use if unobserved at time of procurement.

DeCew concludes that there is not sufficient moral justification for the use of drug testing as a general deterrent to drug use and abuse that may affect job performance and public safety. She believes that, except under very specific circumstances, that negative ethical, moral, and legal consequences of invasive drug screening outweigh the benefit of increased public safety.

Applications

1. As an employee in your future career, what is your position on the use of random or regular, blood, hair, or urine, and voluntary or involuntary drug testing?

2. As an employer in your future career, what is your position on the use of random or regular, blood, hair, or urine, and voluntary or involuntary drug testing?

3. As a member of the public who could be affected by unsafe conditions in the workplace due to drug abuse, what policy would you favor regarding drug testing, and why?

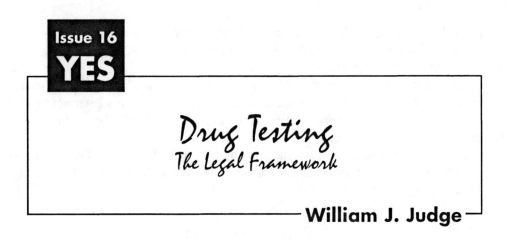

Drug Testing
The Legal Framework

William J. Judge

Introduction

Drug testing is a sensitive subject. Thousands of lawsuits have been filed by individuals who believe that their constitutionally protected rights were violated when forced to submit to a drug test or who feel that they were falsely accused of alcohol or drug use and, as a result, suffered some loss. Because of the contentious nature of employee drug and alcohol testing, not only employers, but collection sites, laboratories, and medical review officers performing drug or alcohol tests are "at risk" of loss resulting from errors or omissions in the performance of the various tasks. A verified positive drug or alcohol test can immediately affect the donor's career and reputation. Because those terminated for suspected drug use find it particularly difficult to secure other employment, the loss of a job for a positive drug test is tantamount to the death penalty of employment.

There is, however, another side to the testing question. Too often employers ignore the problem of drug or alcohol use at work or fail to take reasonable steps to detect drug use. An employer that fails to detect drug or alcohol use can face liability if a drug-or-alcohol-using employee injures someone while performing his or her duties. Today, the best insurance for employers may be in taking action to prevent accidents triggered by drug or alcohol use by employees.

Employers, collection site operators, laboratories, and other service providers are at risk of lawsuit even if they performed their tasks properly. Steps can be taken, however, that limit the risk of loss inherent in the performance of these various tasks. *While there can be no guarantee that lawsuits will not occur*, these steps are designed to *minimize* the risk of a lawsuit and to *maximize* the likelihood of success if sued.

Those thinking of implementing an employee drug program have many questions: "Is it wisest to utilize drug testing as a means of detecting problems or as a deterrent to employee drug or alcohol use?" "Isn't drug testing too controversial?" "Will I be sued if I choose to test my employee or independent workers?"

Clearly, drug testing is controversial and complex. It is, however, a far safer means of dealing with the problem of drug and alcohol use by employees than to do nothing. *To ignore the problem is to invite disaster.*

Background

Employee drug and alcohol use continues to cost American businesses billions of dollars annually. This cost is incurred through increased absenteeism, tardiness, theft, on-the-job injuries, and reduced productivity. Many employers fail to recognize that drugs and alcohol are in their workplace. But one recent survey shows that as many as 64 percent of the employed individuals questioned (50 percent full-time) are admitted current users. As many as 20.1 percent of those full-time employees questioned admitted using marijuana *on the job*.

While existing evidence is anecdotal or the result of unscientific study, it would be difficult to deny that drugs and alcohol have an impact on one's ability to safely perform assigned tasks. One example is tragically illustrative. In 1987 outside Chase, Maryland, a Conrail/Amtrak train accident killed 16 people and injured scores of others. The Conrail engineer admitted smoking marijuana just before the collision.

A number of companies have found a significant reduction in on-the-job accidents after employee drug and alcohol programs were instituted. Utah Power and Light Company conducted an exhaustive study of its employee drug use prevention program and concluded that the reduction in the number of on-the-job vehicle accidents saved it $281,000 between 1985, when the drug testing program was initiated, and 1987 after deducting testing costs. Georgia Power Company's analysis of its testing program resulted in an estimated savings of between $294,000 and $1.7 million by discharging and replacing 198 employees who had failed for-cause drug tests between 1983 and 1987. The overwhelming majority of employers with drug and alcohol programs point to improved workplace safety as a significant benefit from drug testing.

Increasingly, employers are including employee drug testing in their programs as a way to further limit the risks posed by employee drug and alcohol use. While the propriety of drug testing continues to be debated, evidence of the positive impact of testing is emerging. Recent studies of employer drug and alcohol testing programs demonstrate that the costs of employee drug and alcohol use can be contained. These costs can be further reduced by recognizing the value drug testing can have as a defense to workers' compensation claims.

Government Action

The federal government and several state governments have recognized the value of employee drug programs. Currently, nine federally mandated drug-free workplace initiatives are under way, and an additional program was recently proposed by the Department of Energy for employees of private contractors. These initiatives include drug testing for employees of businesses regulated by the six agencies of the Department of Transportation, for private employers contracting with the Department of Defense, and for employees of contractors regulated by the Nuclear Regulatory Commission. In addition, the Anti-Drug Abuse Act of 1988 requires certain federal contractors and grant recipients to establish employee drug awareness programs and to exercise "good faith" to maintain a drug-free workplace. A number of states have adopted similar legislation.

Some states have targeted specific areas where employee drug or alcohol use has been shown to have a particularly damaging effect. The states of Arkansas and Louisiana have enacted legislation that defines drug or alcohol use or being "under the influence of intoxicants" as misconduct and that either prohibits an employee discharged for such misconduct from receiving unemployment benefits or limits the amount that can be collected. The state of Florida, Georgia, and Missouri have recently enacted laws that limit or eliminate the workers' compensation benefits of an injured drug-alcohol-positive employee. The states of Iowa and Ohio also enacted laws recently that deny benefits for injuries "caused by" the use of intoxicants. The state of Texas now requires all employers who have 15 or more employees and who maintain workers' compensation insurance coverage to "adopt a policy designed to eliminate drug abuse and its effects in the workplace."

Litigation Risk

As noted above, drug testing is controversial. Following the initiation of employee drug testing by the federal government in 1988, more than 60 lawsuits were filed attempting to enjoin the government from proceeding. Such a high level of controversy can be explained by recognizing that drug testing sets two fundamental interests on a collision course—the individual's right of privacy against the employer's responsibility to provide and maintain a safe workplace. The courts were faced with the task of balancing those two interests.

The balance has for the most part favored the need to maintain safety over the limited privacy interest of the workers. This period of resolving the dispute between two interests can be viewed as the first phase in the evolution of legal issues posed by employee drug testing.... [T]wo additional phases of legal issues are living with drug testing day to day and the proper employer response to a positive drug test....

To limit these risks, an employer should take time to thoroughly examine the various regulations issued by the federal agencies mandating testing and state laws that restrict such actions. Additionally, every employer should have an appreciation for the legal framework within which drug testing functions. Becoming a legal scholar is not necessary, but you and your supervisors will better appreciate the serious nature of the decisions to be made. There is no substitute for training and education—*You must be prepared!*

Legal Issues Related to Drug Testing...

Phase One: "Can You Test?"

The first "phase" of legal issues arising out of employee drug testing stems from the question, "Can you test employees for drugs?" Essentially what is being asked is whether drug testing is legal—can employers do it? The simple answer is yes. But there are no simple answers in the field of drug testing. Whether an employer can legally require employees to submit to drug testing depends upon the answer to many complex—some still unanswered—questions. Among the many issues facing employers as they begin to develop a drug testing program are the following questions:

1. Is the program constitutional?

2. Must the employer bargain with the union?

3. Must the employer follow both federal and state law?

Is the Program Constitutional? The constitutionality—or legality—of an employer's drug testing program involves the debate between the individual's claimed right of privacy and the employer's demand that the employee submit to drug testing. The resolution of this debate, and the constitutionality of the employer's drug testing program, depends upon who that employer is (government or private employer), who is subject to testing (safety-sensitive employees or all employees), when those subject to testing will be tested (only when there is "suspicion" or randomly), how the testing will be performed, and what will be done with the results. The answer to these questions will be used by a court to determine the legality of an employer's drug testing program. The first question that a court reviewing the program must answer, however, is whether the Constitution even applies.

State Action Required. The restrictions of the United States Constitution *only* apply to *state actors*. Who are state actors? State actors are the government, one of its agencies, or a private company or individual acting at the direction of the government (i.e., in compliance with a federal or state law or as a subcontractor). *Otherwise, individuals and private employers are not state actors!* Why is this important? Only state actors are limited by the Constitution. The concept of privacy exists only if the Constitution applies. Therefore, unless the employer requiring the employee or applicant to submit to a drug test is a state actor, there will be no limits on who, when, how, or where an individual may be tested, because without state action the right of privacy does not exist. An employee of a strictly private employer cannot bring a lawsuit based upon the right of privacy and hope to convince the court to enjoin the testing because the prerequisite state or federal action does not exist.

The Fourth Amendment.   Employers compelled by government agencies to institute a drug testing program are bound by the limits of the United States Constitution. The United States Supreme Court in 1989 concluded that private employers implementing drug testing "at the behest of" the federal government are "state actors" to whom the Constitutional limitations apply. The regulations upheld by the Court in *Skinner v. Railway Executives Association* are similar to those which will serve as the basis of most employer programs. It is appropriate, therefore, to have some sense of the Constitution's application to drug testing.

First, it must be understood that a drug test is a search. Therefore, the limitation on government searches found in the Fourth Amendment to the Constitution apply. The Fourth Amendment provides in part as follows:

> [T]he right of the people to secure in their persons, houses, papers and effects, against unreasonable search and seizure shall not be violated....

Essentially, this means we all have the right to be left alone. Whether privacy exists as a matter of law depends upon a subjective and an objective test. Subjectively, the individual asserting the right must be able to demonstrate that he is treating the subject of the search (e.g., a work locker or desk, a purse, a home) privately. If anyone and everyone is allowed access to a work locker, any limited privacy that may have existed is considered to be waived. Objectively, it must be shown that we as a society (through the courts as our representative) would agree that it was reasonable for the individual to treat the subject of the search privately. One who keeps illicit drugs in a work locker cannot reasonably expect to be protected from a search for such items. Privacy, therefore, may exist, but under the circumstances of the case it may not be protectable.

If both tests are met, then the court will conclude that the concept of privacy exists. The court must then decide if the privacy, under the circumstances, is protectable. The search is protectable only if the government fails to prove the reasonableness of the search.

No government agent can require an individual to submit to a search unless reason exists for that search and the search is conducted in a reasonable manner. The obvious question, then, is what is a reasonable search? To be legal, a search must be reasonable at its inception and as carried out. To be reasonable at its inception, the government must establish a legitimate interest in the search. For example, the Supreme Court in *Skinner* concluded that the Federal Railway Administration's interest in maintaining the safety of rail travel was legitimate and justified the need for its drug testing regulations.

If the search is found to be needed, the method used to conduct the search must also be found to be reasonable. The Court in *Skinner* found the methods adopted by the Federal Railway Administration to, likewise, be reasonable. The Court was convinced that the scientific methods employed along with the steps taken to ensure the individual's sense of dignity established the reasonableness of the search.

If privacy is shown to exist and the government also proves it has a legitimate need for the search (drug tests) and that the method of searching is reasonable, how does the court decide who wins? The judge must balance the competing interests (Refer to Fig.1).

Figure 1

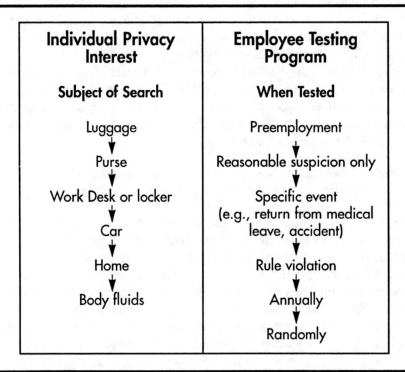

Individual Privacy Interest	Employee Testing Program
Subject of Search	**When Tested**
Luggage	Preemployment
↓	↓
Purse	Reasonable suspicion only
↓	↓
Work Desk or locker	Specific event (e.g., return from medical leave, accident)
↓	↓
Car	
↓	Rule violation
Home	↓
↓	Annually
Body fluids	↓
	Randomly

The left column in Fig. 1 represents circumstances where privacy can exist. As you proceed down the column from the situation where luggage is subject to a search to the search of a home or bodily fluids, your expectation that privacy is protectable by a court is enhanced. Simply put, your home is more protectable than your luggage or your purse, and you expect the courts, when asked, to take appropriate action (i.e., issue an injunction) to protect your privacy. If the government wishes to search your home, significant proof of a reasonable need must be shown. Less proof is required to search your purse.

When the search is a drug test at work, it can be seen that the privacy interest is not as protectable as that at home. The privacy expectation is limited. When balanced against the government's significant need to protect safety at work, the majority of courts have found in favor of the government and upheld the testing regulations. But as you proceed down the right side of the column in Fig. 1, going from preemployment and reasonable suspicion testing to random testing, the level of invasion into the individual's privacy is enhanced; random testing is the ultimate invasion into privacy. Why? Because, generally under the Fourth Amendment a search is not reasonable unless based upon some level of suspicion. By definition, random testing involves no suspicion. But the United States Supreme Court in *Skinner* made it clear that where the government interest to be protected is sufficient, drug testing can occur even where no level of suspicion exits.

Issue 16
NO

Drug Testing
Balancing Private and Public Safety

Judith Wagner DeCew

Recent increases in the use of illegal drugs and problems related to that use have raised a variety of public health and safety concerns and have led many to propose drug testing as one the the best ways to combat the proliferation of drug use. Although my focus is testing for drugs, it is worth noting that similar calls for increased testing have arisen due to the spread of the human immunodeficiency virus (HIV) and the threat it poses to those exposed to it. Clearly, these public health and safety concerns conflict with the privacy claims of those being targeted for testing. Nevertheless, many view the public safety threat as serious enough to override completely any individual privacy interests. Indeed, public opinion polls indicate that there is wide spread support for a variety of testing programs, even those that are random and mandatory.[1]

But it is misleading to view a public policy decision about when and how to conduct drug tests as a simple choice between privacy and public safety. What is less often mentioned is that the issues surrounding testing programs are far more complex than the foregoing suggests. It is both difficult and unwise to reach conclusions about whether testing programs are justified without specifying what type of testing is being proposed (e.g., blood, urine), what is being tested for (e.g., alcohol, drugs, HIV infection), who is initiating the tests (e.g., government agencies, employers, insurance companies), the goals of the tests and the likelihood that they will reduce or eradicate the problem, the harm that would result without the tests, the cost of the proposed testing program, the accuracy of the type of test under consideration, whether confirmatory tests will be added, whether the testing will be mandatory or voluntary, whether the tests will be random or will selectively target particular groups, whether an identifiable showing of suspicion or performance decline will prompt the tests, and how test results will be used and distributed. Furthermore, one must assess which goals of a particular drug-testing program are achievable, and must balance those against the consequences of the testing. The crucial question is to determine when that balance provides adequate moral justification for the testing.

My aim is to address many of these issues by setting out the various arguments and constitutional considerations both in favor of and against certain testing programs. While it should be clear from the above list of concerns relating to drug and HIV tests that broad generalizations are difficult to make, I shall discuss how major public health and safety goals can be addressed seriously while still taking precautions to protect privacy vigorously. Drug abuse should not be tolerated in the workplace or when it threatens the safety of others. But care must be taken to limit the extent to which drug testing intrudes on people's privacy. The ideal is to use the technology selectively, with adequate moral justification, and with enough safeguards and precautions to ensure that testing is done thoughtfully and responsibly.

Arguments in Favor of Drug Testing

Both the government and private employers argue that they have a significant interest in testing citizens and employees for a wide variety of reasons: (1) to fight the "drug war" by weeding out users and curbing drug use; (2) to insure safety by revealing conditions that pose a serious threat to co-workers or the public; (3) to maintain an unimpaired and effective work force; (4) to identify those who will be unable to work in the future; (5) to reduce the costs of employee health care plans; and (6) to maintain public confidence in the integrity and trustworthiness of their operations. Insurers argue in addition that testing is necessary because it is fundamentally unfair to require relatively healthy policyholders to subsidize the costs of health care and life insurance benefits for those with high mortality risks, and because banning insurer testing might leave the industry financially unable to afford to offer individual insurance policies at all.[2] Taken together, these provide strong political, moral, and economic reasons to consider seriously the option of drug testing in some form.

Moreover, the alarming levels of drug abuse in America are estimated to be very costly. The illegal narcotics traffic of about $27 to $110 billion each year correlates with the rising crime rate. In fact, studies showing that "drug use is very much a characteristic of serious and violent offenders" and that "increasing or reducing the level of drug abuse is associated with a corresponding increase or reduction in criminality" may have provided the earliest theoretical justification for initiating drug testing programs.[3] A further consequence is increased medical expenses and rehabilitation costs for drug users.

It has also been claimed that the industrial costs of drug abuse are enormous:

> In human terms they include lost jobs, injuries, illnesses, and deaths. In economic terms they include property damage, tardiness, absenteeism, lost productivity, quality control problems, increased health insurance costs, increased worker's compensation costs, the cost of replacing and training new employees, and employee theft.[4]

According to government estimates, drug abuse cost employers in the United States $33 billion in 1985. More recently, government officials have claimed that these costs are as high as $60 to $100 billion.[5]

Drug testing is taken seriously as a partial solution to the growing drug problem because of the purported results of urinalysis programs instituted by many agencies and employers. The Barcelona Olympics renewed the testing controversy and focused public attention on the athletes who had been disqualified for failing drug tests and on official claims that the tests do deter athletes from taking performance-enhancing drugs. Private companies report that the effects of drug testing programs include increased employee productivity, enhanced job efficiency; significant declines in lost work time and accident rates, and decreased hazards to other employees and the public. If correct, these findings suggest that employer-initiated testing is an efficient way of addressing employee drug abuse and may be a useful deterrent in other contexts as well.

Indeed, drug testing is now commonplace for many workers. In 1986 President Reagan authorized testing all federal job applicants and ordered random testing of federal employees in positions referred to as "safety sensitive." Random urinalysis is utilized for job applicants and sometimes current employees at numerous private businesses, including IBM, DuPont, Exxon, Lockheed, Federal Express, AT&T, the *New York Times*, some Wall Street firms, and over 25 percent of Fortune 500 companies as well.[6] Testing in the trucking industry, for rapid transit and airline workers, law enforcement officials, and athletes is widespread. And recent court cases continue to address the constitutionality of testing teachers, postal workers, customs officials, criminal suspects, prisoners, and many others. The tests are so pervasive that according to the National Institute on Drug Abuse (NIDA) as many as 15 million working Americans had their urine tested for illegal drugs in 1990.[7] Interestingly, these high numbers increase the amounts of money involved, and so have made drug testing a very profitable business.

Threats to Privacy

Despite its popularity, there is good reason to question the justifiability of drug testing. Supreme Court Justice Antonin Scalia, for example, has referred to the practice as a "needless indignity." Drug testing clearly intrudes on individual privacy in a number of distinct ways. One central concern is the technological and physical intrusiveness into a person's biological functions in the actual procedures used for collecting samples. If a blood test is used, it necessarily involves puncturing the skin. If a urinalysis is utilized, the sample must sometimes be gained under direct observation to guard against drug-free substitutions and falsification of results. The additional psychological intrusion of urinating on demand, under surveillance, is not minimal. And critics point out that there are less intrusive ways to identify drug abusers—mainly, observation to detect impairment.

Moreover, besides confirming or disconfirming the presence of drugs in the body, analysis of blood and urine samples may reveal numerous physiological facts about the party being tested that he or she may not want shared with others. Tests can reveal such conditions as the use of contraceptives, pregnancy, epilepsy, manic depression, diabetes, schizophrenia, and heart trouble, for example.

Revelations of this sort are particularly troubling because they raise the privacy question concerning how the results of drug tests are handled. In some testing programs, individuals are not even notified that their samples will be tested. If they are notified and then are informed of the results, it is usually not clear who else has access to the results and what controls there are for maintaining the confidentiality of the information the test reveals. Disclosure of information from drug tests can be embarrassing, can lead to loss of employment and financial loss, discrimination, and further disclosures. There is a serious worry that the individual loses control over any information gained from the tests. Moreover, it is not unreasonable to maintain that employees, for example, should be free from scrutiny during their nonworking hours as long as their activities are not affecting their performance.

Further Arguments against Testing

Opponents of drug testing also focus on the limitations of the testing procedures, arguing that the tests are highly inaccurate. One worry is the sensitivity of the tests. Many types of tests, opponents argue, yield inaccurate results as often as 60 percent of the time. Even if the tests are more highly accurate, they claim, innocent parties will be harmed because most tests produce a large number of false positives, results indicating drug use when there has been none. Such false positives can arise from the use of medications, or passive inhalation of marijuana smoke, for example. Critics worry, moreover, that the technology employed for many drug tests allow false negatives as well, and they cite the human error of lab personnel that further implicates the accuracy of results.

A related issue involves the problems of interpreting the results of drug tests. Most tests set a threshold level that is deemed to establish drug use. But there are few standards for determining how or where that level should be set. Moreover, a true positive may indicate an isolated instance of drug use in the past, not a habitual pattern; interpretation of results does not usually differentiate the two or reveal when the drug was used.

Another serious concern is that the tests cannot establish whether a subject is under the influence of a drug at the time the test is administered, and the tests are incapable of determining if and how much drug use impairs the individual's performance level or actually affects his or her behavior. There is general agreement in the scientific community that "testing does not discriminate between drug use that impairs performance and drug use that does not impair performance. It does not even determine impairment at the time of the test."[8] At best, what is established is whether a person's body contains traces of chemicals that may indicate previous use. Short of this, tests may merely indicate involuntary exposure or an error in procedure. Notably, then, test results may only show non-performance-related conditions that are arbitrary for determining employment or the quality of performance.

Finally, critics worry that tests justified for people in safety sensitive positions can be abused because of the malleability of the term "safety sensitive." Legislators or employers may expand the definition so that it becomes a camouflage for unprincipled random testing.

Tests and Accuracy Concerns

The most commonly administered drug tests are conducted through urinalysis, in part because these are less intrusive than blood tests and in part because they are less expensive to administer. Urinalysis tests can be divided into two types. The most frequently used are administered as presumptive screening tests. The most common involves the enzyme multiplied immunoassay technique (EMIT), others the radioimmunoassay (RIA) and the thin layer chromatography (TLC) tests. These tests are intended to be used easily, rapidly and inexpensively, to identify specimens that most likely contain the sought-after substances. One limit of immunoassay tests is that they are designed to detect only one drug or metabolite of a few closely related ones. The (sometimes erroneous) assumption is that a positive test identifies a user—of marijuana, cocaine, or amphetamines, for example—and a negative test shows a nonuser. Although relatively inexpensive, the screening tests are recognized to be nonspecific and insensitive.

For these programs that add confirmatory tests, a second and more accurate procedure. gas chromatography—mass spectrometry (GC/MS) assessment is also used. In these cases, a sample is reported positive only if both the screening and confirmatory tests are positive. But confirmatory tests are complex, slow to complete, and more expensive than immunoassay tests. A single (GC/MS) tests costs $75 or more. And it is worth noting that confirmatory methods for some drugs are not readily available.

The reliability of the immunoassay screening test is undermined by many factors alluded to above. The high rate of false positives cited by critics can arise from temperature changes in the sample or the presence of substances other than the ones being sought. Positive cannabinoid results have been obtained from urine samples of people who have taken anti-inflammatory drugs such as ibuprofen (Advil, Motrin, etc.) or naproxen, and similar medications might affect the results of tests for barbiturates. Cold remedies such as Contac or Sudafed can suggest the presence of amphetamines, and positive tests for morphine can be obtained from taking drugs containing codeine, including many popular cough syrups. A metabolite of cocaine was measured in a subject who had one cup of an herbal tea which was alleged to have contained decocainized coca leaves, but in fact had about 5 mg. of cocaine per tea bag,[9] thus critics conclude,

> a positive urine test, regardless of the absolute concentration of the sample, provides no information on the amount of drug ingested or inhaled, the time or duration of exposure, or the behavioral effect of the drug. A positive test, if confirmed, may establish exposure, but it does not confirm drug abuse or intoxication, either at the time the sample was obtained or any time prior to that; conversely, a negative test does not rule out abuse or intoxication.[10]

False positive and negative test results indicate the importance of conducting confirmatory tests on samples. But the cost and time required limit the extent to which confirmatory tests are used. Moreover, even a combination of screening and confirmatory tests is susceptible to glaring deficiencies. The threshold or cutoff value that separates positive and negative test results varies depending on the amount of the drug being tested for. If the cutoff is set too low, then a confirmatory test may not actually confirm the result of the initial screening test. If the cutoff is set too high, some positive specimens may be missed, but confirmations will be more reliable. "Decisions on choosing cutoffs depend on how many false negatives, false positives, and unconfirmed test results are economically and scientifically acceptable."[11] When testing donors for blood banks, clearly allowing more false positives is preferable to allowing any false negatives. But in other contexts the balance is less clear, and value judgments may differ more widely.

Another difficulty is that for those who wish to work at it there are ways to defeat the tests. Those who practice timed abstinence or who ingest large amounts of fluids can dilute the concentration of a drug in urine to below the cutoff amount. Adding, salt, vinegar, bleach, liquid soap, blood, or another interfering substance can adulterate samples and produce false negative results that do not rule out abuse.

Quality control in the lab also calls into question the accuracy of test results. Critics claim that technicians are often given minimal training. There can be procedural mishaps as simple as misidentifying a sample, and technicians may not know how to interpret the findings. Signs of a single instance of marijuana use, for example, can persist in urine samples for days or even weeks, but lab technicians might not recognize the importance of including such information along with a positive result. Private laboratories claim that their work is 95 to 99 percent accurate, but they have given little documentation for their claims, nor have the results of proficiency testing for labs been made available.[12]

To the extent drug tests produce false negatives, they are ineffective in identifying users. For those who test positive falsely, the implications for reputation, employment, and freedom may be grave indeed. It is widely agreed that blood tests more accurately measure evidence of intoxication or abuse for alcohol and other drugs. Because concentrations in the blood are usually proportional to concentrations in the brain, blood tests will also be more likely to measure performance capacity with great reliability. In addition, blood tests are taken directly from individuals by lab personnel, so with trustworthy technicians, tampering with specimens is almost impossible. But analyses of blood specimens are also more difficult, complex, and costly. Moreover, because blood concentrations peak and decrease very rapidly, and back calculations in time are rarely possible for most drugs, there is often just a short window of time when a blood test will be useful.

Reviewing the Threat to Public Safety

Given the many difficulties associated with drug tests, it is worth reconsidering the extent of the evidence that urine tests, even with confirmatory testing, will result in improvement in health, safety, and performance. While such claims are made regularly, it is difficult to find confirmatory data. It is also difficult to assess the extent of the deterrent effect of drug test programs. Many in the medical field argue bluntly that "[o]bjective biomedical science tells us that urine testing is of no value in coping with illicit drug use."[13]

Even for transportation accidents, where it is claimed there is evidence that drug impairment plays a major role, evaluations of the findings are unclear. After nearly every plane or rail crash there is (often sensational) publicity about drug tests for pilots and engineers. It is rare, however, for the data to show evidence that employees were impaired by drugs other than alcohol, or that random urine drug testing would have prevented the accident. It has been pointed out that "[f]or testing to be fully effective, every worker would have to be tested daily for every drug that might impair performance, the results would have to be available before he started work, and he would have to be under constant surveillance while at work to make sure he did not use a drug while working."[14]

It is worth noting that marijuana accounts for a huge majority of positive findings nationwide—perhaps as many as 90 percent—because it is the most widely used illegal drug and because it persists in urine for a month or more, compared to two days for most drugs. Yet because of its persistence, many of those true positive drug tests have little or no implication for performance difficulty. Finally, a 1989 NIDA report contradicted claims of increasing illegal drug use. According to the report, illegal drug use has been decreasing for ten years, and the decline accelerated over the latter five of those years.[15]

Thus the correlation between drug use and unsafe or risky job performance is not definitely established. Nevertheless, there are studies that show a significant correlation between positive drug tests and poorer scores on certain general measures of job performance, such as absenteeism and dismissal for other reasons. In addition, studies of airline pilots under simulated conditions indicate diminished ability to perform various maneuvers with prior drug use, including marijuana. Thus there is at least some evidence of correlation between drug use and performance, particularly in one safety sensitive occupation, suggesting a possible rule for appropriately targeted drug tests. One challenge, then, is to determine when drug testing will actually contribute to the goals of public health and safety.

Constitutional Guidelines and the Courts

The first two cases on drug testing to reach the Supreme Court were argued in 1988. From the decisions issued the following year, it is clear that the Court held that urine tests are a significant intrusion into a fundamentally private domain.[16] Since then, virtually every court that has addressed the issue has found that urinalysis and blood tests intrude on privacy as a search and seizure forbidden under the Fourth Amendment. Courts have mainly focused on the privacy invasions involved, first, in the process of urination and the manner in which the specimen is obtained, and second, in the individual's interest in safeguarding the confidentiality of the information contained in the sample. While drug tests might also violate the Fifth Amendment guarantee against self-incrimination, the Fourteenth Amendment protection of due process, and the constitutional privacy interests, courts have nevertheless taken the privacy claims of the Fourth Amendment to be the most forceful constitutional threats.

Courts have been somewhat divided over how intrusive unobserved urine testing is. But they have generally agreed that compulsory urinalysis infringes on and individual's expectation of privacy both in the process and in the loss of control over information. Nevertheless, case law currently indicates that some drug screening is constitutionally permissible. Fourth Amendment protection is not absolute, and the courts have traditionally used a two-part test to decide when the government has infringed on an individual's Fourth Amendment privacy. First, the individual must show a "subjective expectation of privacy," and second, the expectation must be "one that society considers reasonable."[17]

The key, then, is the determination of when drug tests are "reasonable." No court has held testing to be a violation of the Fourth Amendment when there is a showing of "reasonable suspicion" that the individual has been using illegal drugs. But the Supreme Court also allowed testing of any customs officials in positions directly involving the interdiction of drugs or where firearms were required to be carried in the line of duty. The evolving legal standard is that reasonable suspicion be required except for random testing upheld for public employees in safety sensitive positions, law enforcement positions, or where employees have access to classified materials.

It is not surprising that courts have taken Fourth Amendment privacy seriously in the context of drug tests. Historically, stomach pumping, strip searches, and body cavity checks to gain evidence has been judged unconstitutional. By analogy, although United States banks are surely concerned to insure that their employees are not embezzlers, that does not entitle them to search all bank employees and their homes on the chance that they may uncover a dishonest employee.[18]

It is troubling, however, that many courts have refused to address concerns about testing error, and have avoided discussions of the implications of false positives and false negatives. Moreover, protection against warrantless and unreasonable searches does not apply in the private sector, and most private sector drug testing programs have survived legal challenge thus far. Nonconstitutional state regulations are largely absent. The few that have been enacted form a patchwork of conflicting guidelines. Some, such as Utah's, promote employer interests by allowing random testing of all employees. Others have been more sensitive to employee interests, but the great majority of states have no guidelines at all. Still, the model of the courts embracing a basic concern with protecting Fourth Amendment privacy may indicate that those initiating testing programs that do not take sufficient care to address privacy intrusions will face an increasing risk of liability.

Ethical Justifications

Certainly there is a very real problem of drug abuse in this country. Yet drug testing in the workplace may not be the most effective way of tackling the problem. I have explained the various privacy interests at stake for test subjects, including the intrusion of the testing procedure, the revelation of additional medical information, and the difficulties arising from false results and from mismanagement of the information gained. I have also reviewed concerns over the accuracy of screening tests, the difficulty of interpreting results, the expense and difficulty of confirmatory tests, the lack of information on performance ability, and concerns that tests may not ferret out those who are a threat to others. These considerations lead to worry that drug tests cannot adequately protect others from harm as intended. They also provide compelling arguments that widespread and random drug testing is unnecessarily intrusive, unwise, and inefficient.

It might seem, therefore, that we have reached the inevitable conclusion that drug testing is never morally justifiable. I believe such a conclusion would be too hasty, however. That a practice is difficult to justify does not make it impossible to justify in all cases. The key moral issues involve determining when the interests of others are significant enough to outweigh the threats to test subjects and when the achievable goals outweigh the negative consequences of testing. Although I cannot address every conceivable case, I believe that in carefully circumscribed circumstances, drug testing can be defended as morally justifiable. But even then, I will defend testing only when administered with stringent procedural safeguards.

Some cases seem absolutely clear. My sense is that most would agree that tests should be permissible and perhaps even mandated for potential blood donors. The expectation is that donated blood will be clean, and the interests of those needing transfusions are highly significant. The condition is often life-threatening, and the risk of harm to the recipient is immediate and certain. Moreover, such testing is not random, but targets only those wishing to donate blood.

In less clear cases, what considerations can override the privacy invasions and other deleterious consequences of testing? The practice can be justified if there is a substantial and demonstrable likelihood that a significant drug problem exists, and if the testing program targets those potentially causing the problem in the hope that it can be alleviated. That is, I believe the concerns with testing enumerated above are significant enough to require substantial evidence of an existing drug problem and a reasonable expectation of resolving it, before testing becomes morally defensible.

If there is probable cause or reasonable suspicion to believe there is a drug use problem, such as substantial evidence of frequent use or abuse of drugs by a group or individual over a significant amount of time, and if it can be shown likely to be affecting the safety of customers (e.g., passengers), co-workers, or products, then random testing and follow-up to single out those risking the welfare of others gains ethical force. Thus I support, for instance, the Supreme Court's decision in *Skinner v. Railway Labor Executives Association* to allow tests of railway workers where there was evidence of frequent alcohol and drug use and a demonstrated connection between use and accidents. In that particular case it seemed that the safety threat was clear, substantial (at minimum 23 percent of the railway workers were found to be "problem drinkers"), and the subjects formed a targeted group that, if it became drug-free, could decrease the railway accident rate significantly.

Additionally, when individuals or groups show some evidence of performance impairment and the likelihood of a serious accident or defective product is considerably heightened by it, drug testing may also be morally justified. Even if it is not certain that the impairment is due to drug use, the individual's behavior can be worrisome enough to defeat claims that they must not be intruded upon. The presumption of a person's innocence is, in such cases, rightly called into question. A drug test, administered with procedural safeguards, can help determine if drug use is indeed contributing to the performance difficulty observed. In sum, the studies concerning difficulties with drug tests do not rule out testing when some causal showing, performance impairment, or reasonable suspicion of drug use exists.

In contrast, however, absent such evidence, drug testing programs instituted to accomplish general deterrence of drug use, or based on generalized claims about the need to fight the "war on drugs," do not carry sufficient moral justification to outweigh all the negative consequences and difficulties of drug testing. With no showing of a significant problem there is too little evidence that there will be any deterrent effect or any progress made to combat drug use. Thus I find insufficient ethical justification for the Supreme Court's judgment in *National Treasury Employees v. Von Raab*, which upheld random testing of customs workers by virtue of the job they held, even though there was almost no evidence of a drug problem either by individuals or across a section of the group of customs workers.

One difficulty of mandating testing for persons in positions that count as safety sensitive is that it is difficult to assure that this is an accurate, not merely expedient, classification. Moreover, people holding positions where they are required to carry firearms or have access to classified material have already been subjected to extensive background checks. The Court in *Raab* appealed to a generalized compelling interest that customs employees not use drugs even when off duty, and to the extraordinary safety and national security hazards of drug use among customs officials. But combined with the admission that customs is largely drug-free and that previous drug use was not the reason for establishing the testing program, those appeals lose moral force. The actual purposes cited for the testing were to deter drug use among employees in the specified positions and to keep drug users from being promoted into such positions. It was claimed that customs officials who use drugs are more susceptible to bribery and that those in jobs where they may use firearms depend uniquely on their judgment and dexterity, both of which could be compromised by drug use. One major difficulty, however, was that there was at best a potential for harm to others, yet no clear threat of harm. Second, there was virtually no evidence that any customs officials had a drug problem and so no reason to suppose that there was any need to deter any of them, or that testing could reduce drug use. There was minimal likelihood the testing program would have any impact at all.

I have argued that several criteria must be met for drug testing programs to be deemed morally justifiable. The most basic is that a significant drug problem must actually be apparent, through a causal showing, performance impairment, or other reasonable suspicion. We might well consider, therefore, whether a less objectionable alternative focusing more directly on performance can effectively protect the public from harm. Some have argued, for example, that state-of-the-art employee assistance programs, combined with proper education of supervisory personnel, can be as effective as or more effective than drug testing in minimizing harm to others.

This is a provocative suggestion, and it may be that, when fully developed, the implementation of such programs ultimately will be able to supersede drug testing even in the cases where I have defended it. At present, however, there are a number of difficulties with advocating such programs in place of any drug testing at all. First, the educational process of supervisors is critical, and it could take much time to develop and implement it adequately. It would be a mistake to underestimate the scope of the education necessary for such programs to be successful. Second, employee assistance programs could be economically more costly and thus less feasible than drug testing programs. Small businesses, for example, may find it prohibitive to introduce adequate employee assistance programs for only a few isolated cases. Third, it is difficult to see how to mandate procedural safeguards for employees when the programs are individualized and run by supervisory personnel. Some may worry about what recourse or appeal mechanism an employee has if a supervisor is distrustful or is erroneously convinced of an employee's abuse. Drug testing programs have the virtue, perhaps of being more easily subject to federal regulations protecting test subjects' interests uniformly.

Ideally and more characteristically, however, employee assistance programs are set up so supervisory personnel only refer employees for assessment by health care professionals and for treatment recommendations. The object of these assistance programs is not intended to be a determination of wrongdoing. Rather, the goal is to provide treatment recommendations to employees who are chemically dependent or substance abusers, with the assurance of continued employment if treatment is successful. Perhaps the most notable difficulty with these programs is the lack of hard evidence that a high percentage of chemically dependent employees are actually identified and then treated.

Procedural Safeguards and Recommendations

Even in the narrowly circumscribed cases when drug testing can ethically be justified in my view, I believe it is necessary to mandate precautions to protect privacy and minimize error. To be effective, these should be embodied in federal guidelines that are backed up with sanctions for violations and that recommend combining test results with follow-up assessments of performance.

To reiterate, we should mandate that drug tests be conducted only after there is evidence of a reasonable probability of drug abuse. Reasonable suspicion might be indicated if there is perceived impairment, deficient output or performance, major unexplained change in attitude, or other behavior arousing suspicion. When reasonable suspicion is required to justify testing, there is less intrusion into worker's privacy, the testing program is less vulnerable to constitutional attack, and supervisors are forced to oversee more fully the performance of those in their charge.

Even when fully justified, drug testing plans should be explained in writing, and those who might be tested should be made aware of the reasons for the testing program. They will then know whether the testing will involve direct observation, whether it will be voluntary or mandated as a condition of employment, and so on. We might also require that employees be informed in advance whether a testing program is to be random or required as a condition of employment.

Due to the inadequacies and inaccuracies of various types of tests, we should require that whoever initiates a testing program give confirmatory tests for those with positive results. If the initial screening is selective, as I have argued it should be, the cost of confirmatory testing will not be prohibitive. People testing positive should be allowed an opportunity to explain the test results and to have the sample retested in an independent laboratory.

We can hope that the testing technology being developed by Roche, Abbott, and others will continue to improve. Methods are being discovered to discern from a test if a common medication has been the cause of a false positive result. The possibility of less intrusive and more accurate tests—using saliva or hair samples, for example—is also under investigation. In the meantime, it seems reasonable to require laboratories to justify the thresholds used for determining positive and negative readings on tests. Laboratories ought also to be required to state the length of time the drug remains in the system, the test's inability to determine performance limitations, and similar relevant information. This will set the results in perspective and will help explain what they mean. It might also be reasonable to mandate laboratory procedures such as requiring documentation of all handling of a sample and requiring all samples to be divided into two containers, one for analysis and one for freezing in case the results are contested later.

Finally, detailed guidelines must be set up to protect the confidentiality of the information gained from tests. It seems that with computer data banks of medical information it may be almost impossible to guarantee confidentiality. But it can certainly be a legal requirement, with strong sanctions for noncompliance, that test results not be used for any purpose other than that originally articulated, and that test information not be released without permission to anyone other than the individual tested. Confidentiality can be further enhanced by requiring "anonymous" testing, which marks samples by coded numbers rather than names.

This may appear to be a burdensome list of requirements to impose on testing programs. But the requirements not only protect individual privacy, they also encourage the government and employers to use testing only when it is most likely to be helpful in averting public harm. Time, energy, and money not used on widespread random tests could then be better spent on monitoring performance through observation, controlling alcohol abuse on the job, and limiting illegal drug traffic in the United States.

My goal has been to recognize the benefits of drug testing when there is probable cause or clear substantial evidence of abuse, with likely correlation to a safety threat and a reasonable possibility of achieving the desired effects. Mass testing without suspicion is intrusive, inefficient, often inaccurate, and a waste of resources. I have suggested restrictions aimed at maximizing privacy and accuracy of results while still allowing identification of those who use illegal drugs.

References

1.   See, for example, the data cited in Michael R. O'Donnell, "Employee Drug Testing—Balancing the Interests in the Workplace: A Reasonable Suspicion," *Virginia Law Review* 74 (1988): 969–1009, at 971–72

2.   Nancy Perkins, "Prohibiting the Use of the Human Immunodeficiency Virus Antibody Test by Employers and Insurers." *Harvard Journal on Legislation* 25 (1988): 275–315, at 297–303.

3.   Cathryn Jo Rosen and John S. Goldkamp, "The Constitutionality of Drug Testing at the Bail Stage," *Journal of Criminal Law and Criminology* 80 (1989): 114–76 at 117.

4.   Edward S. Adams, "Random Drug Testing of Government Employees: A Constitutional Procedure." *University of Chicago Law Review* 54 (1988): 1335–72, at 1337, citing Thomas Geidt.

5.   John Horgan, "Test Negative," *Scientific American* 262 (March 1990): 18–19, at 18.

6.   Adams, "Random Drug Testing," p. 1337. Steven Wisotsky claims testing is practiced at as many as 80 percent of Fortune 500 companies, in his "A Society of Suspects: The War on Drugs and Civil Liberties." *Policy Analysis* 180 (1992): 1–49, at 12.

7.   Horgan, "Test Negative," p. 18.

8.   Alan R. Westin et al., "College and University Policies on Substance Abuse and Drug Testing," *Academe* 78, no. 3 (1992): 17–23, at 20.

POSTSCRIPT

Should All Employers Be Allowed to Drug Test Their Employees?

As a follow-up to the discussion of whether or not to allow random drug testing, one needs to ask what should be done with people who test positive for drugs. Should they be fired or helped? Is the purpose of drug testing to eliminate workers who use drugs or to help them? Do companies have the right to punish workers for activities engaged in away from the job? Aside from the legal issues, how reliable are drug tests?

Many questions surround the legalities of drug testing. Over the years, the courts have been divided over whether or not drug testing is reasonable and whether or not it constitutes a search under the Fourth Amendment. Most courts have concluded that a mandatory urine, blood, or breath test can be considered a search under the Fourth Amendment; the focus now is on the extent to which drug searchers may be unreasonable.

Advocates of random drug testing argue that testing at the workplace will prevent illicit drug use and associated problems. Proponents believe that it is not a violation of civil rights when the government acts to protect all citizens from the problems of illicit drug use. But drug tests are not always accurate. To avoid a positive result, some drug users submit another person's urine or put salt and detergent in their own samples, which affects the accuracy of the test. People on both sides of the argument contend that more reliable tests are needed if drug testing is to be allowed.

Drug testing raises other questions: How should drug test results be recorded at work? Should testing be implemented at the work site or at a "neutral" location? Who should be allowed access to employees' files regarding test results? How could employees be assured of their privacy? In addition, will job discrimination of employee stigmatization come about from positive test results?

An excellent overview of drug use in the workplace is presented in Michael D. Newcomb's "Prevalence of Alcohol and Other Drug Use on the Job: Cause for Concern or Irrational Hysteria?" *Journal of Drug Issues* (Summer 1994). The merits of drug testing are discussed in John Honour's article "Testing for Drug Abuse," *The Lancet* (July 6, 1996). The prevalence of drug testing is reviewed in "Prevalence of Drug Testing in the Workplace," by Tyler Hartwell et al., *Monthly Labor Review* (November 1996). The legality of the Fourth Amendment, especially as it relates to testing political candidates for drugs, is discussed in the article "Fourth Amendment—Mandatory Drug Testing—Eleventh Circuit Upholds Suspicionless Drug Testing for Political Candidates," *Harvard Law Review* (vol. 110, 1996).

Debate Presenter Form

Follow the guidelines for debate presenters contained in the introduction of this text and those given to you by your instructor. Use the format below to organize the material for your debate. Remember to include all relevant citation information and to present the related information in your own words. Give credit to authors when you cite a quote and be as thorough as possible when writing about your points so you will be prepared for your debate.

Reference citation #1.

Author: _____

Title: _____

Date: _____

Source: _____

_____

Content from reference citation #1: _____

_____

_____

_____

_____

_____

_____

_____

_____

_____

_____

_____

Reference citation #2:

Author: _____

Title: _____

Date: _____

Source: _____

_____

Content from reference citation #2: _____

_____

_____

_____

_____

_____

Reference citation #3:

Author: _____

Title: _____

Date: _____

Source: _____

_____

Content from reference citation #3: _____

_____

_____

_____

_____

Audience Preparation Form

Follow the guidelines for preparing to be an informed audience member on the day of the debate included in the introduction to this text. After reading both sides of the debate from this chapter, answer the following questions. Be as thorough as possible so that you will be able to make a contribution to the debate by asking informed questions or making provocative comments. This form is usually due on the day of the debate.

State the issue in your own words. Do not plagiarize the text. Demonstrate that you understand the topic and it's relevant arguments.

_____

_____

_____

_____

_____

Discuss two points on the "yes" side of the debate.

Point #1: _____

_____

Point #2: _____

_____

Discuss two points on the "no" side of the debate.

Point #1: _____

_____

Point #2: _____

_____

What is your opinion on this topic?

_____

_____

_____

_____

_____

_____

_____

What has contributed to the development of your views about this topic?

_____

_____

_____

_____

_____

_____

_____

_____

What information would be necessary to cause you to change your thinking about this topic?

_____

_____

_____

_____

_____

Debate Response Form

Follow the guidelines for responding to the debates in the introductory chapter of this text. Complete this form and submit your answers at the class following the debate. Try to be thorough and convince your instructor that you were an active listener during the debate.

List a quote from a debate presenter that you think was important and explain why you think this comment was significant.

_____

_____

_____

_____

Which side of the debate do you think made the most convincing arguments, why?

_____

_____

_____

_____

_____

After hearing the debate, in what way has your thinking been affected?

_____

_____

_____

_____

_____

_____

_____

ISSUE 17

Should Tabacco Products Be More Closely Regulated?

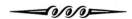

YES Margaret Kriz, *Where There's Smoke....*

NO John Hood, *Anti-Smoking War Could Deny Consumers Choice*

Antismoking activists promote the idea that protecting public health is more important than the right of smokers to choose to use tobacco. Margaret Kriz agrees. She describes three factors that have set in motion proposals to further regulate the tobacco industry. These include the conclusion that second-hand smoke is a carcinogen, nicotine is addictive, and smoking in public has come under attack. Additionally, a movement to restrict availability of cigarettes to children has developed.

Limits on advertising, increased penalties for illegal sale of tobacco products to minors, and restrictions on public smoking are all indicators that non-smoker's rights are prevailing. Kriz cites these developments as indicators that the politics of tobacco are starting to shift toward protection of public health.

Arguing in favor of smoker's rights, John Hood suggests that the real issue is the right of consumers to have free choice of all products, not just tobacco. Also, Hood argues that regulation of tobacco by the commissioner of the Federal Drug Administration places whoever runs the FDA in a position to control the behavior of fellow humans with respect to choices regarding tobacco.

Allowing the FDA to control tobacco is a huge step in the direction of empowering this agency to regulate a great number of products that the average American deserves to express free choice in buying. Hood asks, "Where do we stop?" He provides some examples of food, drink, and drug restrictions that he believes would logically follow increasing the power of the FDA to control tobacco products.

Health and safety issues are hard to regulate and to do so is intrusive on our freedom of choice. No group of individuals is eminently qualified to restrict the choices of others according to Hood.

Applications

1. What other product restrictions can you think of that would be similar to the limitations that have been and will be placed on tobacco products? Discuss your ideas about the future of these products and their restrictions.

2. Do you think the government has the right to protect us from our bad decisions? Explain.

3. Do we have the right to perform behaviors that are not good for us? Even ones that could cause death or cost the public a great deal of money?

Issue 17
YES

Where There's Smoke...

Margaret Kriz

In mid-March, a team of investigators from the Health and Human Services Department's Food and Drug Administration (FDA) made history when, for the first time on record, they were allowed to go to a tobacco processing plant and watch cigarettes being made.

The federal regulators, who are investigating whether tobacco companies manipulate the levels of nicotine in cigarettes, got their rare glimpses first at a Philip Morris Co., Inc.'s tobacco processing plant in Richmond, Va., and later at an RJR Reynolds Tobacco Co. factory in Winston-Salem, N.C.

The visits were unprecedented. Tobacco cultivation and cigarette production and advertising are almost totally unregulated by the federal government, despite growing medical evidence linking cigarette smoking to cancer and heart and lung disease in smokers and nonsmokers.

The American Medical Association estimates that 460,000 Americans die from tobacco-related illnesses each year and that tobacco-related illnesses cost the U.S. health care system more than $80 billion a year.

"We regulate all kinds of minor risks, in the form of additives, pesticides and other products that may affect one person in a million," said Scott D. Ballin, a vice president of the American Heart Association and chairman of the Coalition on Smoking OR Health (which represents Ballin's group, the American Cancer Association and the American Lung Association). "Yet we don't regulate tobacco, which kills far more people. It shows the total inconsistencies in the way we apply the law to this product."

As an FDA official put it, "The cheese in Philip Morris's Kraft (General Foods Inc.) division goes through infinitely more regulation than their cigarettes."

During the three decades since Surgeon General Luther L. Terry issued the landmark report that first linked cigarettes to lung cancer, the tobacco industry has wielded enormous political and economic clout with the American public and in Washington.

Americans have been seduced by advertisements that feature scantily clad bathers, rugged cowboys and, now boldly independent smokers who risk riding on an airplane wing just to enjoy their cigarettes.

More important, David A. Kessler, the FDA's commissioner, suggests that the industry may have hooked its customers by delivering an addictive dose of nicotine in each cigarette.

As the scientific evidence against cigarettes mounted, the tobacco companies tried to neutralize criticism in Washington by pouring millions of dollars into the political war chests of their allies on Capitol Hill and other potentially helpful lawmakers.

But 1994 has proved to be the dawning of a new era of public scrutiny and government oversight of the nation's tobacco industry. Among the signs of change:

In February, McDonald's Corp. banned smoking in its restaurants, joining the growing movement against smoking in public places. Several other restaurant chains promptly followed suit.

Days later, the Defense Department banned smoking at all U.S. military facilities around the world.

In March, Congress passed an education package that prohibits smoking in public schools.

On March 25, the Labor Department issued a preliminary proposal to restrict smoking in all workplaces.

On April 13, the tobacco industry released a long-guarded list of chemicals and other substances that are added to cigarettes. The public disclosure came after a reporter for National Public Radio obtained a copy of the list.

On April 14, the top executives of the seven largest U.S. tobacco companies made history of their own by testifying before Congress for the first time, undergoing six hours of sharp questioning on the health effects of tobacco and business practices within the industry by members of the House Energy and Commerce Subcommittee on Health and the Environment.

In the past two months, Congress and the news media have also focused on internal tobacco company studies that reportedly prove that tobacco is addictive and that the industry has controlled the levels of nicotine in cigarettes. In fact, two former scientists for Philip Morris told Congress on April 28 that after they found evidence in 1983 that nicotine was addictive in test animals, their studies were halted and the results suppressed by company officials.

As the wall of secrecy crumbled, the editorial boards of major newspapers became increasingly critical of the tobacco industry. *The New York Times* has published eight anti-smoking editorials so far this year, and an editorial in *USA Today* described the tobacco company executives who testified on Capitol Hill as "clowns."

A Three-Front War

The fabric of change has been woven primarily from three threads:

- A 1993 scientific study by the Environmental Protection Agency (EPA), which classified secondhand, tobacco smoke as a carcinogen that causes lung cancer and other illnesses in nonsmoking adults and children.

- An FDA investigation, announced in February, into whether nicotine is addictive and should be regulated as a drug.

- The growing grass-roots movement to limit smoking in public and to restrict children's access to cigarettes. It's fueled by the EPA study and by a 1986 Surgeon General's report on the damaging health effects of secondhand smoke.

Riding the wave of public opinion, Congress is considering increasing the 24-cent-a-pack excise tax on cigarettes to $1.25 a pack to pay for health reform. The Clinton Administration supports a 75-cent tax; the industry is fighting all increases.

Congress is also weighing legislation that would ban smoking in public buildings and expand the FDA's authority to regulate all phases of the cigarette industry.

Nevertheless, the tobacco industry hasn't lost its touch.

Forced into a defensive position, it's accusing the Clinton Administration and anti-smoking forces in Congress of trying to impose a total ban, which public opinion polls shows is vastly unpopular.

The industry warns that such a prohibition would result in a black market for cigarettes and further restrictions on prized personal liberties.

Regulation of the tobacco industry "would result in a product that is too expensive to buy, too inconvenient to use and that you can't tell anybody about," Walker Merryman, a vice president of the Washington-based Tobacco Institute, said. "They can't get away with saying that is not prohibition."

But antismoking activists argue that safeguarding public health is more important than preserving the personal freedoms of smokers.

Besides, they ask, does a smoker really have freedom of choice if nicotine is addictive?

"We just want to face reality," said Henry A. Waxman, D-Calif., the chairman of the Health Subcommittee. "The reality is, tobacco kills people. Nicotine is addictive. Advertising influences kids. Environmental tobacco smoke is dangerous. And if we're a rational society we should be doing things to counteract that."

That message seems to be selling well back home, said Rep. Richard J. Durbin, D-Ill., who authored the 1988 ban on smoking on domestic airline flights and who supports current legislation to restrict smoking.

"Many people like myself have challenged the tobacco companies and found that when you went back home, there were more people supporting you than criticizing you," said

Durbin, whose father died of lung cancer when Durbin was 14. "But the tobacco lobby is still a powerhouse. They are not to be underestimated, even though they're under fire today."

A Changeover on Capitol Hill

When it comes to regulating the tobacco industry, Congress has a long history of pulling its punches. In response to the 1964 Surgeon General's report on smoking and cancer, for example, lawmakers merely required manufacturers to print a health warning on cigarette packages.

"It was an awful piece of legislation, essentially designed in conjunction with the industry to put this mild warning on the package, but to stop the federal regulatory agencies from doing anything more," said antismoking activist Michael Pertschuk, a co-director of the Washington-based Advocacy Institute, which trains public-interest lawyers. Pertschuk was on the staff of the House Interstate and Foreign Commerce Committee when the law was written.

By 1969, lawmakers were willing to go a step further by prohibiting tobacco advertisements on television and radio.

That's about where things stood for more than a decade. Then, in 1984, Jim Repace, a little-knows physicist at EPA, independently developed a risk assessment that estimated that secondhand tobacco smoke was causing lung cancer in nonsmokers, too.

Intrigued by Repace's findings, Reagan Administration appointee Joseph A. Cannon, who headed EPA's air pollution office, gave the National Research Council some seed money to develop a more complete study of what has come to be called passive smoking. The fruits of the council's labor became the scientific underpinnings of Surgeon General C. Everett Koop's highly publicized 1986 report that linked passive smoking to lung cancer.

By then, Repace had been reassigned to EPA's newly formed indoor air pollution office, where he pushed for the agency to conduct its own comprehensive scientific study of the health effects of cigarette smoke on nonsmokers.

The conclusions, released in January 1993 by outgoing EPA administrator William K. Reilly, were startling. Exposure to secondhand smoke, the study estimated, causes 3,000 lung cancer deaths among nonsmokers each year and dramatically increases the childhood incidence of asthma, bronchitis, pneumonia and ear infections. The study also said that at least 43 of the hundreds of chemicals added to cigarettes cause cancer in test animals.

"That report was a turning point and began this whole round of scrutiny." EPA administrator Carol Browner said in an interview. "It clearly demonstrated what everyone has suspected for a long time: People who choose not to smoke are at risk, and they deserve to be protected."

The Clinton Administration followed up on the report with a guide that advised parents to help enact restrictions on smoking in their communities and school districts "to make their children's environment smoke-free."

The Tobacco Institute promptly sued EPA, charging that Congress never gave the agency the authority to issue the study. Rep. Thomas J. Bliley Jr., R-Va., a longtime defender of the tobacco industry, also charged that EPA had skewed the science used to back up its risk estimates.

Despite the industry's protests, the EPA report triggered a domino effect with the Administration. The Defense Department's smoking ban and the Labor Department's proposal to restrict smoking in workplaces are both based on the EPA study.

On Capitol Hill, the EPA risk assessment gave Waxman the scientific ammunition he sought to impose national smoking restrictions. His bill to regulate smoking in public buildings is being considered by his subcommittee but faces tough opposition from tobacco-state lawmakers—including Bliley, the subcommittee's ranking Republican.

"The tobacco industry has invested an enormous amount of time and money in influencing our subcommittee," a member of the subcommittee's staff said. "They've been gearing up for this fight for a long time."

A Question of How, Not Whether?

In 1988, the Coalition on Smoking OR Health filed one in a long series of petitions pushing the FDA to regulate cigarettes.

This time the coalition argued that low-tar, low-nicotine cigarettes should be controlled under the nation's drug laws. It argued that by altering tar and nicotine levels in cigarettes, tobacco companies were marketing a product that promised to mitigate disease—that is, to lower the chances that a smoker would contract lung cancer and heart disease.

That interpretation would place such cigarettes under the purview of the 1938 Federal Food, Drug and Cosmetic Act, which requires the FDA to regulate as drugs products that fall within one of two legal definitions: products that are used to treat or mitigate diseases or that affect the structure or function of the body.

The coalition's petitions went nowhere until 1990, when Kessler took the reigns of the agency. Kessler worried, however, that regulating only low-tar, low-nicotine cigarettes would be sending the wrong message to the American public.

In fall 1992, the FDA shifted gears. Three FDA lawyers approached Kessler with a new approach for tackling the tobacco industry: Rather than attacking cigarettes, they said, the government should regulate nicotine as a drug.

Citing tentative evidence that nicotine is addicting and that cigarette companies tinker with the levels of nicotine in cigarettes, they reasoned that nicotine could be regulated as a substance that alters the structure of function of the body.

In a Feb. 25 letter to Ballin, Kessler went public with the FDA's new strategy. "Evidence brought to our attention is accumulating that suggests that cigarette manufacturers may intend that their products contain nicotine to satisfy an addiction on the part of some of their customers," Kessler wrote, "In fact, it is our understanding that manufacturers commonly add nicotine to cigarettes to deliver specific amounts of nicotine."

Some of the accusations were confirmed at the April 14 hearing of Waxman's subcommittee. Under questioning, a Philip Morris executive admitted that the company had suppressed studies showing that animals could become addicted to nicotine and acknowledged that the company packs its low-tar cigarettes with tobacco that contains a higher concentration of nicotine than its regular cigarettes.

While the FDA's lawyers continue to gather evidence against nicotine, its policy makers are beginning to plot their next step.

Under the law, the FDA commissioner can limit the use or ban a drug that isn't safe. But the aggressive Kessler is seeking broader jurisdiction. At a March 25 hearing of Waxman's subcommittee, Kessler asked for Congress's help in handling the nicotine problem, acknowledging that "if nicotine were removed, the nation would face a host of issues involving the withdrawal from addiction that would be experienced by millions of Americans."

In response, Rep. Mike Synar, D-Okla., introduced legislation that would grant the FDA broad authority over nearly every aspect of cigarette production. "It's no longer a question of whether tobacco is going to be regulated under FDA." Synar said in an interview. "It's a matter of how FDA will regulate it."

Protection v. Prohibition

Julia Carol, a co-director of Americans for Nonsmokers' Rights in Berkeley, Calif., is drawing a cartoon for the group's newsletter. It depicts a sleeping giant beginning to awaken, with a little bird musing, "He's awake, but now where's he going?"

The sleeping giant is the federal government, which has long shunned the role of overseer of the nation's tobacco industry. Into that void rushed an army of community activists, who from coast to coast have successfully championed hundreds of local restrictions on smoking in public and bans on cigarette vending machines.

"The most successful element of the whole tobacco control issue is the nonsmokers' rights issue," Carol said. "Forget the rhetoric. Forget the TV shows. Forget the articles. Look at what's really changed in America: What you find is that nonsmokers' issues are making headway."

While the tobacco industry has successfully used campaign contributions to influence federal and state lawmakers, "the tobacco industry is not very effective at the grass-roots level," the Advocacy Institute's Pertschuk said. "They're carpetbaggers. They're men in suits from outside when they come into a local community. Local city councils are not as shielded from their neighbors as the state legislatures."

With Congress and the Clinton Administration increasingly interested in regulating the tobacco industry, however, many antismoking activists worry that lawmakers and policy makers in Washington may inadvertently undercut the progress that's been made at the local level.

Local activists fear that the labor Department's attempts to regulate smoking in workplaces, for example, could result in cumbersome regulations that are hard to enforce and preempt more-aggressive local laws.

More troublesome, Carol said, are pro-tobacco lawmakers in the states who are pushing mild smoking-control measures to preempt tougher action at the local level. She described state legislators, who are becoming increasingly dependent on campaign money from the tobacco industry, as the weakest link in the group's efforts to limit smoking.

The current round of tobacco industry bashing could also create a backlash against the nonsmokers' rights movement, Carol warned.

"We've allowed the debate to get shifted to the question of "Should cigarettes be prohibited?" she said. "That is how the media is interpreting the whole FDA issue, which in my opinion is extremely dangerous. Americans do not like being told what to do, and they will vote for someone else not to be told what to do."

In fact, tobacco companies are escalating the public relations war by portraying themselves as the underdogs against Washington, antismoking activists warn. "The new mantra against anybody who is for sensible regulation of tobacco products,: said Rep. Ron Wyden, D-Ore., "is that they are prohibitionists."

The Shifting Tide

It's incontestable, the Tobacco Institute's Merryman argues, that the Clinton Administration is more hostile to the tobacco industry than any other Administration in the nation's history.

"First the Clintons announced the smoking ban in the White House," Merryman said. "Then Ira Magaziner's health care group leaked the fact that they wanted to propose a $2 a pack tax increase to fund health care. Clinton settled at 75 cents, but it was a very clear signal that there was a free ride at the federal level for anybody who wanted to hammer on tobacco."

Most Members of Congress, Merryman contended, haven't been converted by the antismoking forces. "I think there's been more attention in the media than on the Hill to these issues," he said. "I don't think there is any significantly increased animosity toward the tobacco industry on the Hill."

In fact, a group of tobacco-state Members recently wrote President Clinton, warning that unless his proposed cigarette tax increase was cut to 48 cents a pack, they wouldn't support his health care reform package.

"It certainly is going to be impossible for Democrats in the Southeast to run for reelection with that tax hanging around their necks," Merryman said. "They simply cannot support it. And if the White House decides that it needs three dozen House Members from the Southeast for health care plan, then it can't pursue a 75-cent tax increase."

The nation's six tobacco states—Georgia, Kentucky, North Carolina, South Carolina, Tennessee and Virginia—still present a powerful force in Congress. They elect 55 House

Members, many of whom have posts on key congressional committees. The industry has also been channeling campaign contributions to members of several crucial committees.

"Most of the major legislation has to go through the Health Subcommittee, where the tobacco lobby has quite a group of friends," Durbin said. "They've also really worked on the Rules Committee, which they understand is key to their future."

The southern bloc isn't the only impediment to the current legislative efforts to control tobacco. Labor unions worry that Waxman's measure to control smoking in all public buildings will divert government resources from their campaign to limit worker exposure to more-dangerous chemical fumes.

Southern lawmakers also point out that the state governments have become dependent on tobacco taxes to finance important police and school programs. Federal smoking control measures and a hefty increase in the federal excise tax are likely to shrink state tobacco revenues, they say.

But the once-impenetrable front of tobacco-state lawmakers may be showing a few cracks. "Public sentiment is turning against the tobacco-state legislators, and they know it," Wyden said. "The politics are starting to shift."

The change is evident in the lawmakers themselves. Only 43 Members of Congress—37 in the House and 6 in the Senate—admitted to being regular smokers in a June 1993 survey by *Roll Call*, a newspaper that covers Capitol Hill. That's half the number of smokers it counted four years earlier.

As fewer voters smoke, even southern lawmakers have dropped their arguments that smoking is safe. "I think it's generally accepted on the Hill that smoking is bad for your health," Virginia's Bliley said. "I think you'd be better off if you didn't smoke, healthwise, just as if you didn't drink, and probably if you didn't eat a lot of red meat. No one can say that smoking is good for your health."

But Bliley, who has 15,000 tobacco-related jobs in his district, argues that regulating smoking should be left to individual businesses, not the government. Antismoking activist Ballin said that one way to soften the blow from new tobacco controls and higher tobacco taxes would be to earmark some of the tax revenues to help tobacco farmers convert to different crops.

At the same time, federal subsidies to the tobacco industry are coming under closer scrutiny, according to Durbin, who chairs the Appropriations Subcommittee on Agriculture, Rural Development, Food and Drug Administration and related Agencies. He said that he's systematically challenging a different tobacco subsidy each year, and this year hopes to zero out the $4 million budget for research into tobacco production.

And Durbin predicted that federal aid to the tobacco industry will come under attack during next year's debate over the farm bill. "We spend $25 million—$30 million a year subsidizing the tobacco allotment program," he said. "There are a lot of us that think that is totally inconsistent with our health message that tobacco is dangerous."

Some in Congress see the battle to control tobacco use as a long-term campaign. Synar acknowledged that the best hope for passage of his FDA bill this year would be to attach it as an amendment to a crucial piece of legislation. Waxman is still fighting for subcommittee votes for his smoking restrictions.

Both lawmakers predicted, however, that the growing public concern about the health hazards associated with smoking will eventually break the tobacco industry's hold on Congress and pave the way for tougher federal controls on tobacco.

The Heart Association's Ballin said that the key to beating the tobacco industry lies at the local level. "Members of Congress and someone running to unseat a Member need to be asked where they stand on tobacco control," he said. "Maybe not this year, but in the future that could make a difference."

Anti-Smoking War? Could Deny Consumers' Choice

— **John Hood** —

Are tobacco products regulated? The average person would no doubt answer yes. In the past two decades, at least 600 local laws have been passed across the country to require non-smoking areas in workplaces, schools, government buildings, public facilities, and restaurants. Every state legislature has taken action against smoking in one form or another. On the federal level, tobacco advertising is heavily regulated—banned from broadcast and saddled with labeling requirements in print. Manufacturers must also live with significant reporting requirements for ingredients and additives. And the Occupational Safety and Health Administration (OSHA) proposed a new rule in March that would ban smoking in virtually all indoor workplaces, including bars and restaurants.

But to many regulators and anti-smoking activists, these numerous restrictions seem almost irrelevant. Former U.S. Surgeon General Antonia Novello once said that tobacco was "the least regulated consumer product" in the country. Tobacco is "a product that is virtually unregulated for health and safety," says Scott Ballin, vice president for public affairs at the American Heart Association. Ballin and other activists have been pressing the U.S. Food and Drug Administration (FDA) for years to assert regulatory authority over tobacco—a move that, given current FDA requirements about the "safety" of products, would almost certainly result in banning virtually all tobacco products. FDA Commissioner David Kessler has recently suggested to a congressional subcommittee that his agency does, indeed, have such authority, given so-called "new" information about the use of tobacco as a drug.

Naturally, tobacco companies, farmers, and smokers' rights groups will fight such a move tooth and nail. Indeed, cigarette manufacturer Philip Morris has already filed a multimillion-dollar libel suit against ABC-TV's "Day One" program for its allegations that tobacco companies add nicotine to cigarettes to foster addiction among consumers.

At stake, however, is not simply the survival of the tobacco industry or tobacco farmers. The real issue is freedom of choice by consumers of all products, not merely cigarettes. Kessler recognizes this implication and stated to Congress that "it is fair to argue that the decision to start smoking may be a matter of choice. But once they have started smoking regularly, most smokers are in effect deprived of their choice to stop smoking." The commissioner is arguing that he, as head of the FDA, must step in to help consumers who can't otherwise help themselves. His intention may be genuine benevolence, but the result of such new regulation would codify and extend the powers of an agency that already limits the freedom of individual consumers to make their own decisions.

A Risky Decision

Are smokers the prisoners of nicotine and therefore of the companies that supply their "fix"? Kessler reports that even smokers who develop serious health conditions, presumably as a result of their smoking, remain "in the grip of nicotine." After surgery for lung cancer, he says, almost half of smokers resume smoking. Among smokers who suffer a heart attack, 38% resume smoking while they are still in the hospital.

Overall, Kessler argues that 15 million of the 17 million Americans who try to stop smoking every year fail. But the fact remains that since 1964, more than 40 million people have stopped smoking permanently without any outside intervention or assistance. Over the past decade, domestic consumption of tobacco has dropped both in share (37% of Americans were smokers in 1981, 30% in 1991) and in products (U.S. smokers consumed 640 billion cigarettes in 1981, 500 billion in 1991). Perhaps one reason for this is that, according to statistics from the U.S. Department of Health and Human Services, levels of tar and nicotine have fallen by almost 70% since the 1950's, in nicotine's case, from 2.5 milligrams per cigarette to less than 1 milligram. This fact is difficult to square with conspiracy theories about manufacturers spiking cigarettes with nicotine to keep smokers addicted.

Indeed, the evidence that manufacturers do this is essentially that manufacturers *could* do this. Kessler's case, and that of other anti-smoking partisans, centers almost entirely around patents obtained by tobacco companies for processes which replace nicotine lost during manufacturing. When confronted with strong industry denials that spiking has occurred—as well as evidence showing that there is less nicotine than in the original tobacco leaves from which they are made—Rep. Henry Waxman (D-Calif.) claimed that manufacturers were only playing semantic games. Deliberately restoring some of the nicotine lost during manufacturing is still "playing around with nicotine levels," he said. But tobacco industry officials reply that previous attempts to introduce nicotine-free cigarettes have flopped, and that the presence of the substance clearly affect a smoker's enjoyment of the product.

However, the crucial question in evaluating Kessler's argument is not just whether tobacco companies spike cigarettes, but what should be the operative definition of "addiction." Many of us use the term addiction in loose fashion. We sometimes say we're addicted to coffee, to chocolate, to Cajun cooking, to television. In every case, what we mean is that we value highly the experience of consuming a product or participating in an activity that provides us pleasure, and even that we would be willing to sacrifice other valuable goods— be they money or time—to continue our consumption. Some of these addictions have a physical component, such as the caffeine in coffee. Others do not.

Using the broadest definition of addiction, most Americans might legitimately be termed "addicts." They could give up their addictions, but it would be distressing for them to do so. Not only are there millions of people who have tried and failed to quit smoking—there are also millions of people who have tried and failed to stop eating fatty foods and sweets, to give up coffee and sodas, to exercise regularly, or to limit the time they spend watching TV. In every case, one can argue that there are health issues at stake (in the case of TV, perhaps mental health issues). At most, tobacco's risks differ only by degree, not by kind; certainly the health risks of alcohol abuse, high-fat diets, and a sedentary lifestyle are themselves most serious. The Center for Science in the Public Interest claims that 445,000 Americans die prematurely each year from poor diet and lack of exercise, compared with 420,000 per year from tobacco use. Alcohol abuse kills around 100,000.

In *Smoking: Making the Risky Decision*, published in 1993, Duke University researcher Kip Viscusi challenges the notion that smokers, as distinguished from people who engage in other personally or socially destructive behavior, are not to be trusted to make their own decisions. "We make choices throughout our lives that are costly to reverse—getting married, choosing a profession, selecting a place to live, and purchasing a car. The fact that reversing such decisions is costly does not imply that such choices are incorrect." Viscusi's research has found that smokers tend to accept and tolerate higher levels of risk in other areas, such as choice of career. They also tend to overestimate, not underestimate, the risks associated with smoking, reflecting the effectiveness decades of public service and campaign on the evils of tobacco.

As long as there are lower-nicotine cigarettes, nicotine patches, chewing gum, and fortitude, some smokers will limit their risk, others will eliminate altogether by quitting, and still others will choose to continue their habit, most of them knowing the risks they are assuming. Viscusi notes that survey data showing most smokers want to quit but can't are about as reliable as surveys showing that most people want to move to the country or change jobs, even though they never do: "Survey statements in which individuals indicate that they would like to quit smoking, for example, might mean that they would like to smoke without risk. However, the fact that they have continued to smoke, even with the availability of chewing gum with nicotine suggests that these statements...should not always be taken at face value."

Obviously, the debate on smoking regulation would change dramatically with the introduction of solid evidence that significant numbers of *nonsmokers* are harmed by tobacco smoke. But...such evidence does not yet exist. Indeed, if the risk the consumption of a substance poses on innocent bystanders is to be the criterion for banning the substance, then bringing back the prohibition of alcohol would be a much higher priority than banning cigarettes, given the former's undeniable role in many of the 44,000 traffic fatalities each year. So far, the highest number of second-hand smoke fatalities the EPA can come up with—by massaging the data well beyond believability—is 3,000 a year. (See also, "Facts Catch Up With 'Political' Science," *CR*, May 1993).

So, the new war against tobacco, predicated on the idea that cigarettes are nothing more than the delivery system for a highly addictive drug, must be waged on behalf of paternalism, not concern for bystanders. To justify a major expansion of federal regulatory authority, Kessler and the Congress should have to prove that smokers cannot help themselves and do not recognize the risks associated with their behavior—and that regulation would resolve these problems.

Muzzling Information

Unfortunately, Kessler does not really have to prove these points. Once Congress decides that the FDA has authority to regulate cigarettes, the burden of proof for all health and safety issues shifts to manufacturers and consumers. The government doesn't have to prove that tobacco kills innocent bystanders, or that nicotine can be reduced without affecting the quality of tobacco products, or that new tobacco products are unsafe, to make rulings. Instead, tobacco companies will have to prove that their products are "safe," which under the FDA definition means essentially risk-free, an admittedly impossible standard to meet for these products.

Based as it is on the "guilty until proven innocent" standard, the FDA's scrutiny of new pharmaceuticals has already deprived consumers of products from which they might have obtained great benefit. The average cost of developing a new drug approaches $360 million, according to the U.S. Office of Technology Assessment. A good amount of this cost reflects regulatory compliance. Firms have to field separate applications, running up to 1,000 pages each, for different treatments by the same drug. The approval process can last up to 12 years. In recent years, the FDA has stymied efforts to bring drugs to market that could have treated patients suffering from Alzheimer's disease, angina, hypertension, gastric ulcers, heart conditions, and AIDS.

The agency has also limited or prohibited advertising of health claims that it doesn't believe are conclusively proven by scientific research. So, despite the fact that many researchers think the regular ingestion of aspirin may help prevent heart attacks, the FDA forbids aspirin manufacturers from telling consumers this. The agency has made similar rulings regarding health claims for some *foods* containing vitamins—such as vitamin E, Vitamin C, and betacarotene—but not for *supplements* containing the same vitamins. These restrictions prevent many consumers from discovering and evaluating information that could help them make healthier choices. As former Federal Trade Commission economist Paul Rubin says, "the FDA behaves as if it has a general aversion to provision of information to consumers by manufacturers."

The FDA "is charged with regulating 'false and misleading' advertising and product labeling. However, the agency has substantial discretion in fulfilling this mission," Rubin adds. "While advertising which is clearly false should be eliminated, the agency uses its mandate to enforce an extremely broad interpretation of misleading [advertising] and thereby muzzles the flow of valuable information to consumers."

Kessler says that because extension of the FDA's authority to tobacco would likely result in an immediate ban, Congress should impose stiff regulations directly on the industry that stop short of an outright ban.

But even enacting legislation to give the FDA specific powers to regulate nicotine content, the manufacturing process, and the introduction of new tobacco products would represent a massive increase in the agency's power over the average American. Once let loose on tobacco, the FDA will probably never be restrained by subsequent legislation, as the drafter of the current anti-smoking bill, Rep. Mike Synar (D-Okla.), has admitted. "We wanted to get the jurisdiction over tobacco into the FDA," he says. "It was simple politics. Once we got the product in there, we wouldn't have to do anything legislatively again."

The question must be asked: Where do we stop? Will the FDA also regulate the fat content of steaks, or require that caffeine be removed for all soft drinks (obviously this can be done, given the prevalence of caffeine-free brands today)? And it's not just the FDA that will be emboldened by congressional action here. Efforts by OSHA, EPA, and other regulators will intensify. Regulatory scrutiny of personal behavior will move beyond the workplace as well. Already courts in 11 states have ordered parents to stop smoking or risk losing custody of their children. Will parents next be forced to comply with diet, exercise, or other behavioral guidelines?

At the core of the new war on tobacco is the notion that federal agencies must not only provide information about the risks of what consumers choose to do, but also substitute their judgment to prevent consumers from choosing the "wrong" things.

Health and safety issues are not so cut and dried. Many popular activities have varying levels of risks and benefits, and consumers differ dramatically in how tolerant they are of risk and how highly they value pleasure or satisfaction. No team of regulators is qualified to make blanket judgments about what is and isn't a good choice for consumers. And when government makes such judgments, the consequences can be significant—ranging from lost satisfaction and pleasure to, in the case of drug approvals, lost lives.

The FDA should become less intrusive, not more. Consumers have good reason to make decisions for themselves, given their disparate interests and needs in marketplace of one-quarter billion Americans. Given the opportunity and accurate, timely information, most consumers will make choices that maximize their happiness. The FDA's role, like that of other federal agencies, should be to provide such information and let individual Americans, even smokers, take it from there.

Debate Presenter Form

Follow the guidelines for debate presenters contained in the introduction of this text and those given to you by your instructor. Use the format below to organize the material for your debate. Remember to include all relevant citation information and to present the related information in your own words. Give credit to authors when you cite a quote and be as thorough as possible when writing about your points so you will be prepared for your debate.

Reference citation #1:

Author: _____

Title: _____

Date: _____

Source: _____

_____

Content from reference citation #1: _____

_____

_____

_____

_____

_____

_____

_____

_____

_____

_____

_____

_____

_____

Reference citation #2:

Author: _____

Title: _____

Date: _____

Source: _____

_____

Content from reference citation #2: _____

_____

_____

_____

_____

_____

Reference citation #3:

Author: _____

Title: _____

Date: _____

Source: _____

_____

Content from reference citation #3: _____

_____

_____

_____

_____

418

Audience Preparation Form

Follow the guidelines for preparing to be an informed audience member on the day of the debate included in the introduction to this text. After reading both sides of the debate from this chapter, answer the following questions. Be as thorough as possible so that you will be able to make a contribution to the debate by asking informed questions or making provocative comments. This form is usually due on the day of the debate.

State the issue in your own words. Do not plagiarize the text. Demonstrate that you understand the topic and it's relevant arguments.

_____

_____

_____

_____

_____

Discuss two points on the "yes" side of the debate.

Point #1: _____

_____

Point #2: _____

_____

Discuss two points on the "no" side of the debate.

Point #1: _____

_____

Point #2: _____

_____

What is your opinion on this topic?

_____

_____

_____

_____

_____

_____

_____

_____

What has contributed to the development of your views about this topic?

_____

_____

_____

_____

_____

_____

_____

_____

What information would be necessary to cause you to change your thinking about this topic?

_____

_____

_____

_____

_____

_____

Debate Response Form

Follow the guidelines for responding to the debates in the introductory chapter of this text. Complete this form and submit your answers at the class following the debate. Try to be thorough and convince your instructor that you were an active listener during the debate.

List a quote from a debate presenter that you think was important and explain why you think this comment was significant.

_____

_____

_____

_____

Which side of the debate do you think made the most convincing arguments, why?

_____

_____

_____

_____

_____

After hearing the debate, in what way has your thinking been affected?

_____

_____

_____

_____

_____

_____

✑ Appendix ✑

List your name on the appropriate side below if you plan to be a presenter on this topic. Note that signing here constitutes a commitment on your part to be prepared to present valid and reliable information supporting your side of this debate.

Are there valid psychological reasons for physician assisted suicide?

Yes	No